THE YEAR IN
INTERVENTIONAL
CARDIOLOGY
2003

THE YEAR IN INTERVENTIONAL CARDIOLOGY

2003

Edited by

A P BANNING and **P J DE FEYTER**

CLINICAL PUBLISHING

OXFORD

Distributed worldwide by
CRC Press

Boca Raton   London   New York   Washington, DC

Clinical Publishing

an imprint of Atlas Medical Publishing Ltd

Oxford Centre for Innovation
Mill Street, Oxford OX2 0JX, UK

Tel: +44 1865 811116
Fax: +44 1865 251550
Web: www.clinicalpublishing.co.uk

Distributed by:

CRC Press LLC
2000 NW Corporate Blvd
Boca Raton, FL 33431, USA
E-mail: orders@crcpress.com

CRC Press UK
23–25 Blades Court
Deodar Road
London SW15 2NU, UK
E-mail: crcpress@itps.co.uk

A catalogue record for this book is available from the British Library

ISBN 1 904392 14 8
ISSN 1478-0178

**The publisher makes no representation, express or implied, that the dosages in this
book are correct. Readers must therefore always check the product information and
clinical procedures with the most up-to-date published product information and data
sheets provided by the manufacturers and the most recent codes of conduct and
safety regulations. The authors and the publisher do not accept any liability for any
errors in the text or for the misuse or misapplication of material in this work**

Commissioning Editor: Jonathan Gregory
Project Manager: Carolyn Newton
Typeset by Footnote Graphics Limited, Warminster, Wiltshire
Printed in Spain by T G Hostench SA, Barcelona

Contents

Contributors

ADRIAN BANNING, MD, FRCP, FESC, Department of Cardiology, John Radcliffe Hospital, Oxford, UK

EMANUELE BARBATO, MD, Cardiovascular Center, OLV Hospital, Aalst, Belgium

DAN BLACKMAN, MD, MRCP, Department of Cardiology, John Radcliffe Hospital, Oxford, UK

MALCOLM I BURGESS, MRCP, Cardiothoracic Centre, Liverpool, UK

PIM J DE FEYTER, MD, PhD, Erasmus Medical Centre, Rotterdam, The Netherlands

CARLO DI MARIO, MD, FACC, FESC, San Raffaele Hospital, Milan, Italy

ANGELA HOYE, MB ChB, MRCP, Thoraxcentrum, Rotterdam, The Netherlands

MICHAEL V KNOPP, MD, PhD, Department of Radiology, The Ohio State University, Ohio, USA

PHILIP MACCARTHY, BSc, PhD, MRCP, Department of Cardiology, King's College Hospital, London, UK

EUGÈNE P McFADDEN, FRCP, FESC, FACC, Thoraxcentrum, Erasmus MC, Rotterdam, The Netherlands

L KRISTIN NEWBY, MD, MHS, Duke Clinical Research Institute, Durham, North Carolina, USA

ITALO PORTO, MD, Department of Cardiology, John Radcliffe Hospital, Oxford, UK

SUNIL V RAO, MD, Duke Clinical Research Institute, Durham, North Carolina, USA

BENNO RENSING, MD, FESC, Department of Cardiology, St Antonius Hospital, Nieuwegein, The Netherlands

RODNEY H STABLES, MA DM, FRCP, Cardiothoracic Centre, Liverpool, UK

FABIO SGURA, MD, San Raffaele Hospital, Milan, Italy

MARTYN THOMAS, MD, FRCP, Department of Cardiology, King's College Hospital, London, UK

NEAL UREN, MD, MRCP, Department of Cardiology, New Royal Infirmary, Edinburgh, UK

ERIC VAN BELLE, MD, PhD, FESC, FACC, Service de Cardiologie B et Hémodynomique, Hôpital Cardiologique, Lille, France

MARK WI WEBSTER, MB ChB, FRACP, Cardiac Catheterization Laboratories, Green Lane Hospital, Auckland, New Zealand

WILLIAM WIJNS, MD, PhD, FESC, FAHA, Cardiovascular Center, OLV Hospital, Aalst, Belgium

FELIX ZIJLSTRA, MD, PhD, Department of Cardiology, University Hospital, Groningen, The Netherlands

Preface

Has there ever been a more exciting time to be an interventional cardiologist? I doubt it. In the last year, we have seen dramatic and monumental progress in the practice of interventional cardiology.

Drug-eluting stents have been at the forefront as the spectre of restenosis which has hung over interventional cardiologists since balloon angioplasty began. The possibility that we can shake ourselves free of this is clearly an enormous step forward. Increasingly, we now have the tools to tackle major interventional challenges that have been the topic of debate for many years including left main disease, multivessel angioplasty, and implementation of primary angioplasty for emergency therapy of acute myocardial infarction.

This book has drawn together authors from around the world to reflect on literature published in 2002 and in the first six months of 2003. It builds on the success of last year's volume which provided a valuable resource for both clinicians and clinical investigators alike.

In Part I, Dr Sunil Rao and Dr Kristin Newby discuss how risk stratification, particularly using troponin estimation, continues to become a more exact science. It is clear that we can now determine which patients are at highest risk when they present to hospital. For many of these patients, intervention will reduce their risk significantly. Felix Ziljlstra then reflects on his enormous personal experience in primary angioplasty from the Zwolle Group. In the US and in Europe, primary angioplasty is replacing thrombolysis as the treatment of choice for acute myocardial infarction and data are presented which justifies this change in practice. Benno Rensing reflects on the published data for intervention in stable and non-ST elevation acute coronary syndromes. This group represents the biggest volume of work for most interventional centres. Rod Stables was one of the lead investigators in the stent or surgery (SOS) trial. With his colleague, Dr Malcolm Burgess from Liverpool in the UK, they reflect on the data comparing surgical and percutaneous revascularization.

The second part of the book is dedicated to interventional technique. William Wijns and his colleague Emanuele Barbato look at the data comparing direct stenting with pre-dilatation and subsequent stenting. Direct stenting saves time in suitable lesions and there has been great discussion as to whether other benefits may be inferred by avoiding a preceding balloon dilatation. Eugene McFadden then reviews the increasing data for pressure and flow measurement. With drug-eluting stents, we will be increasingly tempted to treat less severe lesions. Pressure wire measurement allows accurate determination of the functional significance of stenosis and also gives immediate data on the consequences and adequacy of stent implantation. It seems likely that these techniques will continue to expand their indications in the coming years. Although stent design has perhaps been rather neglected during discussions in the last few years, it remains a critical issue. In the future, optimal stents will have maximum flexibility whilst inducing a minimal intimal reaction. It is likely that this will be combined with a biologically inert polymer that will moderate release of perhaps two or three biologically active and synergistic drugs.

In Part Three, Mark Webster from Green Lane in Auckland reviews the data on statin therapy. Optimal use of plaque modifying agents clearly has potential in preventing progressive disease, particularly in those at highest risk. Perhaps the highest risk group we treat are diabetics and Eric Van Belle from France reviews the progress that intervention has made in this subgroup of patients. It was not so long ago that intervention was discouraged in diabetics with LAD disease. Surgery was felt to be absolutely necessary. Perhaps it is in this group particularly where the new developments in intervention will see their greatest application.

In Part Four, new developments in intervention are raised. Advances in brachytherapy are discussed by Philip McCarthy and Martin Thomas from King's College Hospital in London. Results from brachytherapy seem to be increasingly reliable and as we are already seeing some patients who have had drug-eluting stents presenting with restenosis, we should not discard this technique too early. The issue of 'no reflow' and how to protect the distal coronary bed is reviewed by Dan Blackman. The use of distal protection devices, particularly in vein graft intervention, is clearly an enormous step forward. No reflow has dogged interventional cardiologists for many years and increasing scrutiny of the mechanisms contributing to no reflow will hopefully provide a solution to this multifactorial problem. Dr Porto and I have reviewed the recent data on drug-eluting stents. Data from the RAVEL studies and the early Paclitaxel data is summarized. Neal Uren examines the role of intravascular ultrasound. Clearly, this has been a crucial part of the development of drug-eluting stents. Data about malposition of stents can only be obtained from intravascular ultrasound; it therefore seems likely that lessons obtained from this technique will remain a crucial part of the development of interventional cardiology. Carlo di Mario and Fabio Sgura review data on atherectomy. Lesions which cannot be dilated by balloons remain problematic particularly as the average age of the interventional population continues to increase. Although it is possible that debulking as a strategy may be starting to dwindle, there do appear to be persistent niche applications for these devices. Finally, Dr Knopp gives a short review on contrast agents and their use in interventional cardiology. Although many of us rarely think about this issue, recent developments have occurred which can make cases safer, particularly when we are administering large contrast loads to patients undergoing complex interventional procedures.

Overall, this book gives an up-to-date and thorough review of many of the topics of interest for interventionalists in 2003. It seems likely that 2004 will be at least as exciting a year for us and I hope this book will provide a useful resource.

Adrian Banning and Pim J de Feyter

Part I

Strategy

1

Risk stratification in acute coronary syndromes

Introduction

Acute coronary syndromes (ACS) range in severity from unstable angina to acute ST-segment elevation myocardial infarction (MI). The underlying pathophysiology of the different manifestations of ACS is similar, with coronary artery plaque rupture and platelet adherence, activation and aggregation forming the basis for varying degrees of artery occlusion. Incomplete occlusion results in the clinical syndrome of unstable angina, whereas complete occlusion leads to cardiac myocyte necrosis and MI. The variation in presentation mirrors the risk of recurrent infarction or death. Therein lies the importance of risk stratification. It serves to facilitate both communication between the doctor and the patient by providing prognostic information, and selection of therapies that maximize benefit and minimize harm.

Given that the clinical presentation is what is first encountered, the cornerstone of risk stratification is the history and physical examination. Indeed, the value of baseline clinical characteristics has been confirmed by several investigators [1,2]. Demographic characteristics such as age and previous history of ischaemic heart disease, and presenting characteristics such as blood pressure, heart rate and Killip class are all critical for the initial risk assessment.

After the initial history and physical examination, the 12-lead electrocardiogram (ECG) is the first objective risk stratification tool available. The ECG serves as the basis for the first therapeutic decision point. The presence of ST-segment elevation separates patients into a category in which the prompt administration of reperfusion therapy, either fibrinolytic medications or primary percutaneous coronary intervention, can improve both short- and long-term survival [3,4]. Patients without persistent ST-segment elevation fall into the category of non-ST-segment elevation ACS. For this heterogeneous group of patients, a combination of ECG findings and laboratory data provide incremental prognostic value above that which is gained from the history and physical.

The importance of both baseline and serial measures of markers of myocardial necrosis (particularly creatine kinase [CK]-MB and the troponins) in risk stratification of both ST-segment elevation MI and non-ST-segment elevation ACS patients has been firmly established [5]. However, because both markers are cleared renally, the significance of CK-MB and/or troponin elevation in patients with decreased renal function was previously uncertain. Furthermore, elevation of proteins such as C-reactive protein and B-type natriuretic peptide that are unrelated to myocardial necrosis but are related to 'upstream' events in the atherosclerotic cascade may also help to risk stratify patients with ACS. Finally, clinicians must wrestle with the issue of how to integrate all of the information available – history, physical examination, ECG and laboratory data – for appropriate triage.

The following articles published over the past year were selected to highlight recent developments in each of these areas. Their findings may point the way to the prognostic evaluation of the ACS patient in the years to come.

The prognostic and therapeutic implications of increased troponin T levels and ST depression in unstable coronary artery disease: the FRISC II invasive troponin T electrocardiogram substudy.

E Diderholm, B Andren, G Frostfeldt, *et al. Am Heart J* 2002; **143**: 760–7.

B A C K G R O U N D . In patients with ACS, elevation of cardiac troponin is associated with a worse outcome. The presence of ST-segment depression on the initial ECG is also a poor prognostic sign. However, little information exists as to the relation between the combination of both risk indicators and the outcome of an early invasive strategy in

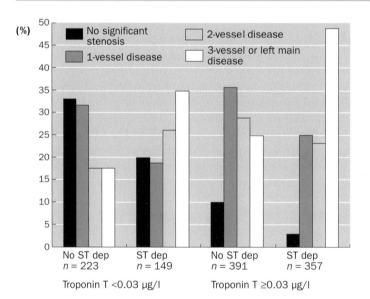

Fig. 1.1 Angiographic extent of coronary artery disease by troponin T level and presence or absence of ST-segment depression. Source: Diderholm *et al.* (2002).

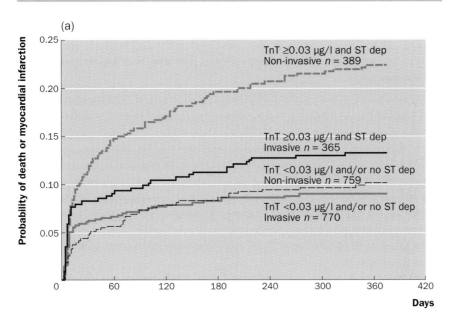

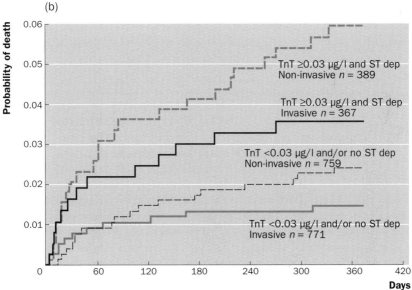

Fig. 1.2 Probability of 1-year death or myocardial infarction (a) and death (b) among early invasive or conservative strategies based on troponin T levels and presence or absence of ST-segment depression. Source: Diderholm *et al.* (2002).

patients with acute cardiac ischaemia. Using data from 2457 patients enrolled in the
Fast Revascularization during InStability in Coronary disease (FRISC) II trial, Diderholm
and colleagues investigated whether troponin T level, alone or in combination with the
presence of ST-segment depression, was associated with the angiographic extent of
coronary artery disease and could identify patients with differential benefit from an early
invasive strategy.

INTERPRETATION. Patients with both troponin elevation and ST-segment depression
were older, had more cardiac risk factors and were more likely to have left ventricular
dysfunction than those with either risk indicator alone. Fig. 1.1 shows the angiographic
extent of coronary artery disease in patients according to the presence or absence of
troponin elevation and ST-segment depression. Almost 50% of patients with both risk
indicators had either 3-vessel disease or left main disease. Fig. 1.2 demonstrates that an
early invasive strategy was associated with a lower rate of 1-year death and death or
recurrent MI regardless of the presence of troponin elevation or ST-segment depression.
Patients with both risk indicators had the greatest absolute benefit from an early invasive
strategy (1-year rate of death or MI 22.1% with non-invasive strategy vs 13.2% with
invasive strategy).

Comment

This study shows that among patients with unstable coronary disease, the presence of
both troponin elevation and ST-segment depression is associated with a higher rate
of death or recurrent MI compared with the presence of either risk marker alone. For
these high-risk patients, an early invasive strategy results in a profound reduction in
adverse events and should be the preferred therapeutic approach.

Troponin T and quantitative ST-segment depression offer complementary prognostic information in the risk stratification of acute coronary syndrome patients.
P Kaul, L K Newby, Y Fu, et al. J Am Coll Cardiol 2003; **41**: 371–80.

BACKGROUND. As mentioned earlier, both cardiac troponin and the initial ECG are
valuable for risk stratification. The ECG, however, is readily available and responsive to
cardiac ischaemia, whereas troponin takes a finite time to increase. In this study,
Kaul et al. used quantitative ST-segment data from 959 patients enrolled in the troponin
substudy of the Platelet IIb/IIIa Antagonism for the Reduction of Acute Coronary
Syndrome Events in a Global Organization Network (PARAGON)-B trial to determine
whether ST-segment depression offered complementary information in assessing the
risk of 6-month death or MI, and whether time to evaluation affected the prognostic
value of either risk indicator. Patients were grouped into three categories based on the
degree of ST-segment depression (none, 1 mm and ≥2 mm) and into two categories
based on troponin > or <0.1 ng/ml. The rate of the primary end-point was highest

among patients with both elevated troponin and ST-segment depression ≥2 mm (8.4% for troponin-negative/no ST depression vs 28.6% for troponin-positive/ST depression ≥2 mm). When troponin level was analyzed as a continuous variable, even low levels of troponin elevation were associated with an increased risk for the primary end-point compared with no detectable troponin (Fig. 1.3). In the time to evaluation analysis, ST-segment depression that occurred over 6 h after symptom onset was associated with a higher risk than if it occurred within 6 h of symptom onset (Table 1.1). Conversely, troponin elevation occurring within 6 h of symptom onset was associated with a higher risk of adverse events compared with later elevation. Treatment with the glycoprotein IIb/IIIa inhibitor lamifiban significantly reduced the rate of 6-month death/MI among patients with troponin elevation >0.1 ng/ml, but not significantly among those with varying degrees of ST-segment depression.

INTERPRETATION. Both troponin and degree of ST-segment depression offer complementary information in risk assessment for patients with non-ST-segment elevation ACS. In this study, cardiac troponin appeared to be a better marker of which patients would benefit from glycoprotein IIb/IIIa inhibition.

Comment

The lessons of this analysis are that both the ECG and laboratory assessment of myocardial cell necrosis are important in risk stratification, but that the time from

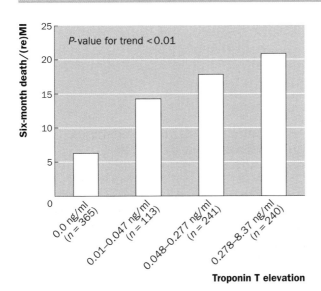

Fig. 1.3 Six-month death or myocardial (re)infarction according to troponin T levels. Source: Kaul *et al.* (2003).

Table 1.1 Prognostic significance by time to electrocardiogram or time to troponin T

	Electrocardiogram		Troponin T	
	<6 h (*n* = 743)	>6 h (*n* = 144)	<6 h (*n* = 421)	>6 h (*n* = 532)
Distribution of ST-segment depression				
None	38%	48%	–	–
1 mm	46%	44%	–	–
≥2 mm	16%	12%	–	–
Association with 6-month death or MI				
1 mm	1.2 (1.4, 4.2)	4.2 (1.1, 15.9)	–	–
≥2 mm	2.1 (1.2, 3.7)	7.3 (1.3, 42.0)	–	–
Distribution of troponin T				
Negative	–	–	70%	53%
Positive	–	–	30%	46%
Association with 6-month death or MI				
Positive	–	–	2.4 (1.4, 4.2)	1.5 (0.92, 2.5)
Duration of pain (min)	30 (20, 120)	210 (38, 618)	30 (20, 64)	60 (25, 120)

MI, myocardial infarction.
Source: Kaul *et al.* (2003).

symptom onset to the appearance of either risk indicator is important. The presence of ST-segment depression ≥2 mm over 6 h after symptom onset was associated with more than three times the risk than if it occurred earlier. In contrast, early troponin elevation is associated with a higher risk than late troponin elevation and appears to facilitate treatment decisions with regard to the administration of aggressive antiplatelet therapy.

Troponin T levels in patients with acute coronary syndromes, with or without renal dysfunction.

R J Aviles, A T Askari, B Lindahl, *et al. N Engl J Med* 2002; **346**: 2047–52.

BACKGROUND. Cardiac troponins are useful for both the diagnosis of ACS and assessing prognosis. However, they are cleared renally, therefore, their value in risk stratification among patients with renal dysfunction is unknown. Aviles and colleagues used data from 7033 patients enrolled in the Global Use of Strategies to Open Occluded Coronary Arteries (GUSTO)-IV trial to examine the association between troponin elevation, renal dysfunction and 30-day death or MI. Renal function was assessed using the Cockcroft–Gault formula to calculate creatinine clearance. Seven hundred and eighty-three patients had abnormal renal function defined as a creatinine clearance <58.4 ml/min; 20% of these patients had troponin levels ≥0.1 ng/ml. The association between troponin elevation and the primary end-point was assessed among patients grouped by quartiles of increasing renal function, as well as by using creatinine clearance as a continuous variable. Table 1.2 shows the unadjusted and adjusted odds of the primary end-point for patients with and without troponin elevation grouped by quartiles of increasing renal function. Troponin elevation was associated with a significantly increased risk of 30-day death or MI regardless of renal function. Fig. 1.4 shows the relationship between creatinine clearance as a continuous measure and the odds of the primary end-point among patients with troponin elevation ≥0.1 ng/ml.

INTERPRETATION. Among patients with signs and symptoms of ACS, troponin elevation is predictive of short-term adverse events regardless of renal function. This risk persists even after adjustment for other potential confounders.

Table 1.2 Unadjusted and adjusted outcomes for troponin positive (≥0.1 ng/ml) vs troponin negative (<0.1 ng/ml) by quartile of creatinine clearance

Quartile of creatinine clearance	Unadjusted odds ratio (95% confidence interval)	Adjusted odds ratio (95% confidence interval)
First	2.5 (1.9, 3.3)	2.5 (1.8, 3.3)
Second	1.6 (1.2, 2.3)	1.8 (1.3, 2.6)
Third	1.3 (0.9, 2.0)	1.4 (0.9, 2.1)
Fourth	2.0 (1.2, 3.5)	2.3 (1.3, 4.1)

Source: Aviles *et al.* (2002).

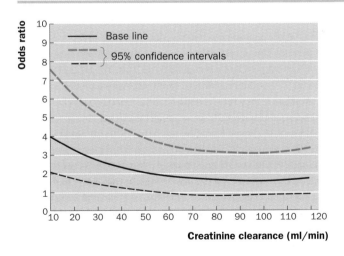

Fig. 1.4 Adjusted odds ratio (solid line) with 95% confidence intervals (dashed lines) for death or myocardial infarction by estimated creatinine clearance. Source: Aviles *et al.* (2002).

Comment

This important study shows that troponin elevation in patients with reduced renal function and suspected ACS should not be ignored or ascribed solely to decreased clearance. When applying these findings to clinical practice, it is important to remember that all of the patients in GUSTO-IV had signs and symptoms consistent with ACS. That is, the history is important when assessing the troponin level among patients with renal dysfunction. Furthermore, very few patients in this trial had markedly reduced creatinine clearance. Whether the prognostic value of troponin elevation is similar in this group remains to be seen.

N-Terminal pro-brain natriuretic peptide on admission for early risk stratification of patients with chest pain and no ST-segment elevation.

J Jernberg, M Stridsberg, P Venge, B Lindahl. *J Am Coll Cardiol* 2002; **40**: 437–45.

BACKGROUND. Patients with chest pain account for a significant proportion of accident and emergency visits. Many of these patients will have non-diagnostic ECGs, thereby making this important risk stratification tool less helpful. Reliable early identification of low-risk patients would theoretically expedite discharge and lead to cost savings. Brain natriuretic peptide (BNP) is a circulating hormone secreted by the ventricles in response to wall tension and has been shown to be associated with poor outcome in patients with non-ST-segment elevation ACS |6|. BNP is one of the products of cleavage of the pro-hormone proBNP. The other product is N-terminal proBNP (NT-proBNP), which may be a better marker of left ventricular dysfunction |7|. Jernberg *et al.* sought to determine the relationship between NT-proBNP and long-term mortality among patients with chest pain and a non-diagnostic ECG. The NT-proBNP was measured at admission for 775 patients admitted to the coronary care unit with chest pain. Patients were excluded if they received pre-hospital thrombolytic therapy, had ST-segment elevation on the admission ECG, or were previously enrolled in the study. Patients were divided into four groups based on the initial ECG: (1) normal ECG, (2) ST-segment depression, (3) pathological changes other than ST-segment depression or left bundle branch block, and (4) left bundle branch block. The median NT-proBNP level was 400 ng/l. Patients in the highest quartile of NT-proBNP were older, had longer time from onset of pain to admission, and more often elevated troponin and ST-segment depression ≥ 0.05 mV on the admission ECG. Patients ultimately diagnosed with acute MI had the highest levels of NT-proBNP, whereas those with a diagnosis of non-cardiac chest pain had the lowest levels. Fig. 1.5 shows the cumulative probability of death for patients in the four quartiles of NT-proBNP. In the multivariable analysis, NT-proBNP level at admission was an independent predictor of mortality. This persisted across patients with and without elevated troponin levels and regardless of the admission ECG findings.

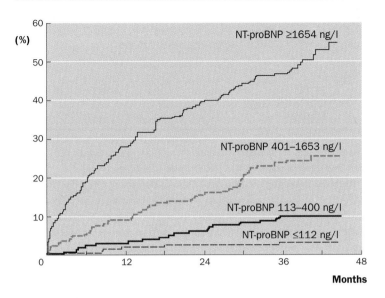

Fig. 1.5 Cumulative probability of death by levels of NT-proBNP. NT-proBNP ≤112 ng/l (light solid line); NT-proBNP 113–400 ng/l (heavy solid line); NT-proBNP 401–1653 ng/l (dashed line); NT-proBNP ≥1654 ng/l (dotted line). Source: Jernberg *et al.* (2002).

INTERPRETATION. A single measurement of NT-proBNP at admission substantially improved the risk stratification of patients with symptoms consistent with ACS in this study. Although the mechanism by which this marker is related to risk is unclear, it may be an indicator of either temporary or pre-existing left ventricular dysfunction in patients with cardiac ischaemia.

Comment

This study points to the important role of the neurohormonal system in ACS. Left ventricular function is one of the most important prognostic indicators in patients with acute ischaemic syndromes. NT-proBNP level may be an easily obtained and sensitive reflection of left ventricular dysfunction and, therefore, may become another tool to guide triage and treatment decisions.

Prognostic implications of abnormalities in renal function in patients with acute coronary syndromes.

J Al Suwaidi, D N Reddan, K Williams, *et al. Circulation* 2002; **106**: 974–80.

BACKGROUND. Patients with end-stage renal disease (ESRD) have high 1-year mortality |8|. Approximately half of the deaths in this population are attributable to cardiovascular causes. Whether mild to moderate degrees of renal dysfunction are also associated with increased risk of adverse outcomes is unclear. Al Suwaidi *et al.* combined data from four clinical trials of ACS (GUSTO IIb, GUSTO III, Platelet Glycoprotein IIb/IIIa in Unstable Angina: Receptor Suppression Using Integrilin Therapy [PURSUIT] and PARAGON A) to compare patients with and without baseline renal dysfunction and to determine the relation between reduced baseline renal function and 30- and 180-day all-cause mortality. Baseline creatinine data were collected for patients enrolled in the four trials. Per protocol, patients with a creatinine >2 mg/dl were excluded from GUSTO IIb, PURSUIT and PARAGON A. Using creatinine clearance calculated using the Cockcroft–Gault formula, patients were grouped according to the presence or absence of abnormal baseline renal function defined as a creatinine clearance <70 ml/min. Using creatinine clearance as a continuous variable, the relation between renal function and outcomes was assessed using Cox regression. Of the 10 951 patients with ST-segment elevation, 41% had renal insufficiency at enrolment. Among the patients with non-ST-segment elevation ACS, 42% had renal insufficiency at baseline. Patients with abnormal renal function were older, more often female and were more likely to have cardiac risk factors than those with normal renal function. Table 1.3 shows the rates and unadjusted and adjusted hazard ratios of 180-day mortality among patients with and without reduced renal function. As creatinine clearance increased, the rate of 180-day death and the hazard ratio for 180-day death decreased regardless of ST-segment status.

INTERPRETATION. Mild to moderate renal dysfunction is common among patients with ST-segment elevation and non-ST-segment elevation ACS. These patients also have more cardiac risk factors than those with normal renal function. After adjusting for these potential confounders, the presence of abnormal baseline renal function is associated with a significant increase in short- and long-term mortality.

Comment

This study highlights two important issues for patients with ACS. First, patients with even mild to moderate degrees of renal dysfunction are at high risk for adverse outcomes and therefore deserve aggressive evaluation. Secondly, more research is needed into the biological mechanisms by which abnormal renal function affects cardiovascular outcomes.

Table 1.3 Mortality at 180 days among patients with acute coronary syndromes by tertiles of creatinine clearance

	Non-ST-segment elevation			ST-segment elevation	
	PURSUIT	**GUSTO IIb**	**PARAGON A**	**GUSTO IIb**	**GUSTO III**
Creatinine clearance					
First tertile	11.3%	12.8%	10.6%	16.2%	19.0%
Second tertile	5.0%	4.5%	5.6%	5.1%	6.0%
Third tertile	2.5%	2.5%	2.2%	2.5%	3.2%
Unadjusted hazard ratio	0.72	0.70	0.74	0.64	0.67
(95% confidence interval)	(0.69, 0.75)	(0.67, 0.74)	(0.67, 0.81)	(0.61, 0.69)	(0.65, 0.69)
Adjusted hazard ratio	0.80	0.81	0.83	0.79	0.79
(95% confidence interval)	(0.65, 0.97)	(0.66, 0.99)	(0.50, 1.38)	(0.72, 0.88)	(0.76, 0.83)

Source: Al Suwaidi *et al.* (2002).

Scores for post-myocardial infarction risk stratification in the community.

M Singh, G S Reeder, S J Jacobsen, S Weston, J Killian, V L Roger. *Circulation* 2002; **106**: 2309–14.

BACKGROUND. **Using data from large multicentre clinical trials and cohort studies, several investigators have devised risk scores to predict outcomes in patients with acute MI. Although there is some overlap in the clinical information used to derive these scores, their applicability to populations other than the original derivation sample is unknown. This is particularly true of scores generated from patients enrolled in clinical trials who may be highly selected. Furthermore, not all scores include an index of left ventricular function. Singh *et al.* evaluated the generalizability of the Thrombolysis in Myocardial Infarction (TIMI) risk score (derived from the TIMI trials of non-ST-segment elevation and ST-segment elevation MI) and the Predicting Risk of Death in Cardiac Disease Tool (PREDICT) score (derived from a cohort study of patients with acute MI) and also sought to determine if the addition of ejection fraction added to the prognostic value of either score. The validation population for this study comprised patients with a confirmed discharge diagnosis of acute MI from Olmstead County, Minnesota. Clinical data were obtained from hospital records by trained abstractors. Patients were stratified according to the presence of ST-segment elevation on the initial ECG. Using logistic regression, the authors determined the discriminant accuracy of each score and the incremental value of adding ejection fraction to each score. As shown in Table 1.4, the**

discriminant accuracy of the TIMI score was better for patients with ST-segment elevation ACS; the PREDICT score was consistently better than the TIMI score across both strata. Ejection fraction added incremental value to the discriminant value of the PREDICT score.

INTERPRETATION. When applied to a community-based patient population, the PREDICT score, which includes measures of co-morbidity (the Charlson Index), performed better than a score derived from a selected trial population. The addition of ejection fraction to the score significantly improved the discriminant accuracy.

Comment

This study underscores the limitations of some clinical trial data to community-based patient cohorts. Patients in clinical trials can be highly selected and may not necessarily reflect the entire patient population affected by ischaemic heart disease. For example, elderly patients, patients with renal insufficiency and patients with other medical illnesses are often excluded from or under-represented in clinical trials |9|. For this reason, the PREDICT score that includes the Charlson Index would be expected to have better discriminant value than a score derived from a clinical trial population. In addition, left ventricular function is a powerful prognostic indicator and should be considered when assessing the risk of any patient with ACS.

Table 1.4 Predictive accuracy of various acute coronary syndrome risk scores

	C-statistic (95% confidence intervals)		
	TIMI	TIMI + Charlson	PREDICT
Non-ST-segment elevation			
Death			
1-month	0.59 (0.53, 0.66)	0.72 (0.65, 0.78)	0.78 (0.73, 0.84)
1-year	0.61 (0.56, 0.66)	0.76 (0.72, 0.81)	0.81 (0.77, 0.85)
Death or myocardial infarction			
1-month	0.59 (0.53, 0.65)	0.68 (0.62, 0.74)	0.73 (0.67, 0.79)
1-year	0.62 (0.57, 0.67)	0.74 (0.70, 0.78)	0.78 (0.74, 0.82)
ST-segment elevation			
Death			
1-month	0.73 (0.67, 0.79)	0.78 (0.72, 0.83)	0.81 (0.76, 0.87)
1-year	0.73 (0.67, 0.79)	0.76 (0.70, 0.81)	0.78 (0.73, 0.83)
Death or myocardial infarction			
1-month	0.71 (0.65, 0.76)	0.76 (0.70, 0.81)	0.79 (0.74, 0.84)
1-year	0.71 (0.69, 0.76)	0.74 (0.69, 0.79)	0.77 (0.72, 0.81)

Source: Singh et al. (2002).

Is blood glucose an independent predictor of mortality in acute myocardial infarction in the thrombolytic era?

N N Wahab, E A Cowden, N J Pearce, M J Gardner, H Merry, J L Cox; ICONS Investigators. *J Am Coll Cardiol* 2002; **40**: 1748–54.

BACKGROUND. It has been established that patients with diabetes mellitus are at high risk for developing ischaemic heart disease |10,11|. Patients with and without known diabetes may present with hyperglycaemia during an ACS. Glucose level on admission has been associated with adverse outcomes among patients with ACS |12|, but many of these studies were conducted prior to the era of reperfusion therapy. Given that the treatment of acute MI and diabetes mellitus has changed significantly over the last decade, Wahab and colleagues undertook this study to determine the association between admission blood glucose level and in-hospital outcomes in the modern era. They defined hyperglycaemia as a random blood sugar >198 mg/dl per the guidelines issued by the American and Canadian Diabetic Associations. Using clinical data from 1664 consecutive patients hospitalized with acute MI and followed in a prospective-cohort disease management study, the authors stratified the sample into four groups: (1) no hyperglycaemia, no diabetes; (2) hyperglycaemia, no diabetes; (3) no hyperglycaemia, diabetes; (4) hyperglycaemia, diabetes. Table 1.5 shows the baseline characteristics of the four patient groups. The majority of patients had neither hyperglycaemia nor diabetes. Using this as the reference group, multivariable logistic regression was used to determine the association between admission glucose level and the occurrence of in-hospital and 1-year mortality. Fig. 1.6 shows the outcomes of each group; Table 1.6 shows the independent predictors of in-hospital mortality.

Table 1.5 Baseline characteristics by diabetes and glycaemic status

	Group 1 (n = 1078)	Group 2 (n = 135)	Group 3 (n = 169)	Group 4 (n = 282)
Age (years)	64.7	69.9	68.6	68.2
Male (%)	69	51	63	57
Glucose (mmol/l)	7.3	21.0	8.6	19.0
Creatinine (mmol/l)	110.5	133.8	125.7	125.8
Smoker (%)	65	53	61	58
Hypertension (%)	45	50	63	65
Hyperlipidaemia (%)	33	24	44	37
Prior MI (%)	24	26	34	33
Prior heart failure (%)	7	19	17	20
Peripheral vascular disease (%)	3	0.7	6	4

Group 1, no previous diagnosis of diabetes and random blood glucose ≤198 mg/dl (11 mmol/l). Group 2, no previous diabetes and random blood glucose >198 mg/dl. Group 3, known diabetes and random blood glucose ≤198 mg/dl. Group 4, known diabetes and random blood glucose >198 mg/dl. Source: Wahab *et al.* (2002).

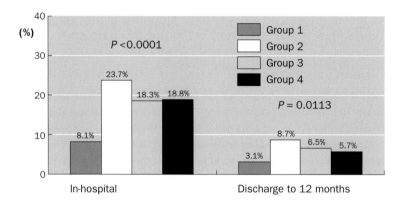

Fig. 1.6 Mortality according to diabetes and glycaemic status. Group 1, no previous diagnosis of diabetes and random blood glucose ≤198 mg/dl (11 mmol/l). Group 2, no previous diabetes and random blood glucose >198 mg/dl. Group 3, known diabetes and random blood glucose ≤198 mg/dl. Group 4, known diabetes and random blood glucose >198 mg/dl. Source: Wahab *et al.* (2002).

Table 1.6 Independent predictors of in-hospital mortality

	Odds ratio (95% confidence interval)
Group 1	1.00
Group 2	2.44 (1.42, 4.20)
Group 3	1.87 (1.05, 3.34)
Group 4	1.91 (1.16, 3.14)
Peripheral vascular disease	4.33 (1.88, 9.96)
Insulin on admission	2.05 (1.07, 3.92)
Age (per 10 years)	1.89 (1.58, 2.24)
Prior heart failure	1.81 (1.09, 3.00)
Prior myocardial infarction	1.95 (1.28, 2.98)
Female	1.66 (1.31, 2.43)
Creatinine (per 10 mmol/L)	1.04 (1.02, 1.05)
Aspirin on admission	0.53 (0.33, 0.86)
Angiotensin converting enzyme inhibitor on admission	0.46 (0.26, 0.79)
Beta-blocker on admission	0.25 (0.14, 0.44)
Digoxin on admission	0.13 (0.04, 0.47)
Statin on admission	0.06 (0.01, 0.46)

Source: Wahab *et al.* (2002).

Hyperglycaemia was associated with poor outcome even among patients without known diabetes mellitus.

INTERPRETATION. This study has several important findings. First, 8% of the patients presented with elevated blood glucose but did not have a prior diagnosis of diabetes. Secondly, these patients were older, had multiple cardiac risk factors, and were more likely to have a history of prior congestive heart failure. Thirdly, they had higher in-hospital and 1-year mortality relative to patients with known diabetes with and without hyperglycaemia.

Comment

It is likely that non-diabetic individuals with hyperglycaemia had undiagnosed diabetes of varying duration. This may have predisposed them to prolonged vascular damage from the glucose intolerant state and may have, in part, accounted for their poor outcomes. In any case, this study highlights the importance of evaluating hyperglycaemic patients with ACS for impaired glucose tolerance and diabetes mellitus. It also underscores the need for better screening for diabetes in the community.

Benefit of an early invasive management strategy in women with acute coronary syndromes.

R Glaser, H C Herrman, S A Murphy, *et al. JAMA* 2002; **288**: 3124–9.

BACKGROUND. Several studies have described the differential effect of gender on the outcomes of non-ST-segment elevation ACS. For example, a meta-analysis of glycoprotein IIb/IIIa inhibitor trials showed no benefit in women |13|, and an invasive strategy led to worse outcomes in women in two clinical trials |14,15|, but better outcomes in an observational study |16|. Glaser *et al.* examined data from the Treat Angina with Aggrastat and Determine Cost of Therapy with an Invasive or Conservative Strategy–Thrombolysis in Myocardial Infarction (TACTICS–TIMI) 18 trial to determine sex-related differences in baseline characteristics and outcomes in ACS, and to determine if women had better rates of death, MI or ACS rehospitalization at 6 months with an early invasive strategy. Of the 2220 patients analysed, 757 were women. The women enrolled were older and more often had a history of hypertension, but less often had elevation in cardiac markers. There was no difference in the distribution of TIMI risk scores between men and women. A similar proportion of men and women underwent coronary angiography during the hospitalization; Table 1.7 shows the degree of coronary artery disease in men and women. Overall, women more often had no significant coronary artery disease and less often had left main disease. Table 1.8 shows the odds ratios for clinical outcomes in men and women after adjustment for important covariates. Women had a 28% reduction in the primary end-point when treated with an early invasive strategy. This benefit was greater among women with elevated troponin levels.

INTERPRETATION. The findings reported by Glaser *et al.* run counter to those from the Fast Revascularization during InStability In Coronary Artery Disease (FRISC II) randomized trial. Whereas the female patients in TACTICS–TIMI 18 and FRISC II less often had significant coronary artery disease, the invasive strategy was associated with better outcomes in TACTICS–TIMI 18, but not in FRISC II. Two differences in the trials may explain this disparity. The CABG mortality was significantly lower in TACTICS–TIMI 18 compared with that in FRISC II (1.2 vs 9.9%). In addition, the mean time to angiography in FRISC II was 5 days compared with a much earlier time frame in TACTICS-TIMI 18 (within 48 h).

Comment

This study shows that an early invasive strategy, including a platelet glycoprotein IIb/IIIa inhibitor and coronary stents, was associated with a similar benefit in women and men. This benefit was enhanced in women with elevated troponin levels. The early invasive strategy should be pursued in women with ACS who have elevated levels of troponin.

Table 1.7 Degree of coronary artery disease (%)

	Women	Men
Angiography performed	75	76
Invasive strategy only	97	98
Conservative strategy only	50	54
Diseased coronary vessels		
All patients		
None	17	9
1 vessel	31	24
2 vessels	26	28
3 vessels	25	39
Left main	7	10
Invasive strategy only		
None	18	10
1 vessel	31	23
2 vessels	25	29
3 vessels	26	37
Left main	7	9
Conservative strategy only		
None	14	7
1 vessel	32	25
2 vessels	31	25
3 vessels	23	43
Left main	7	12

Source: Glaser *et al.* (2002).

Table 1.8 Odds ratios for 180-day clinical outcomes by invasive or conservative strategy in women and men

	Invasive	Conservative	Odds ratio (95% confidence interval)	
			Unadjusted	Adjusted
Women	(n = 395)	(n = 362)		
Death	3.8%	3.6%	1.06 (0.50, 2.26)	0.94 (0.37, 2.44)
Death or myocardial infarction	6.6%	9.7%	0.66 (0.39, 1.12)	0.45 (0.24, 0.88)
Death, myocardial infarction, rehospitalization	17.0%	19.6%	0.84 (0.58, 1.21)	0.72 (0.47, 1.11)
Men	(n = 719)	(n = 744)		
Death	3.1%	3.5%	0.87 (0.40, 1.55)	0.75 (0.36, 1.56)
Death or myocardial infarction	7.6%	9.4%	0.80 (0.55, 1.15)	0.68 (0.43, 1.05)
Death, myocardial infarction, rehospitalization	15.3%	19.4%	0.75 (0.57, 0.99)	0.64 (0.47, 0.88)

Source: Glaser *et al.* (2002).

Prognostic value of isolated troponin elevation across the spectrum of chest pain syndromes.

S V Rao, E M Ohman, C B Granger, *et al. Am J Cardiol* 2003; **91**: 936–40.

B A C K G R O U N D . For patients presenting with chest pain, the significance of troponin elevation in the absence of CK-MB elevation or other high-risk clinical features is unclear. Rao *et al.* determined the association between isolated troponin elevation and 30-day death or recurrent MI in patients with ACS and in patients with low-risk chest pain. They used combined data from the GUSTO IIa and PARAGON B troponin substudies, and data from the Chest Pain Evaluation by Creatinine Kinase-MB, Myoglobin, and Troponin I (CHECKMATE) study. The former population was considered high-risk based on clinical features, whereas the latter population was low-risk. The patients were grouped according to baseline marker status (Tn+/CKMB+; Tn+/CKMB−; Tn−/CKMB+; Tn−/CKMB−). Data from the GUSTO IIa and PARAGON trials were combined using a meta-analytic technique and data from CHECKMATE were considered separately. Using two validated statistical models (one for the high-risk population and one for the low-risk population) that included adjustment for ECG findings, the authors generated adjusted odds ratios for the primary outcome with patients negative for both markers as the reference group. As Fig. 1.7 shows, troponin

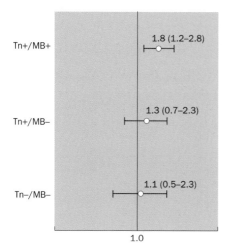

Fig. 1.7 Adjusted odds ratios and 95% confidence intervals for 30-day death or MI by marker status in the high-risk acute coronary syndrome population (left) and low-risk chest pain unit population (right). Patients negative for both CK-MB and troponin are the reference group. Source: Rao *et al.* (2003).

elevation at baseline without concomitant CK-MB elevation was associated with a significantly higher odds of 30-day death or MI in both the high- and low-risk patients.

INTERPRETATION. This study further confirms the prognostic value of troponin across the continuum of chest pain syndromes. In both high- and low-risk patients, isolated troponin elevation was significantly associated with adverse 30-day outcomes. This suggests that patients with troponin elevation, even without CK-MB elevation, should be monitored closely in either a step-down or intensive care unit setting.

Comment

The study by Rao *et al.* adds to the literature on risk stratification by showing that troponin may be a superior marker of risk over CK-MB for patients with suspected ACS. Whether low-risk patients with isolated troponin elevation would benefit from aggressive antiplatelet and invasive therapy remains to be seen.

Conclusion

As these important articles demonstrate, risk stratification in ACS continues to evolve. The cornerstone of risk assessment remains the history and physical examination. The presence of renal insufficiency and hyperglycaemia (even in the absence of diagnosed diabetes) appear to be important markers of adverse outcomes, which are often under-appreciated. Other measures of risk, the cardiac troponins, in particular, appear to offer incremental prognostic information to the baseline ECG. Although their utility in patients with renal dysfunction was questioned, there are now data to support their use in the risk stratification of ACS patients with mild to moderate renal insufficiency. Troponin appears in the blood only when and if cardiac myocyte necrosis has occurred, therefore, newer neurohormonal markers such as NT-proBNP may offer additional useful information. Finally, clinicians must take into account left ventricular function and other medical co-morbidities when evaluating patients with ACS in order to obtain a more comprehensive risk assessment.

References

1. Lee KL, Woodlief LH, Topol EJ, Weaver WD, Betriu A, Col J, *et al.* Predictors of 30-day mortality in the era of reperfusion for acute myocardial infarction. Results from an international trial of 41,021 patients. GUSTO-I Investigators. *Circulation* 1995; **91**: 1659–68.

2. Boersma E, Pieper KS, Steyerberg EW, Wilcox RG, Chang WC, Lee KL, *et al.* Predictors of outcome in patients with acute coronary syndromes without persistent ST-segment elevation. Results from an international trial of 9461 patients. The PURSUIT Investigators. *Circulation* 2000; **101**: 2557–67.

3. The GUSTO Investigators. An international randomized trial comparing four thrombolytic strategies for acute myocardial infarction. *N Engl J Med* 1993; **329**: 673–82.

4. Weaver WD, Simes RJ, Betriu A, Grines CL, Zijlstra F, Garcia E, *et al.* Comparison of primary coronary angioplasty and intravenous thrombolytic therapy for acute myocardial infarction: a quantitative review. *JAMA* 1997; **278**: 2093–8.

5. Heidenreich P, Allogiamento T, Melsop K, McDonald KM, Hlatky M. The prognostic value of troponin in patients with non-ST elevation acute coronary syndromes: a meta-analysis. *J Am Coll Cardiol* 2001; **38**: 478–85.

6. de Lemos JA, Morrow DA, Bentley JH, Omland T, Sabatine MS, McCabe CH, *et al.* The prognostic value of B-type natriuretic peptide in patients with acute coronary syndromes. *N Engl J Med* 2001; **345**: 1014–21.

7. Hunt PJ, Richards AM, Nicholls MG, Yandle TG, Doughty RN, Espiner EA. Immunoreactive amino-terminal pro-brain natriuretic peptide (NT-PROBNP): a new marker of cardiac impairment. *Clin Endocrinol* 1997; **47**: 287–96.

8. Kasiske BL, Ravenscraft M, Ramos EL, Gaston RS, Bia MJ, Danovitch GM. The evaluation of living renal transplant donors: clinical practice guidelines. Ad Hoc Clinical Practice

Guidelines Subcommittee of the Patient Care and Education Committee of the American Society of Transplant Physicians. *J Am Soc Nephrol* 1996; 7: 2288–313.

9. Lee PY, Alexander KP, Hammill BG, Pasquali SK, Peterson ED. Representation of elderly persons and women in published randomized trials of acute coronary syndromes. *JAMA* 2001; **286**: 708–13.

10. Mak KH, Moliterno DJ, Granger CB, Miller DP, White HD, Wilcox RG *et al.* Influence of diabetes mellitus on clinical outcome in the thrombolytic era of acute myocardial infarction. GUSTO-I investigators. Global utilization of streptokinase and tissue plasminogen activator for occluded coronary arteries. *J Am Coll Cardiol* 1997; **30**: 171–9.

11. Cho E, Rimm EB, Stampfer MJ, Willett WC, Hu FB. The impact of diabetes mellitus and prior myocardial infarction on mortality from all causes and from coronary heart disease in men. *J Am Coll Cardiol* 2002; **40**: 954–60.

12. Capes SE, Hunt D, Malmberg K, Gerstein HC. Stress hyperglycaemia and increased risk of death after myocardial infarction in patients with and without diabetes: a systematic overview. *Lancet* 2000; **355**(9206): 773–8.

13. Boersma E, Harrington RA, Moliterno DJ, White H, Theroux P, Van de WF, *et al.* Platelet glycoprotein IIb/IIIa inhibitors in acute coronary syndromes: a meta-analysis of all major randomised clinical trials. *Lancet* 2002; **359**(9302): 189–98.

14. Lagerqvist B, Safstrom K, Stahle E, Wallentin L, Swahn E, FRISC II Study Group Investigators. Is early invasive treatment of unstable coronary artery disease equally effective for both women and men? FRISC II Study Group Investigators. *J Am Coll Cardiol* 2001; **38**: 41–8.

15. Fox KA, Poole-Wilson PA, Henderson RA, Clayton TC, Chamberlain DA, Shaw TR, *et al.* Interventional versus conservative treatment for patients with unstable angina or non-ST-elevation myocardial infarction: the British Heart Foundation RITA 3 randomised trial. Randomized Intervention Trial of unstable Angina. *Lancet* 2002; **360**(9335): 743–51.

16. Mueller C, Neumann FJ, Roskamm H, Buser P, Hodgson JM, Perruchoud AP, *et al.* Women do have an improved long-term outcome after non-ST-elevation acute coronary syndromes treated very early and predominantly with percutaneous coronary intervention: a prospective study in 1,450 consecutive patients. *J Am Coll Cardiol* 2002; **40**: 245–50.

2

Percutaneous coronary intervention for acute ST-elevation myocardial infarction

Introduction

Primary coronary angioplasty has become the reperfusion treatment of choice in many hospitals throughout the world. New findings and developments further improve clinical outcome for many of these patients with ST-elevation myocardial infarction. Adjunctive pharmacotherapy is complex and consists of several classes of drugs aimed at thrombosis and ischaemia.

Anti-ischaemic therapy with nitrates and beta blockers and anti-thrombotic therapy with anti-thrombin and anti-platelet agents play a crucial role before, during and after the acute intervention.

Some of these drugs such as aspirin, clopidogrel and (low molecular weight) heparin should be given to most, if not all, patients, and many other drugs will be needed in many or most patients, with the difficult task to tailor appropriate therapy to the needs of the individual patient. Many other aspects of primary angioplasty therapy have shown rapid developments, in particular the use of stents, with currently enrolling studies focusing on drug-eluting stents, angioplasty therapy in hospitals without surgical capabilities, the complex interaction between time from symptom-onset to treatment and clinical outcome, and some remaining issues of the old debate of angioplasty versus lytic therapy. The interventional cardiology community will continue to plan and conduct trials that will further improve our possibilities to care for patients with acute ST-elevation myocardial infarction. Crucial steps in this direction of the last year include:

1. The use of intravenous beta blockade to improve procedural safety and clinical outcome in primary angioplasty patients;

2. The reporting of the large, multicentre CADILLAC trial that defines the relative benefits of stenting and abciximab in 2681 patients enrolled at 76 centres in 9 countries

3. The Atlantic C-PORT (Cardiovascular Patient Outcomes Research Team) trial, a real-world comparison of angioplasty versus lytic therapy at 11 community hospitals, after completion of a formal primary angioplasty development program;

4. A carefully performed retrospective analysis of 1336 unselected primary angioplasty patients to study in detail the relation of time to treatment and mortality.

5. A randomized comparison of angioplasty versus pre-hospital thrombolytic therapy in 840 patients in mobile emergency care units affiliated with 27 tertiary hospitals in France, important in particular as the outcome after lytic therapy is strongly related to the time delay between symptom onset and start of therapy.

6. A quantitative review of all 23 randomized trials performed so far, showing impressive and consistent benefits of the interventional approach towards ST-elevation myocardial infarction in a wide range of settings.

In summary, it requires regular extensive reading to keep in touch with the rapidly evolving field of primary angioplasty.

Effects of prior beta-blocker therapy on clinical outcomes after primary coronary angioplasty for acute myocardial infarction.

K J Harjai, G W Stone, J Boura, et al. *Am J Cardiol* 2003; **91**: 655–60.

BACKGROUND. Beta blockers are recommended for the management of acute myocardial infarction (AMI), as well as for secondary prevention. The anti-ischaemic and anti-arrhythmic effects improve survival and reduce the risk of re-infarction in patients with AMI. However, the influence of pre-treatment with beta-blockers on clinical outcomes in patients treated with primary angioplasty had not been described. In a setting with a heightened sympathetic state, characterized by chest pain, ischaemia, necrosis and acute reperfusion, effective blunting of sympathetic activity by beta-blockers may attenuate the harmful effects of adrenergic stimulation.

INTERPRETATION. The clinical, angiographic and outcome data of 2537 patients enrolled in the Primary Angioplasty in Myocardial Infarction trials (PAMI 1, PAMI 2 and Stent PAMI) were studied. Patients were classified as beta-patients if they received beta-blocker therapy before primary angioplasty ($n = 1132$) or no-beta patients if they did not ($n = 1405$). Beta-patients were younger, had higher systolic blood pressure and heart rate, and were more likely to be in Killip class I at admission. They had lower left ventricular ejection fraction, greater door-to-balloon time, greater likelihood of having a left anterior descending artery culprit lesion, but a similar incidence of Thrombolysis in Myocardial Infarction (TIMI) 3 flow after primary angioplasty (92.6 vs 92.7%, $P = 0.91$). The beta group had fewer procedural complications, in particular arrhythmias, and better clinical outcome at 30 days and 1 year compared to the no beta patients, see Table 2.1.

Table 2.1 Outcome of patients treated with versus without beta-blockers prior to primary angioplasty for acute myocardial infarction

	Beta group	P	No beta group
Procedural complications	23%	<0.0001	34%
In-hospital mortality	1.8%	0.0035	3.7%
MACE	5.5%	0.027	7.8%
1-year mortality	4.9%	0.055	6.7%

Major adverse cardiac event (MACE) = death, re-infarction, ischaemia-driven target vessel revascularization or disabling stroke during the index hospitalization.
After adjustment for baseline differences, beta patients had a lower in-hospital mortality, odds ratio 0.41, 95% confidence interval 0.20–0.84, $P <0.01$ and trend toward lower 1-year mortality, odds ratio 0.72, 95% confidence interval 0.47–1.08, $P = 0.11$.
Source: Harjai *et al.* (2003).

Comment

These data clearly demonstrate the benefit of beta-blocker treatment prior to primary angioplasty for AMI. Owing to a large reduction in arrhythmias, complications during the procedure are markedly reduced. For every ten patients treated, one catheterization laboratory event is prevented. Furthermore, the data strongly suggest an improved in-hospital and 1-year outcome, although it should be kept in mind that these data come from a *post hoc* analysis, not a randomized, controlled trial. Nevertheless, beta-blockers should become more popular on the way to the catheterization laboratory for patients with acute ST-elevation myocardial infarction.

Comparison of angioplasty with stenting, with or without abciximab, in acute myocardial infarction.
G W Stone, C L Grines, D A Cox *et al. N Engl J Med* 2002; **346**: 957–66.

BACKGROUND. As compared with thrombolytic therapy, primary angioplasty increases patency rates, improves survival and reduces the rates of re-infarction and stroke. However, ischaemia and re-infarction do occur in 5–15% of patients in the first months, and late restenosis or re-occlusion increases morbidity, mortality and costs. Compared with balloon angioplasty, stenting offers the advantage of stabilizing dissections during the acute event and decreases the likelihood of restenosis. Glycoprotein (Gp) IIb/IIIa inhibitors have shown consistent benefits in trials of acute coronary syndrome patients treated with a percutaneous coronary intervention. Several published case series and small or moderately sized randomized trials have suggested improved outcome in patients with acute ST-segment elevation myocardial infarction when treated with stenting and Gp IIb/IIIa inhibitors during the primary angioplasty procedure.

INTERPRETATION. In total, 2681 patients with acute myocardial infarction were enrolled at 76 centres in 9 countries, of whom 78% met the angiographic criteria for stent implantation and underwent randomization. Using a 2-by-2 factorial design, the CADILLAC investigators randomly assigned 2082 patients with AMI, to undergo balloon angioplasty (518 patients), balloon angioplasty plus abciximab (528 patients), stenting with a Multilink Stent (512 patients) or stenting plus abciximab (524 patients). In the balloon-only group, 16% received stents and fewer than 10% no-abciximab patients received abciximab, both when angiographic results were suboptimal. Normal flow was restored in 95–7% of patients and did not vary according to strategy. There was no benefit of abciximab in stented patients, and only a modest effect of abciximab seemed to be present in patients treated with plain old balloon angioplasty. Stenting had a major effect on angiographic restenosis and re-occlusion, see Table 2.2.

Comment

The potential benefits of the adjunctive use of abciximab in AMI patients treated with primary angioplasty are improved flow before and after the procedure, treatment of lesion-associated thrombus and thrombotic embolism and improved clinical outcome, and several previous trials have supported this concept. The results of this much larger CADILLAC trial do not confirm these benefits of abciximab in this setting. Previous studies have used abciximab as pre-treatment and in the CADILLAC trial abciximab was used as adjunctive therapy in the catheterization laboratory after diagnostic coronary angiography. Pre-treatment with a Gp IIb/IIIa inhibitor still holds great promise, particularly when there is a significant delay between diagnosis of acute infarction and first balloon inflation.

The principle finding of the CADILLAC study is that in stent-eligible patients, routine stent implantation results in higher rates of event free survival and better angiographic outcome compared with plain old balloon angioplasty with stenting only as bail-out in case of poor or unsatisfactory balloon results.

Table 2.2 Angiographic follow-up at 7 months in 656 of 900 pre-specified eligible patients (73%)

	Balloon	P	Stent
Diameter stenosis >50%	41%	<0.001	22%
Re-occlusion	11%	0.01	6%

Therapy with abciximab resulted in a lower rate of subacute thrombosis (0.4 vs 1.4%, $P < 0.001$) but blood transfusions were more common in these patients (4.2 vs 1.9%, $P = 0.002$), without a significant impact on 30-day or 6-month mortality and/or re-infarction.
Source: Stone *et al.* (2002).

Thrombolytic therapy versus primary percutaneous coronary intervention for myocardial infarction in patients presenting to hospitals without on-site cardiac surgery; a randomized controlled trial.

T Aversano, L T Aversano, E Passamani, *et al. JAMA* 2002; **287**: 1943–51.

BACKGROUND. Most institutions participating in comparative trials of thrombolytic therapy versus primary angioplasty have been hospitals with on-site cardiac surgery and active elective angioplasty programmes. However, the majority of patients with AMI present to hospitals without such capability. The fact that access to primary angioplasty is restricted despite its superior outcomes has resulted in the development of strategies to overcome this limitation. Transportation to hospitals with full invasive capabilities has been studied in several multicentre randomized trials, and has shown that primary angioplasty after additional interhospital transportation is safe and compatible with excellent clinical outcome. The other potential solution to cope with the limited access to primary angioplasty is to start primary angioplasty programmes in community hospitals without on-site cardiac surgery or sometimes even without elective angioplasty programmes.

INTERPRETATION. The Atlantic C-PORT investigators thought to determine whether treatment of AMI with primary angioplasty is superior to thrombolytic therapy at hospitals without on-site cardiac surgery, in eleven community hospitals in Massachusetts and Maryland. After completion of a formal primary angioplasty development programme, 451 thrombolytic-eligible patients with AMI of less than 12 hours duration, and with ST-segment elevation on the electrocardiogram (ECG), were randomly assigned to receive primary angioplasty ($n = 225$) or accelerated tissue plasminogen activation. The incidence of a composite end-point (death, re-infarction and stroke), was reduced by primary angioplasty at 6 weeks: 11 vs 18%, $P = 0.03$, and at 6 months: 12 vs 20%, $P = 0.03$. The median length of hospital stay was also reduced in the primary angioplasty group: 4.5 vs 6.0 days, $P = 0.02$.

Comment

These data demonstrate that primary angioplasty can be performed safely, promptly and effectively in a community hospital without an elective angioplasty or cardiac surgery programme, provided that, in an extensive development programme, careful attention has been paid to training, logistics and quality control. A systematic primary angioplasty strategy involves a team of healthcare personnel, including the pre-hospital diagnosis and transports system, the emergency department, coronary care unit and cardiac catheterization laboratory. The Atlantic C-PORT trial was a 'real-world' comparison of alternative therapies, and these investigators continue their research effort in the ongoing Atlantic C-PORT primary percutaneous coronary intervention (PCI) registry. This type of information will expand our understanding of the best ways to improve access to primary angioplasty. In many settings patients have to travel to the doctor, in C-PORT the care providers went towards the community, illustrating that there is no single 'recipe' for optimal reperfusion therapy, for acute myocardial infarction.

Relation of time to treatment and mortality in patients with acute myocardial infarction undergoing primary coronary angioplasty.

D Antoniucci, R Valenti, A Migliorini, *et al. Am J Cardiol* 2002; **89**: 1248–52.

BACKGROUND. The benefit of thrombolysis for AMI is strongly dependent on the delay between symptom onset and treatment, but this relation is less clear in patients undergoing primary angioplasty. Many studies have shown that mortality was fairly constant from 2 to 12 h after symptom onset, and a somewhat increased benefit has been described of very early intervention in patients treated within 2 h after symptom onset. This may imply that the additional delay in treatment due to patient transfer from a hospital without invasive facilities to an interventional hospital would have little or no impact on the benefit of primary angioplasty. This would overcome the most important logistic problem of the primary angioplasty strategy, that is delay to therapy.

INTERPRETATION. The investigators hypothesized that the relation of time to treatment to mortality is related to baseline risk of the patient. They tested this in a series of 1336 unselected primary angioplasty patients, stratified into 'low-risk' and 'not low-risk' groups according to the TIMI criteria. The 6 months mortality rate was 9.3% for not low-risk patients and 1.3% for low-risk patients, $P < 0.001$. In low-risk patients there was no relation between time to treatment and outcome. Mortality of not low-risk patients increased from 4.8 to 12.9% with increasing time to reperfusion up to 6 hours. However, in multivariate analysis time to reperfusion was not an independent predictor of mortality. The only independent predictors of mortality were age, diabetes and cardiogenic shock. In conclusion, in not low-risk primary angioplasty patients, there is a strong association between time to treatment and mortality, in low-risk patients this relation does not exist. A potential explanation of these findings is the worse risk profile of patients with a longer delay to treatment.

Comment

These data support the notion that the relation between time to therapy and outcome of thrombolytic therapy and primary angioplasty differs markedly. Some reports have suggested that an additional delay, even of several hours, does not have a clinically relevant impact on the outcome after primary angioplasty. This may not be true for several categories of patients. It has been described that very early (<2 h) reperfusion by primary angioplasty may result in more myocardial salvage and lower mortality, in particular, in patients with large anterior myocardial infarctions. This report suggests that patients aged ≥70 years, with anterior myocardial infarction or heart rate ≥100 beat/min may benefit by measures to reduce time to therapy.

Primary angioplasty versus pre-hospital fibrinolysis in acute myocardial infarction: a randomized study.

E Bonnefoy, F Lapostolle, A Leizorovicz, *et al. Lancet* 2002; **360**: 825–9.

BACKGROUND. Reperfusion therapy in AMI is aimed at complete and sustained patency of the infarct-related artery, obtained as early as possible. Primary angioplasty results in higher patency and lower rates of re-infarction and stroke, compared with thrombolytic therapy. However, in many patients a strategy of primary angioplasty may impose an additional delay that may, in part, attenuate its clinical benefit. Pre-hospital administration of lytic therapy is associated with a time gain of 30 min to 2 h compared with in-hospital administration and can be combined with urgent rescue angioplasty when fibrinolysis is suspected to have failed.

INTERPRETATION. The Comparison of Angioplasty and Prehospital Thrombolysis in Acute Myocardial Infarction (CAPTIM) Study group performed a randomized multicentre trial of 840 patients (of 1200 planned) who presented within 6 h of AMI with ST-segment elevation, initially managed by mobile emergency-care units affiliated with 27 tertiary hospitals in France. All participating hospitals had experience in routine primary angioplasty and had a 24-hour on-call angioplasty team available. The primary end-point was a composite of death, non-fatal re-infarction and non-fatal disabling stroke at 30 days. The median delay between onset of symptoms and (start of intravenous lytic) therapy was 130 min in the pre-hospital-fibrinolysis group and 190 min in the primary angioplasty group (time to first balloon inflation). Rescue angioplasty was performed in 26% in the fibrinolysis group. The rate of the primary end-point was 8.2% in the pre-hospital-lytic group compared with 6.2% in the primary angioplasty group (not significant). Strokes were noted only in the pre-hospital-lytic group and unplanned revascularization (angioplasty or bypass surgery) was performed more frequently in lytic patients, 35 vs 5%, $P < 0.001$.

Comment

A shortcoming of the CAPTIM study is that cessation of funding resulted in a lower than planned recruitment, and the confidence intervals for the primary end-point show that there could be a real difference in the treatment effects. The mortality rates, in particular in the lytic group (4 vs 5% in the primary angioplasty group) were low, and in fact in the lytic group lower than expected. There are several possible explanations, such as the inclusion of a relative low-risk population, short delays from symptom onset to therapy and liberal use of rescue angioplasty. The data suggest that the potential exists for further reductions in the rates of mortality and re-infarction after both primary angioplasty and lytic therapy.

Primary angioplasty versus intravenous thrombolytic therapy for acute myocardial infarction: a quantitative review of 23 randomized trials.

E C Keeley, J A Boura, C L Grines. *Lancet* 2003; **361**: 13–20.

BACKGROUND. **The reperfusion era started with the realization that an occlusive thrombus on top of a ruptured atherosclerotic plaque is the cause of acute ST-segment elevation MI. Over the past decades many trials have been performed, comparing mechanical (primary angioplasty) with pharmacological (fibrinolysis) reperfusion strategies, the initial comparison being intracoronary thrombolytic therapy with plain old balloon angioplasty, followed by a phase in which intravenous thrombolytic therapy was compared with balloon angioplasty and finally comparative trials studying modern (pre-hospital) lytic therapy and primary PCI with stenting and Gp IIb/IIIa inhibitors.**

INTERPRETATION. The aim of this quantitative review was to look at the combined results of 23 randomized trials published to date (Table 2.3). A total of 7739 thrombolytic eligible patients with ST-segment elevation myocardial infarction were randomly assigned to primary angioplasty (*n* = 3872) or lytic therapy (*n* = 3867). Streptokinase was used in twelve trials and fibrin-specific agents in fifteen. Stents were used in twelve trials and platelet Gp IIb/IIIa inhibitors in eight.

Comment

Since the previous systematic review of this topic, published in 1997, several new trials have been undertaken, significantly increasing the total number of patients studied. These new trials reflect the rapid evolution of angioplasty technology and medical therapy. These new trials used modern lytic therapy, stents, Gp IIb/IIIa inhibitors, and addressed important issues such as safety and efficacy of emergent

Table 2.3 Clinical outcome after primary angioplasty compared with lytic therapy in 23 randomized trials

	Primary angioplasty	*P*	Lytic therapy
Death	7%	0.002	9%
Re-infarction	3%	<0.0001	7%
Stroke	1%	0.004	2%
MACE	8%	<0.0001	14%

MACE = combined clinical end-point of death, non-fatal re-infarction and stroke.
These results seen with primary angioplasty remained better than those seen with lytic therapy during long-term follow-up, and were independent of both the type of lytic agent used, and whether or not the patient was transferred for primary angioplasty.
Source: Keeley *et al.* (2003).

interhospital transfer, high-risk subgroup (elderly and shock), angioplasty in hospitals without surgical standby and pre-hospital lytic therapy.

These data, including long-term follow-up, show consistent findings in favour of primary angioplasty and document that this procedure is applicable in a wide range of settings.

Conclusion

Outcome after primary angioplasty can be further improved by meticulous attention to many 'details' of this treatment strategy, and it is becoming more and more clear that this therapy can be delivered to a much larger percentage of myocardial infarction patients than previously thought. The findings of this year's publications can best be summarized in the following 4 statements.

1. Whenever and wherever possible, primary angioplasty has become the preferred reperfusion strategy in patients with ST elevation myocardial infarction irrespective of presence or absence of (relative) contraindications for intravenous thrombolytic therapy. Referral of patients to established heart centres with full capability interventional catheterization facilities is an option for many patients as well as the performance of primary angioplasty in hospitals without cardiac surgery, provided adequate training and preparations and including careful attention to quality control. Our understanding of the best ways to improve access to primary angioplasty will certainly evolve during the coming years.

2. Stenting, 'plaque sealing', seems preferable when technically feasible, provided a suitable coronary anatomy. The value of adjunctive abciximab therapy in patients with a perfect stent result may not be great. This contrast with benefits of glycoprotein IIb, IIIa antagonists when started before the procedure, and suggests that a tailored approach is preferable when this therapy is considered as adjunctive measure during the interventional procedure.

3. Even when new approaches have been shown to offer important benefits, old lessons should not be forgotten; intravenous beta-blocker therapy continues to be an important adjunct in the early hours of acute infarction and should be used to decrease procedural complications during acute interventions.

4. The relation between time to treatment and clinical outcome is one of the fundamental differences between thrombolytic therapy and primary angioplasty. Further studies are needed to help us understand the mechanisms involved and to reconsider how this phenomenon should impact the way we organize the acute care of ST elevation myocardial infarction patients.

References

1. De Luca G, Suryapranata H, Thomas K, van't Hof AW, de Boer MJ, Hoorntje JC, Zijlstra F. Outcome in patients treated with primary angioplasty for acute myocardial infarction due to left main coronary artery occlusion. *Am J Cardiol* 2003; **91**(2): 235–8.

2. Grines C, Patel A, Zijlstra F, Weaver WD, Granger C, Simes RJ; PCAT Collaborators. Percutaneous transluminal coronary angioplasty. Primary coronary angioplasty compared with intravenous thrombolytic therapy for acute myocardial infarction: six-month follow up and analysis of individual patient data from randomized trials. *Am Heart J* 2003; **145**(1): 47–57.

3. Dixon SR, Whitbourn RJ, Dae MW, Grube E, Sherman W, Schaer GL, Jenkins JS, Baim DS, Gibbons RJ, Kuntz RE, Popma JJ, Nguyen TT, O'Neill WW. Induction of mild systemic hypothermia with endovascular cooling during primary percutaneous coronary intervention for acute myocardial infarction. *J Am Coll Cardiol* 2002; **40**(11): 1928–34.

4. Dalby M, Montalescot G. Transfer for primary angioplasty: who and how? *Heart* 2002; **88**(6): 570–2. Review.

5. Bolognese L, Neskovic AN, Parodi G, Cerisano G, Buonamici P, Santoro GM, Antoniucci D. Left ventricular remodeling after primary coronary angioplasty: patterns of left ventricular dilation and long-term prognostic implications. *Circulation* 2002; **106**(18): 2351–7.

6. Stone GW. Primary angioplasty versus 'earlier' thrombolysis – time for a wake-up call. *Lancet* 2002; **360**(9336): 814–16.

7. Bertrand ME, McFadden EP. Late is perhaps not too late for primary PCI in acute myocardial infarction. *Eur Heart J* 2002; **23**(15): 1146–8.

8. Henriques JP, Zijlstra F, Ottervanger JP, de Boer MJ, van't Hof AW, Hoorntje JC, Suryapranata H. Incidence and clinical significance of distal embolization during primary angioplasty for acute myocardial infarction. *Eur Heart J* 2002; **23**(14): 1112–17.

9. Zijlstra F, Ernst N, de Boer MJ, Nibbering E, Suryapranata H, Hoorntje JC, Dambrink JH, van't Hof AW, FW Verheugt. Influence of pre-hospital administration of aspirin and heparin on initial patency of the infarct-related artery in patients with acute ST elevation myocardial infarction. *J Am Coll Cardiol* 2002; **39**(11): 1733–7.

10. de Boer MJ, Ottervanger JP, van't Hof AW, Hoorntje JC, Suryapranata H, Zijlstra F; Zwolle Myocardial Infarction Study Group. Reperfusion therapy in elderly patients with acute myocardial infarction: a randomized comparison of primary angioplasty and thrombolytic therapy. *J Am Coll Cardiol* 2002; **39**(11): 1723–8.

11. Grines CL, Westerhausen Jr DR, Grines LL, Hanlon JT, Logemann TL, Niemela M, Weaver WD, Graham M, Boura J, O'Neill WW, Balestrini C; Air PAMI Study Group. A randomized trial of transfer for primary angioplasty versus on-site thrombolysis in patients with high-risk myocardial infarction: the Air Primary Angioplasty in Myocardial Infarction study. *J Am Coll Cardiol* 2002; **39**(11): 1713–19.

12. Cannon CP. Primary percutaneous coronary intervention for all? *JAMA* 2002; **287**(15): 1987–9.

13. Zijlstra F, Patel A, Jones M, Grines CL, Ellis S, Garcia E, Grinfeld L, Gibbons RJ, Ribeiro EE, Ribichini F, Granger C, Akhras F, Weaver WD, Simes RJ. Clinical characteristics and outcome of patients with early (<2 h), intermediate (2–4 h) and late (>4 h) presentation treated by primary coronary angioplasty or thrombolytic therapy for acute myocardial infarction. *Eur Heart J* 2002; **23**(7): 550–7.

14. Stone GW, Peterson MA, Lansky AJ, Dangas G, Mehran R, Leon MB. Impact of normalized myocardial perfusion after successful angioplasty in acute myocardial infarction. *J Am Coll Cardiol* 2002; **39**(4): 591–7.

3

Percutaneous coronary intervention for stable and non-ST elevation acute coronary syndromes

Introduction

The major development in interventional cardiology over the past year has been the introduction of drug-eluting stents for routine patient care. Angiographic restenosis rates below 10%, even in subsets of patients at high risk for restenosis, will undoubtedly change the practice of interventional cardiology. The far higher price, however, will force cardiologists to restrict application of these devices to patients at high risk for in-stent restenosis.

Moreover, it is probably not necessary to expose all patients to a drug-eluting stent. Certain lesion types are attended with a very low restenosis rate. To treat all patients with these lesions with a drug-eluting stent although only 10% will benefit seems to be rather unnecessary. In these patients a strategy of watchful waiting for clinical restenosis with subsequent deployment of a drug-eluting stent seems a sensible approach.

Because of this, strategies that minimize the chance for in-stent restenosis with bare metal stents will remain of both clinical and economic importance. Several studies have recently been published that address this issue. They are discussed.

Treatment of patients with non-ST elevation acute coronary syndrome (NSTEACS) should include antiplatelet therapy with aspirin and clopidogrel, antithrombotic therapy with unfractionated heparin or low molecular weight heparins and glycoprotein (Gp) IIb/IIIa inhibitor therapy with early angiography in a subset of patients with high-risk characteristics such as ST depression and/or positive markers for myocardial necrosis. In the latter category of patients, Fast Revascularization during Instability in Coronary artery disease II (FRISC II) and Treat Angina with Aggrastat and Determine Cost of Therapy with an Invasive or Conservative Strategy–Thrombolysis in Myocardial Infarction-18 (TACTICS–TIMI 18) trials |1,2| have shown that a strategy of early angiography and subsequent revascularization under an umbrella of Gp IIb/IIIa inhibition plus using stents when possible, improves 30-day outcome compared with a strategy of initial medical therapy. In FRISC II angiography had to be performed within 4 days of admission in the early invasive arm. There was almost no cross-over to angiography in the conservative arm of the study. At 1 year there was a clear survival benefit for the early invasive cohort compared with the non-invasive arm (mortality 2.2 vs 3.9%; relative risk [RR] 0.57, 95% confidence interval [CI] 0.36–0.90). In the TACTICS trial angiography was performed at a mean of 22 h after randomization in the early invasive group. Sixty-one per cent of patients in the early invasive cohort underwent revascularization during initial hospitalization compared with 37% in the conservative group. In the invasive group percutaneous coronary intervention (PCI) was performed at a mean of 25 h from randomization and coronary artery bypass grafting (CABG) at a mean of 89 h from randomization. At 6-month follow-up the incidence of myocardial infarction (MI; 4.8 vs 6.9%, odds ratio [OR] 0.67, 95% CI 0.46–0.96) and death or MI (7.3 vs 9.5%, OR 0.74, 95% CI 0.54–1.0) was significantly lower in the invasive arm of the study. At 6 months no survival benefit was apparent (3.3 vs 3.5%). A third recently published trial that investigated whether an early invasive strategy is better than a conservative treatment is the British Heart Foundation Randomized Intervention Trial of unstable Angina (RITA) 3 randomized trial.

An open question is the optimal timing of 'early angiography' in these high-risk non-ST elevation acute coronary syndrome patients. Can we afford to wait 24–72 h or should we go as far as to treat these high-risk patients as ST elevation myocardial infarction (STEMI) patients with emergency coronary angiography and if possible immediate PCI? The latter scenario would mean setting up or expanding a very costly nationwide 24-hour angiography service similar to the acute infarction angiography services already functioning in many areas. This timing issue has been addressed in a *post hoc* analysis of the Platelet Glycoprotein IIb/IIIa in Unstable Angina: Receptor Suppression Using Integrilin Therapy (PURSUIT) trial and in a small randomized trial from the Czech Republic (see Ronner *et al.* and Spacek *et al.*).

Heparin-coated stent placement for the treatment of stenoses in small coronary arteries of symptomatic patients.

M Haude, T F M Konorza, U Kalnins, *et al. Circulation* 2003; **107**: 1265–70.

BACKGROUND. The role of stents, in particular, heparin-coated stents for the treatment of stenoses in small coronary arteries, is still unclear. Therefore, the authors performed this prospective, randomized trial to evaluate the angiographic and clinical outcome after treatment of stenoses in small coronary arteries (2.0–2.6 mm) of symptomatic patients. They randomly assigned 588 patients to undergo angioplasty (*n* = 195), bare stenting (*n* = 196) or heparin-coated stenting (*n* = 197). The primary end-point was minimal lumen diameter (MLD) at 6 months. With comparable baseline parameters, the two stent arms showed a larger post-interventional MLD, larger acute gain and smaller residual percentage diameter stenosis, although a residual stenosis of

12 ± 16% was achieved in the angioplasty arm, including a 27% cross-over rate to stenting. Eighty per cent of patients had follow-up angiography, which documented a borderline significantly larger MLD and smaller percentage diameter stenosis for the two stent groups (1.34 ± 0.48 mm and 42 ± 20% after angioplasty, 1.47 ± 0.48 mm and 36 ± 20% after bare stenting, and 1.45 ± 0.54 mm and 38 ± 23% after heparin-coated stenting; $P = 0.049$ and $P = 0.038$, respectively), but restenosis rates were not different (32, 25 and 30%). Thrombotic events occurred in 1.0% after angioplasty and 0.5% after bare or heparin-coated stenting. Survival without MI or target vessel revascularization at 250 days was 84.6% (angioplasty), 88.3% (bare stenting) and 88.3% (heparin-coated stenting; log-rank $P = 0.39$).

INTERPRETATION. Compared with angioplasty with provisional stenting, bare and heparin-coated stenting confer superior angiographic results and a non-significant 24% reduction in clinical events, with no difference between bare and heparin-coated stenting in the treatment of stenoses in small coronary arteries.

Comment

Both balloon angioplasty and stenting of smaller vessels are attended with an increased angiographic and clinical restenosis rate compared with interventions in larger vessels |3,4|. The possible superiority of stenting in these smaller vessels has been the subject of seven recently published randomized trials |5–10|. All trials show that both stenting and balloon angioplasty of small vessels is safe with a similar low peri-procedural complication rate as found in larger vessels. Table 3.1 summarizes the main results. The need for stent implantation because of a suboptimal initial result or (threatening) vessel occlusion in the balloon angioplasty arms (provisional stenting) was low in all trials. Indeed a satisfactory balloon angioplasty result was attainable in 75–85% of cases. Angiographic superiority of stenting was found in two of the six trials and clinical superiority in three. It should be noted that the magnitude of clinical treatment benefit (lower target vessel revascularization [TVR] or target lesion revascularization [TLR]) of stenting is likely to be inflated by the reluctance of cardiologists to perform a repeat angioplasty for in-stent restenosis, especially in small vessels and especially in trials with mandatory follow-up angiography. This bias is well described by Brophy et al. |11|.

In all trials at least a trend towards a better outcome with stenting was noticed. It is therefore likely that a formal meta-analysis will show a significant angiographic and clinical benefit for stenting. However, the differences are small and a strategy of provisional stenting with repeat intervention for restenosis only if combined with recurrence of ischaemia therefore seems to be a cost-effective option. In the near future, this might change to provisional drug-eluting stent implantation for small vessels. With that strategy, in-stent restenosis will be avoided and recurrence after balloon angioplasty can then effectively be treated with a drug-eluting stent. Furthermore, over-treatment with these expensive devices with unknown long-term consequences can be prevented.

Table 3.1 Summary of randomized trails comparing stenting and balloon angioplasty in small vessels

Trial	Year	No. of patients	Vessel size	Cross-over (%)		Restenosis rate (>50% DS)			TVR @ 6–8 months		
				Balloon -stent	Stent -balloon	Balloon %	Stent %	P	Balloon %	Stent %	P
Park et al. |7|	2000	120	<3.0 mm	20	0	36	31	NS	18	20	NS
ISAR-SMART |8|	2000	404	2.0–2.8 mm	16.5	4.4	37	36	NS	20	17	NS
BE-SMART |9|	2001	381	<3.0 mm	24	3	47	21	<0.0001	25**	13**	0.006
SISA |10|	2001	351	2.3–2.9 mm	20.3	2.4	33	28	NS	20	18	NS
SISCA |11|	2001	145	2.1–3.0 mm	14.1	4.1	19	10	0.15	23	10	0.04
RAP |12|	2000	426	2.2–2.7 mm			37	27	0.04	22**	12**	0.02
COAST	2003	588	2.0–2.6 mm	27.2	1.8*	32	27*	NS	14	11	NS

*Combined heparin-coated and bare metal stent groups. **TLR = target lesion revascularization, TVR = target vessel revascularization, BE-SMART= be-stent in small arteries, COAST = heparin-coated stent, ISAR-SMART = intracoronary stenting or angioplasty for restenosis reduction in small arteries, RAP = restenosis in arterias perquenas, SISA = stenting in small arteries, SISCA = stenting in small coronary arteries.
Source: Haude et al. (2003).

Effects of gold coating of coronary stents on neointimal proliferation following stent implantation.

J vom Dahl, P K Haager, E Grube, *et al. Am J Cardiol* 2002; **89**: 801–5.

BACKGROUND. Experimental studies suggest a reduced neointimal tissue proliferation in vascular stainless steel stents coated with gold. This prospective multicentre trial evaluated the impact of gold coating on neointimal tissue proliferation in patients undergoing elective stent implantation. The primary end-point was the in-stent tissue proliferation measured by intravascular ultrasound (IVUS) at 6 months comparing stents of identical design with or without gold coating (Inflow). Two hundred and four patients were randomized to receive uncoated (group A, *n* = 101) or coated (group B, *n* = 103) stents. Baseline parameters did not differ between groups. Stent length and balloon size were comparable, whereas inflation pressure was slightly higher in group A (14 ± 3 vs 13 ± 3 atm, *P* = 0.013). Procedural success was similar (A, 97%; B, 96%). The acute angiographic result was better for group B (remaining stenosis 4 ± 12% vs 10 ± 11%, *P* = 0.002). Six-month examinations revealed more neointimal proliferation in group B. Using ultrasound, the neointimal volume within the stent was 47 ± 25 versus 41 ± 23 mm³ (*P* = 0.04), with a ratio of neointimal volume-to-stent volume ratio of 0.45 ± 0.12 versus 0.40 ± 0.12 (*P* = 0.003). The angiographic MLD was smaller in group B (1.47 ± 0.57 vs 1.69 ± 0.70 mm, *P* = 0.04), with a higher late luminal loss of 1.17 ± 0.51 versus 0.82 ± 0.56 mm (*P* = 0.001).

INTERPRETATION. Thus, gold coating of the tested stent type resulted in more neointimal tissue proliferation.

Comment

At least four randomized trials comparing a bare metal stent with a gold-coated stent have been conducted over the past year. Experimental studies had shown that gold coating reduced thombogeneity and elicited less intimal hyperplastic response. This, coupled with a superior visibility, made the gold-coated stent a potential winner. Results of human clinical trials, however, were very disappointing. The InFlow Dynamic gold-coated stent showed more intimal hyperplasia in the current trial and a trend toward a higher angiographic restenosis rate, although this was not statistically significant. A methodological problem with the assessment of angiographic results after gold-coated stents is their enhanced radiopacity. Because of this the automated edge detection software might miss the true vessel edges and this might influence the measurements. To account for this, IVUS analysis was performed in a subset of patients. This imaging modality confirmed the quantitative angiographic data. More intimal hyperplasia was found in the gold-coated stents at follow-up. The study was underpowered to detect significant differences in clinical outcome, although a trend towards a higher TLR was again apparent in the gold-coated stent group. In an earlier, larger trial using the same InFlow Dynamic stent Kastrati *et al.* |**12**| reported a higher clinical as well as angiographic restenosis rate. The results found using the InFlow Dynamic stent were confirmed by Park *et al.* for the gold-coated NIR stent |**13**|. Late loss was again much larger in the gold coated stents (1.4 ± 1.1 vs 1.0 ± 0.9 mm; $P = 0.005$). Angiographic restenosis rate (>50% diameter stenosis at 6-month follow-up angiography) was 47% in the gold-coated stent group compared with 26% in the bare stent group ($P <0.05$). A trend towards a higher TLR was also apparent (23 vs 15%, $P = 0.15$).

Finally, the recently presented 305 patient NIR Top trial failed to show equivalence of gold-coated and bare NIRflex stents. In fact, the primary end-point of MLD at 6-month follow-up was significantly less in the gold-coated stent group, and late loss and binary restenosis rate were significantly higher. Clinical outcomes were not significantly different between the two groups. There is no good explanation for the discrepancy found between animal experiments and human studies, but these four trials taken together toll the knell for gold-coated stents in interventional cardiology.

Evidence for use of coronary stents: a hierarchical Bayesian meta-analysis.

J M Brophy, P Belisle, L Joseph. *Ann Intern Med* 2003; **138**: 777–86.

BACKGROUND. Coronary stents are widely used in interventional cardiology, but a current quantitative systematic overview comparing routine coronary stenting with standard percutaneous transluminal coronary angioplasty (PTCA) and restricted stenting (provisional stenting) has not been published. Electronic databases were searched by using the keywords angioplasty and stent. References from identified articles were also reviewed. In addition, several prominent general medical and cardiology journals were searched and agencies known to perform systematic reviews were consulted. All comparative randomized clinical trials were included, except those involving primary angioplasty for the treatment of acute myocardial infarction (AMI). A specified protocol was followed, and two of the authors independently extracted the data. Outcomes assessed were total mortality, MI, angiographic restenosis, CABG, repeated PTCA and freedom from angina. The results were synthesized by using a Bayesian hierarchical random-effects model. In total, 29 trials involving 9918 patients were identified. There was no evidence for a difference between routine coronary stenting and standard PTCA in terms of deaths or MIs (OR 0.90, 95% CI 0.72–1.11) or the need for coronary artery bypass surgery (OR 1.01, CI 0.79–1.31). Coronary stenting reduced the rate of restenosis (OR 0.52, CI 0.37–0.69) and the need for repeated PTCA (OR 0.59, CI 0.50–0.68). The trials showed a wide range of crossover rates from PTCA to stenting. By use of a multiplicative model, each 10% increase in cross-over rate decreased the need for repeated angioplasty by approximately 8% (OR multiplying factor 1.08, CI 0.98–1.18). Routine stenting probably reduces the need for repeated angioplasty by fewer than 4–5 per 100 treated persons compared with PTCA with

provisional stenting. Studies were not blinded and suggest a bias with a possible overestimation of this benefit.

INTERPRETATION. In the controlled environment of randomized clinical trials, routine coronary stenting is safe but probably not associated with important reductions in rates of mortality, AMI or CABG compared with standard PTCA with provisional stenting. Coronary stenting is associated with substantial reductions in angiographic restenosis rates and the subsequent need for repeated PTCA, although this benefit may be overestimated because of trial designs. The incremental benefit of routine stenting for reducing repeated angioplasty diminishes as the crossover rate of stenting with conventional PTCA increases.

Comment

Provisional stenting, i.e. a strategy of initial balloon angioplasty and stenting only in case of a bail-out situation or suboptimal result, has been specifically tested in at least nine randomized trials |14–23|. The impetus for these trials was cost reduction and avoidance of in-stent restenosis, which is notoriously difficult to treat. Provisional stenting was necessary in 30–50% of patients in these trials. Irrespective of the method of guidance that was used (angiography, quantitative coronary angiography, IVUS, coronary flow reserve) clinical and angiographic outcomes were similar in the routine stenting and the provisional stenting arms of almost all these trials |14,15,17–22|. In the ADVANCE (additional value of the NIR stent for the treatment of long coronary lesions) trial, provisional stenting after balloon angioplasty in long lesions was found to be associated with an excess of peri-procedural MIs |23|. The OPUS-1 (optimum percutaneous transluminal coronary angioplasty versus routine stent strategy trial) was the only trial that showed improved clinical outcome with a routine stenting strategy |16|. Angiographic follow-up was, however, not performed in this trial and therefore no inferences can be made on the mechanism of the treatment effect of routine stenting.

Brophy *et al.* in their extensive meta-analysis of 29 trials again show that routine stenting does not reduce hard clinical events such as death, MI or the need for bypass surgery compared with a strategy of balloon angioplasty with provisional stenting. Routine stenting reduced angiographic restenosis and the need for repeat PTCA, but only modestly. The absolute reduction in need for re-PTCA was found to be 6.8% and this figure is likely to be inflated because of an observed tendency in this analysis to perform repeat PTCA more often for restenosis after balloon angioplasty than for in-stent restenosis. They further elegantly made plausible that a provisional stenting rate of >20–40% does not further improve clinical restenosis rate (Fig. 3.1).

If the benefit of routine stenting is so small why are stents now used in >80% of cases? Several explanations for the fact that interventional cardiologists prefer stenting over balloon angioplasty can be given.

First the availability of stents has dramatically reduced the need for emergency bypass surgery. In the balloon angioplasty era approximately 5% of PTCA procedures ended in the operating theatre with very high morbidity and mortality. Nowadays <1% of cases have to be referred for bypass surgery and most of these can

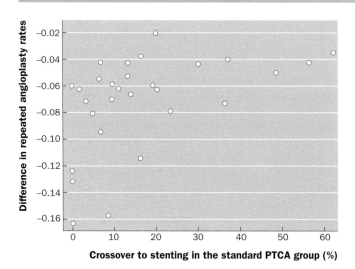

Fig. 3.1 Plot of the difference in repeat PTCA rate between the stenting and balloon angioplasty groups as a function of the cross-over rate from balloon angioplasty to stenting. Each dot represents the findings in 1 of the 29 trials. The graph suggests that the number of re-PTCAs prevented by routine stenting levels off at approximately 5% once a provisional stenting rate of 20–40% is attained. Source: Brophy *et al.* (2003).

be stabilized with stents. Surgery can then be performed on a more elective basis without ongoing ischaemia.

Stent implantation takes less time. It is safe and what you see immediately is what you get. No waiting times are necessary to assess whether the attained balloon result is durable and no deliberations are needed on balloon upsizing or higher inflation pressure to improve on an already reasonable result.

Stent implantation often results in a very appealing, perfect anatomic result. Although it is well known that this does not preclude restenosis, the strong psychological sentiment that what looks beautiful is good and holds promise for the future is also operational in the mind of the interventional cardiologist.

Stenting now allows safe treatment of complex lesions in older patients with more advanced coronary artery disease. Lesions and patients that were not included in the analysed randomized trials. Without stents these patients would not have been candidates for PCI.

Finally, although smaller than perceived by the cardiology community, a treatment benefit with respect to restenosis does exist for stenting. The much-dreaded complication of in-stent restenosis is in fact a rather benign problem which clinically affects only 20% of stented patients. A large part of these can now be treated with brachytherapy or, although not yet definitely proven, with a drug-eluting stent.

Once the price of these devices falls and there are no long-term safety issues, there is no doubt that all patients will be treated with a drug-eluting stent rather than only patients at high risk for restenosis. Until that time a strategy of drug-eluting stent implantation for in-stent restenosis seems a wise strategy from both a cost-effectiveness and a safety perspective.

Randomized trial of a distal embolic protection device during percutaneous intervention of saphenous vein aorto-coronary bypass grafts.

D S Baim, D Wahr, B George, *et al.* and the SAFER trial investigators. *Circulation* 2002; **105**: 1285–90.

BACKGROUND. Stents provide effective treatment for stenotic saphenous venous aorto-coronary bypass grafts, but their placement carries a 20% incidence of procedure-related complications, which potentially are related to the distal embolization of atherosclerotic debris. The authors report the first multicentre randomized trial to evaluate use of a distal embolic protection device during stenting of such lesions. Of 801 eligible patients, 406 were randomly assigned to stent placement over the shaft of the distal protection device, and 395 were assigned to stent placement over a conventional 0.014-inch angioplasty guidewire (control group). The primary end-point – a composite of death, MI, emergency bypass or TLR by 30 days – was observed in 65 patients (16.5%) assigned to the control group and 39 patients (9.6%) assigned to the embolic protection device ($P = 0.004$). This 42% relative reduction in major adverse cardiac events was driven by MI (8.6 vs 14.7%, $P = 0.008$) and 'no-reflow' phenomenon (3 vs 9%, $P = 0.02$). Clinical benefit was seen even when platelet Gp IIb/IIIa receptor blockers were administered (61% of patients), with composite end-points occurring in 10.7% of protection device patients compared with 19.4% of control patients ($P = 0.008$).

INTERPRETATION. Use of this distal protection device during stenting of stenotic venous grafts was associated with a highly significant reduction in major adverse events compared with stenting over a conventional angioplasty guidewire. This demonstrates the importance of distal embolization in causing major adverse cardiac events and the value of embolic protection devices in preventing such complications.

Comment

Treatment of stenosed saphenous vein grafts (SVG) together with chronic total occlusions are the last remaining challenges for interventional cardiology. Athero-sclerotic vein graft lesions are composed of large friable soft plaques often with over-lying thrombotic material. Introduction of guidewires, balloons and stents in these friable lesions carries a very high risk of distal embolization with subsequent MI. Severe microvascular vasoconstriction caused by vasoactive substances release by platelet thrombi also contributes to the myocardial under-perfusion which becomes angiographically evident as the no-reflow phenomenon. MI rates of up to 20% have been reported for SVG interventions. The advocated therapy for no-reflow is intracoronary administration of arteriolar vasodilators such as calcium blockers, adenosine and nitroprusside. Although flow frequently improves, vasodilation tackles only part of the problem. Prevention of embolization of atherosclerotic debris seems necessary, therefore, to prevent procedural myocardial infarcts. This can be achieved with covered stents that trap the debris behind the stent, with a filter device or with a capture/aspiration device as used in the Saphenous vein graft Angioplasty Free of Emboli Randomized (SAFER) trial. In this trial an absolute reduction of the occurrence of the composite end-point of 6.9% was found in the protection device group (Fig. 3.2). This means that 14 patients have to be treated to prevent 1 composite end-point. This was primarily caused by a reduction in non-Q myocardial infarcts. The absolute reduction was 6.1% which means that 16 patients need to be treated to prevent 1 MI. Although these numbers are impressive the device is not perfect. MIs still occur in almost 9% of procedures and in 10% of cases the device could not be used as intended. The problem with most of the current capture and filter devices is that they are poorly steerable and are often difficult to cross the friable lesions especially in a tortuous anatomy. Lesions located very distally or in sequential grafts are also not ideal. A problem specific to the GuardWire device is that the graft has to be occluded during the intervention. Reported occlusion times of 4–10 min might not be tolerable in patients with a stenosis in a large sequential graft. It is not currently known how covered stents perform relative to a capture device. We have to wait for comparative studies.

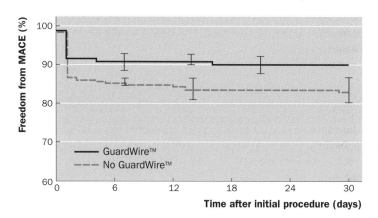

Fig. 3.2 Kaplan–Meier MACE-free survival curves. The curves separate very early and run parallel afterwards, indicating that the treatment benefit of the distal protection device occurs during the procedure. Source: Baim *et al.* (2002).

Another problem is the high restenosis rate after PTCA and stent implantation of SVG lesions. Whether drug-eluting stents are equally effective in vein grafts as they are in native coronary arteries needs to be confirmed.

Undoubtedly devices will become better, easier to use and safer and it might well be that obstructive disease of degenerated vein grafts can be treated in the near future with similar risks and outcome as obstructive native coronary artery disease. Until that time embarking on a SVG intervention should be preceded by serious consideration of other options such as PCI of the native, bypassed, coronary arteries or redo bypass surgery with the use of arterial grafts. If PCI is chosen a distal protection device should be used especially if the patient suffers an acute non-ST elevation coronary syndrome together with (drug-eluting) stents to lower the chance for restenosis.

Interventional versus conservative treatment for patients with unstable angina or non-ST elevation myocardial infarction: the British Heart Foundation Randomized Intervention Trial of unstable Angina 3 randomized trial.

K A Fox, P A Poole-Wilson, R A Henderson, *et al. Lancet* 2002; **360**: 743–51.

BACKGROUND. Current guidelines suggest that, for patients at moderate risk of death from unstable coronary artery disease, either an interventional strategy (angiography followed by revascularization) or a conservative strategy (ischaemia- or symptom-driven angiography) is appropriate. The authors aimed to test the hypothesis that an interventional strategy is better than a conservative strategy in such patients. They carried out a randomized multicentre trial of 1810 patients with non-ST elevation acute coronary syndromes (mean age 62 years, 38% women). Patients were assigned an early intervention or conservative strategy. The antithrombin agent in both groups was enoxaparin. The co-primary end-points were a combined rate of death, non-fatal MI or refractory angina at 4 months; and a combined rate of death or non-fatal MI at 1 year. Analysis was by intention to treat. At 4 months, 86 (9.6%) of 895 patients in the intervention group had died or had a MI or refractory angina, compared with 133 (14.5%) of 915 patients in the conservative group (RR 0.66, 95% CI 0.51–0.85, $P = 0.001$). This difference was mainly due to a halving of refractory angina in the intervention group. Death or MI was similar in both treatment groups at 1 year (68 [7.6%] vs 76 [8.3%], respectively; RR 0.91, 95% CI 0.67–1.25, $P = 0.58$). Symptoms of angina were improved and use of anti-anginal medications significantly reduced with the interventional strategy ($P < 0.0001$).

INTERPRETATION. In patients presenting with unstable coronary artery disease, an interventional strategy is preferable to a conservative strategy, mainly because of the halving of refractory or severe angina, and with no increased risk of death or MI (Figs. 3.3 and 3.4)

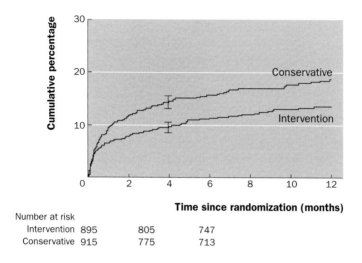

Number at risk

Intervention	895	805	747
Conservative	915	775	713

Fig. 3.3 Cumulative risk of death, MI or refractory angina. SE bars are shown for co-primary end-point by 4 months. Source: Fox *et al.* (2002).

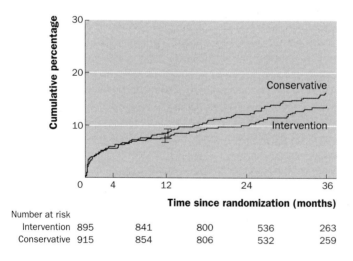

Number at risk

Intervention	895	841	800	536	263
Conservative	915	854	806	532	259

Fig. 3.4 Cumulative risk of death or MI. SE bars are shown for co-primary end-point by 12 months. Source: Fox *et al.* (2002).

Comment

The results of this large randomized trial confirm the benefit of early coronary angiography in non-ST elevation acute coronary syndromes. Coronary angiography was performed a mean of 2 days after randomization in the intervention group. At least one significantly stenosed vessel was found in 78% of patients. PCI was performed in 33% of patients during the index admission and bypass surgery in 12%. This was 7 and 4% in the conservative arm. Stents were used in 88% of PCI patients.

The lack of treatment effect on the end-point of death or non-fatal MI at 1 year in Randomized Intervention Trial of unstable Angina (RITA) 3 might be explained by the definition of MI in RITA 3. A common definition was used for all patients irrespective of the setting the MI occurred (post PCI, post CABG or no intervention). This is in contrast to the definition of MI in TACTICS and FRISC II where more stringent criteria were applied for the diagnosis of MI after PCI or bypass surgery. This might have increased the differences between the invasive and the conservative groups in FRISC II and TACTICS-TIMI 18.

The outcomes of the contemporary FRISC II, TACTICS-TIMI 18 and RITA 3 trials all point in the same direction; In non-ST elevation acute coronary syndrome patients at moderate (RITA 3) to high baseline risk (FRISC II and TACTICS-TIMI 18) an early invasive approach reduces major cardiac events and should be the preferred treatment strategy.

Patients with acute coronary syndromes without persistent ST elevation undergoing percutaneous coronary intervention benefit most from early intervention with protection by a glycoprotein IIb/IIIa receptor blocker.

E Ronner, E Boersma, K M Akkerhuis, et al. Eur Heart J 2002; **23**: 239–46.

BACKGROUND. Many patients with acute coronary syndromes are offered PCI. However, the appropriate indications for, and optimal timing of, such procedures are uncertain. The authors analysed timing of intervention and associated events (death and MI) in the PURSUIT trial in which 9461 patients received a platelet Gp IIb/IIIa inhibitor, eptifibatide or placebo for 72 h. Other treatment was left to the investigators. In total, 2430 patients underwent PCI within 30 days. Four groups were distinguished, who underwent PCI on day 1; on days 2 or 3; at days 4–7 days; or between 8 and 30 days, for eptifibatide- and placebo-treated patients. The four groups treated with placebo demonstrated total 30-day events of 15.9% for day 1 PCI, 17.7, 15.0 and 18.2%, respectively, for successive intervals of later intervention. Later intervention was associated with more pre-procedural events (2.2–13.7%, $P = 0.001$) which was balanced by a decrease in procedure-related events (12.1 to 3.1%, $P = 0.001$), whereas the overall 30-day event rates were similar. Eptifibatide-treated patients with percutaneous coronary intervention on day 1 had the lowest rate of 30-day events (9.2%, $P < 0.05$ vs other groups). In this group, pre-procedural risk was only 0.3%, whereas PCI on eptifibatide treatment was associated with low procedural risk (7.2%). The total 30-day event rate for later PCI in patients receiving eptifibatide was 14.0% on days 2 and 3, 15.0% for days 4–7 and 17.4% for days 7–30, respectively.

INTERPRETATION. Patients treated with a platelet Gp IIb/IIIa receptor blocker, and early PCI (within 24 h) had the lowest event rate in this *post hoc* analysis. Thus 'watchful waiting' may not be the optimal strategy. Rather an early invasive strategy with PCI under protection of a platelet Gp IIb/IIIa receptor blocker should be considered in selected patients. Randomized trials are warranted to verify this issue.

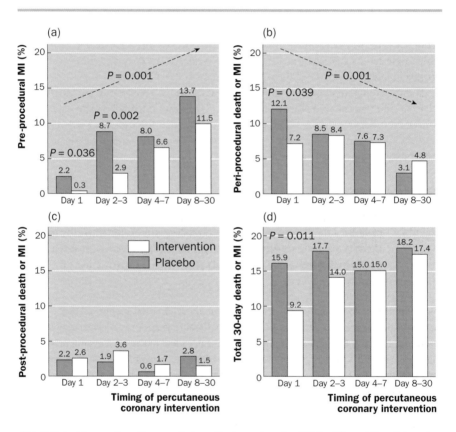

Fig. 3.5 Incidence of cardiac events in patients undergoing PCI in different time intervals from day 0 to 30 after randomization. Patients were randomly assigned to Gp IIb/IIIa receptor blocker (white bars) or placebo (black bars) for 72 h. Events were classified as occurring before the PCI (pre-procedural), from the start of the PCI to 48 h after the PCI (peri-procedural), or from 48 h after the PCI to 30 days follow-up (post-procedural). In each period only 1 event per patient was counted. For the total 30-day event rate also only one event per patient was counted. Source: Ronner *et al.* (2002).

Comment

This *post hoc* analysis of the PURSUIT trial data shows that early PCI in patients admitted with a non-ST elevation acute coronary syndrome prevents the occurrence of pre-procedural events. The addition of a Gp IIb/IIIa receptor blocker before and after the procedure allows an early (higher risk) PCI to be performed just as safe as a PCI that is performed >48 h after admission. Thus, the combination of early (within 24 h) PCI and Gp IIb/III receptor blockade reduced the total 30-day death or MI rate in this analysis (Fig. 3.5). The authors make a strong case that a medical cooling off period is not in the best interest of the non-ST elevation acute coronary syndrome (NSTEACS) patient and that, if feasible, diagnostic angiography and subsequent PCI should be performed on day 1 of admission. The retrospective nature of this analysis, however, should caution us with interpretation. The baseline characteristics of the subgroups differed significantly. Slightly surprisingly, patients who were sent for early angiography had a more favourable risk profile. They were younger, had less often ST depression on the admission ECG and had less peripheral vessel disease. Even in this lower risk population early intervention is beneficial if it is performed early enough under protection of Gp IIb/IIIa inhibition. A randomized trial is necessary to confirm the results of this analysis. Ideally, in this trial patients should be randomized to immediate intervention, intervention within <24 h of admission or intervention >24 h after admission.

Value of first day angiography/angioplasty in evolving non-ST segment elevation myocardial infarction: an open multicenter randomized trial (VINO study).

R Spacek, P Widimsky, Z Straka, *et al. Eur Heart J* 2002; **23**: 230–8.

B A C K G R O U N D . Direct angioplasty is an effective treatment for ST elevation MI. The role of very early angioplasty in non-ST elevation infarction is not known. Thus, a randomized study of first day angiography/angioplasty compared with early conservative therapy of evolving MI without persistent ST-elevation was conducted. One hundred and thirty-one patients with confirmed AMI without ST-segment elevations were randomized within 24 h of last rest chest pain: 64 in the first day angiography/angioplasty group and 67 in the early conservative group (coronary angiography only after recurrent or stress-induced myocardial ischaemia). All patients in the invasive group underwent coronary angiography on the day of admission (mean randomization–angiography time 6.2 h). First day angioplasty of the infarct-related artery was performed in 47% of the patients and bypass surgery in 35%. In the conservative group, 55% underwent coronary angiography, 10% angioplasty and 30% bypass surgery within 6 months. The primary end-point (death/reinfarction) at 6 months occurred in 6.2% versus 22.3% (*P* <0.001). Six-month mortality in the first day angiography/angioplasty group was 3.1% compared with 13.4% in the conservative group (*P* <0.03). Non-fatal reinfarction occurred in 3.1% versus 14.9% (*P* <0.02).

INTERPRETATION. First day coronary angiography followed by angioplasty whenever possible reduces mortality and reinfarction in evolving MI without persistent ST elevation, in comparison with an early conservative treatment strategy.

Comment

The small VINO trial showed that a very early invasive strategy in patients presenting with an ongoing non-ST elevation MI is associated with a reduction in reinfarctions and even with a mortality reduction at 6 months (Fig. 3.6). The investigators reduced the time interval from randomization to angiography to a mean of 6.2 h in the invasive strategy group. Whether this is the reason for the treatment benefit found remains unclear, because a control group with deferred angiography until after a cooling off period was lacking in this trial. Even though Gp IIb/IIIa inhibitors were not used, these very early interventions could be performed safely considering the low reinfarction rate in the invasive arm at 30 days. Although a significant mortality benefit was found at 6 months, one should realize that this is based on only 2 versus 9 fatal events. The VINO trial is a small trial and its promising results must be confirmed in a much larger study.

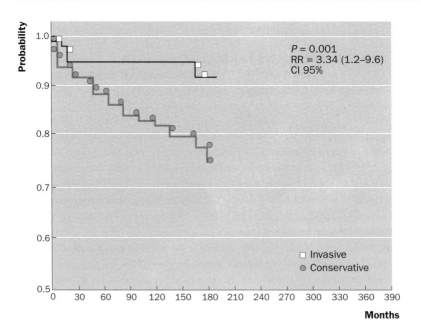

Fig. 3.6 Kaplan–Meier event-free survival curve according to treatment strategy. Source: Spacek *et al.* (2002).

The issue of immediate angiography and PCI or deferral of PCI until after a cooling off period was addressed in the recently presented ISAR COOL study. Four hundred and fifty patients presenting with non-ST elevation myocardial infarction acute coronary syndromes (non-STEMI ACS) with ST depression and/or positive biomarkers for necrosis were randomized to either immediate angiography and PCI or deferred PCI after a period of 24–120 h of cooling off. Patients in both groups were treated with aspirin, clopidogrel and the Gp IIb/IIIa receptor blocker tirofiban. In the early invasive group PCI performed at a median of 2.4 h after randomization. This was 86 h in the cooling off group. At 30 days the incidence of death or non-fatal MI was 11.6% in the cooling off group and 5.9% in the early invasive group. The difference in event rate was completely explained by a far higher pre-procedural event rate in the cooling off group. Peri-procedural and post-procedural event rate was similar in both groups. The ISAR COOL therefore seems to confirm the findings of Ronner et al. in their retrospective analysis of the PURSUIT trial data that deferral of PCI in these patients is not the optimal strategy.

Conclusion

The introduction of drug eluting stents has undoubtedly been the most important recent development in interventional cardiology. Angiographic restenosis rates are reduced to around 5% and restenosis tends to occur at the edges of the drug eluting stents or locally in the stented segment at sites with incomplete stent coverage [24]. Drug eluting stents, however, have not shown a reduction in mortality or myocardial infarction and therefore the clinical benefit of drug eluting stents lies in the reduction of repeat revascularization procedures. Serruys et al. only showed a 4.4% (from 7.1% to 2.7%) absolute reduction in repeat revascularization procedures after they started implanting sirolimus eluting stents in all their patients [25]. A very large percentage of patients therefore received very costly drug eluting stents from which they gained no benefit. Further more, long-term effects of the drugs and polymers on the vessel wall are yet unknown. It therefore seems wise to selectively use these new devices in patients and lesions at high risk for restenosis and treat the majority of patients with the tried and tested provisional stenting strategy. The small number of patients who subsequently need treatment for their (in-stent) restenosis can then be treated with a drug eluting stent.

There is no discussion anymore that high-risk patients presenting with a non-ST elevation acute coronary syndrome, i.e. patients with ST depression and/or positive troponins, benefit from early angiography and revascularization. The question remains, how early is early enough? Ronner et al. in their retrospective analysis of PURSUIT data suggest that same-day angiography and PCI under an umbrella of GpIIb/IIIa blockade is superior to deferred PCI after a period of medical cooling down. This was confirmed in the randomized ISAR COOL trial. Ongoing trials push the envelope even further and test the hypothesis that a strategy of emergency coronary angiography and PCI, similar to primary PCI for acute ST elevation myocardial infarction, is superior to deferred angiography after a cooling down period.

References

1. FRISC II investigators. Invasive compared with non-invasive treatment in unstable coronary artery disease: FRISC II prospective randomized multicenter study. *Lancet* 1999; **354**: 708–15.

2. Cannon CP, Weintraub WS, Demopoulos LA, *et al*. Comparison of early invasive and conservative strategies in patients with unstable coronary syndromes treated with the glycoprotein IIb/IIIa inhibitor tirofiban. *N Engl J Med* 2001; **344**: 1879–87E.

3. Foley DP, Melkert R, Serruys PW. Influence of coronary vessel size on renarrowing process and late angiographic outcome after successful balloon angioplasty. *Circulation* 1994; **90**: 1239–51.

4. Serruys PW, Kay P, Disco C, et al. Peri-procedural coronary angiography after Palmaz-Schatz stent implantation predicts the restenosis rate at six months. *J Am Coll Cardiol* 1999; **34**: 1067–74.

5. Park SW, Lee CW, Hong MK, *et al*. Randomized comparison of coronary stenting with optimal balloon angioplasty for treatment of lesions in small coronary arteries. *Eur Heart J* 2000; **140**: 898–905.

6. Kastrati A, Schomig A, Dirschinger J, *et al*. A randomized trial comparing stenting with balloon angioplasty in small vessels in patients with symptomatic coronary artery disease. *Circulation* 2000; **102**: 2593–8.

7. Koning R, Eltchaninoff H, Commeau P, *et al*. Stent placement compared with balloon angioplasty for small coronary arteries in-hospital and 6-month clinical and angiographic results. *Circulation* 2001; **104**: 1604–8.

8. Doucet S, Schalij M, Vrolix M. Stent placement to prevent restenosis after angioplasty in small coronary arteries. *Circulation* 2001; **104**: 2029–33.

9. Moer R, Myreng Y, Mølstad P, *et al*. Stenting in small coronary arteries (SISCA) trial: a randomized comparison between balloon angioplasty and the heparin-coated be stent. *J Am Coll Cardiol* 2001; **38**: 1598–603.

10. Garcia E, Gomez-Recio M, Moreno R, *et al*. Stent reduces restenosis in small vessels. Results of the RAP study. *J Am Coll Cardiol* 2001; **37**: 17A (abstract).

11. Brophy JM, Belisle P, Joseph L. Evidence for use of coronary stents. A hierarchical Bayesian meta-analysis. *Ann Intern Med* 2003; **138**: 777–86.

12. Kastrati A, Schomig A, Dirschinger J, *et al*. Increased risk of restenosis after placement of gold-coated stents: results of a randomized trial comparing gold-coated with uncoated steel stents in patients with coronary artery disease. *Circulation* 2000; **101**: 2478–83.

13. Park S, Cheol L, Myeong-Ki H, *et al*. Comparison of gold coated NIR stents with uncoated NIR stents in patients with coronary artery disease. *Am J Cardiol* 2002; **89**: 872–5.

14. Rodriguez A, Ayala F, Bernardi V, *et al*. Optimal balloon angioplasty with provisional stenting versus primary stent (OCBAS): immediate and long-term results. *J Am Coll Cardiol* 1998; **32**: 1351–7.

15. Dangas G, Ambrose JA, Rehmann D, et al. Balloon optimization versus stent study (BOSS): provisional stenting and early recoil after balloon angioplasty. *Am J Cardiol* 2000; **85**: 957–61.

16. Weaver D, Reisman M, Griffin J, *et al*. Optimum percutaneous transluminal coronary angioplasty compared to routine stenting strategy trial (OPUS-1). *Lancet* 2000; **355**: 2199–203.

17. Fluck DS, Chenu P, Mills P, *et al*. Is provisional stenting the effective option? The WIDEST study (Wiktor stent in *de novo* stenosis). *Heart* 2000; **84**: 522–8.

18. Serruys PW, de Bruyne B, Carlier S, *et al*. Randomized comparison of primary stenting and provisional balloon angioplasty guided by flow velocity measurement. *Circulation* 2000; **102**: 2930–7.

19. Di Mario C, Moses JW, Anderson TJ, *et al*. Randomized comparison of elective stent implantation and coronary balloon angioplasty guided by online quantitative angiography and intracoronary doppler. *Circulation* 2000; **102**: 2938–44.

20. Lafont A, Dubois-Rande JL, Steg PG, *et al*. The French Randomized Optimal Stenting Trial: a prospective evaluation of provisional stenting guided by coronary velocity reserve and quantitative coronary angiography. FROST Study Group. *J Am Coll Cardiol* 2000; **36**: 404–9.

21. Frey AW, Hodgson JM, Muller C, *et al*. Ultrasound guided strategy for provisional stenting with focal balloon combination catheter: results from the randomized strategy for intracoronary ultrasound guided PTCA and stenting (SIPS) trial. *Circulation* 2002: **102**: 2497–502.

22. Schiele F, Meneveau N, Gilard M, *et al*. Intravascular ultrasound guided balloon angioplasty compared with stent. Immediate and 6-months results of the multicenter, randomized balloon equivalent to stent study (BEST). *Circulation* 2003; **107**: 545–51.

23. Serruys PW, Foley DP, Suttorp M, *et al*. A randomized comparison of the value of additional stenting after optimal balloon angioplasty for long coronary lesions. *J Am Coll Cardiol* 2002; **39**: 393–9.

24. Lemos PA, Saia F, Ligthart JMR, *et al*. Coronary restenosis after sirolimus eluting stent implantation. Morphological description and mechanistic analysis from a consecutive series of cases. *Circulation* 2003; **108**: 257–60.

25. King SB III. Restenosis. The mouse that roared. *Circulation* 2003; **108**: 248–9.

4

Percutaneous coronary intervention versus coronary artery bypass surgery

Introduction

Coronary artery disease is a chronic condition that tends to be inexorably progressive. A comprehensive management strategy may require intervention from risk factor recognition and primary prevention through to terminal care. Coronary revascularization procedures play a major role in the management of symptomatic disease and consume a considerable proportion of healthcare resources allocated for cardiac management. Coronary artery bypass grafting (CABG) provides the historical standard for safety and efficacy in coronary revascularization. Developments in operative technique and adjunctive medication schedules continue to refine this important therapy. There have also been important developments in the field of percutaneous coronary intervention (PCI) – the vast majority of procedures now involving balloon dilatation of flow limiting coronary disease with subsequent implantation of a coronary stent. There has been rapid growth in PCI activity and in most developed countries PCI volume now exceeds that of coronary artery surgery |1,2|.

This growth in PCI activity is supported by a strong evidence base of observational studies and randomized control trials. Comparative trials against coronary surgery were first initiated in the late 1980s when PCI techniques were based on simple balloon dilatation. A 'second generation' of more recent studies has re-addressed this question in the era of routine stent implantation |3,4|. The principal clinical results of one of these studies – the Stent or Surgery (SoS) trial – are presented in this chapter. Also included are important subgroup analyses from other stent versus surgery trials.

There is no doubt that development in PCI equipment and techniques – most notably the advent of coronary stents and improved antiplatelet therapy – has improved clinical results. Despite this, coronary artery surgery remains the gold standard for coronary revascularization. Patients initially managed with surgery demonstrate a markedly reduced need for additional unplanned repeat revascularization and enjoy better relief of their anginal symptoms in the medium term. It would appear, however, that the gap is narrowing and PCI may provide the optimum initial approach in younger patients with less extensive coronary disease, in patients at high surgical risk and for acute presentations. The reduced procedural morbidity, early mobilization and reduced procedural costs associated with PCI revascularization mean that it is likely to enjoy an enduring appeal.

There have been important developments in cardiac surgical technique, particularly the increasing availability of bypass surgery without peri-operative cardiopulmonary bypass and the performance of minimally invasive bypass grafting through limited incisions. A number of key papers published this year, present the results of comparative studies for these newer surgical techniques and coronary stent implantation for isolated significant disease of the left anterior descending coronary artery (LAD). Papers have also appeared describing initial experience with robotic coronary artery surgical techniques. In these procedures, surgeons operate through limited incisions with robotic manipulation of surgical tools. These devices hold the potential for increasing the precision and accuracy of tissue manipulation and anastomosis formation.

Coronary artery bypass surgery versus percutaneous coronary intervention with stent implantation in patients with multivessel coronary artery disease (the Stent or Surgery trial): a randomized controlled trial.

The SOS Investigators. *Lancet* 2002; **360**: 965–70.

BACKGROUND. Results of trials, comparing percutaneous transluminal coronary angioplasty (PTCA) with CABG, indicate that rates of death or myocardial infarction (MI) are similar with either treatment strategy. Management with PTCA is, however, associated with an increased requirement for subsequent, additional revascularization. Coronary stents, used as an adjunct to PTCA, reduce restenosis and the need for repeat revascularization. The aim of the Stent or Surgery (SoS) trial was to assess the effect of stent-assisted PCI versus CABG in the management of patients with multivessel disease. In 53 centres in Europe and Canada, symptomatic patients with multivessel coronary artery disease were randomized to CABG ($n = 500$) or stent-assisted PCI ($n = 488$). The primary outcome measure was a comparison of the rates of repeat revascularization. Secondary outcomes included death or Q-wave myocardial infarction and all-cause mortality. Analysis was by intention to treat. All patients were followed-up for a minimum of 1 year and the results are expressed for the median follow-up of 2 years. Twenty-one per cent ($n = 101$) of patients in the PCI group required additional revascularization procedures compared with 6% ($n = 30$) in the CABG group (hazard ratio 3.85, 95% confidence interval [CI] 2.56–5.79, $P <0.0001$). The incidence of death or Q-wave myocardial infarction was similar in both groups (PCI 9% [$n = 46$], CABG 10% [$n = 49$]; hazard ratio 0.95, 95% CI 0.63–1.42, $P = 0.80$). There were fewer deaths in the CABG group than in the PCI group (PCI 5% [$n = 22$], CABG 2% [$n = 8$]; hazard ratio 2.91, 95% CI 1.29–6.53, $P = 0.01$).

INTERPRETATION. The use of coronary stents has reduced the need for repeat revascularization when compared with previous studies that used balloon angioplasty, although the rate remains significantly higher than in patients managed with CABG. The apparent reduction in mortality with CABG requires further investigation.

Comment

This study confirms that, in the PCI management of multivessel disease, the advent of routine stent implantation reduces the need for repeat revascularization, when compared with the balloon angioplasty era. In this respect, the results are comparable with the previously published similar study, Arterial Revascularization Therapy Study (ARTS) |3|. Stent-assisted angioplasty cannot, however, match surgical revascularization in this respect (see Fig. 4.1). A surprising finding in this study is the apparent mortality advantage with surgical revascularization. There is a very real possibility that this difference represents the play of chance. The study was not powered to detect small differences in mortality and the absolute number of deaths was small. Although there was a trend for improved cardiovascular mortality with coronary surgery, there was a marked disparity in non-cardiovascular death. Of a total of nine cancer deaths, eight were observed in patients randomized to PCI revascularization (see Table 4.1).

As with previous PCI versus surgery trials only a very small proportion (perhaps 3–6%) of patients screened for eligibility were eventually randomized. Trial inclusion and exclusion criteria demanded a patient suitable for revascularization by either means. The resulting patient population tended to demonstrate low surgical risk and ideal anatomy for surgical revascularization. This of course is reflected in the clinical outcomes for surgical patients with very low operative and medium-term mortality and excellent relief of angina.

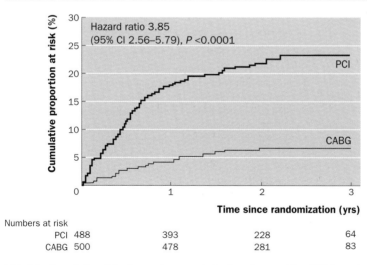

Fig. 4.1 Cumulative risk of repeat revascularization. Source: The SOS Investigators (2002).

Table 4.1 Death by cause during a median 2.0 years' follow up

	PCI ($n = 488$)	CABG ($n = 500$)
Cause of death		
Cardiac	9	4
Other vascular	2	1
Non-cardiovascular	9	3
Unknown	2	0
Total	22	8

For total deaths $P = 0.01$.
Source: The SOS Investigators (2002).

Data from the SoS trial were presented for a median follow-up of 2 years (range 1–4 years). Initial 1-year results from the comparable ARTS study were published in 2001 |3|. The following papers present 2-year results from this important randomized trial and a sub-study analysis of results in patients presenting with stable or unstable symptoms.

Revascularization in multivessel disease: comparison between two-year outcomes of coronary bypass surgery and stenting.

F Unger, P W Serruys, M H Yacoub, *et al. J Thorac Cardiovasc Surg* 2003; **125**: 809–20.

BACKGROUND. **The recent appreciation that stenting has improved the short- and long-term outcomes of patients treated with coronary angioplasty has made it imperative to reconsider the comparison between surgery and percutaneous interventions in patients with multivessel disease. One thousand two-hundred and five patients were randomly assigned to undergo bypass surgery or angioplasty with stent implantation when there was consensus between the cardiac surgeon and interventional cardiologist as to equivalent treatability. The primary clinical end-point was freedom from major adverse cardiac and cerebrovascular events at 1 year. Major adverse cardiac and cerebrovascular events at 2 years constituted a secondary end-point. At 2 years, 89.6% of the surgical group and 89.2% of the stent group were free from death, stroke and MI (log-rank test $P = 0.65$). Among patients who survived without stroke or MI, 19.7% in the stent group underwent a second revascularization, compared with 4.8% in the surgical group ($P < 0.001$). At 2 years, 84.8% of the surgical group and 69.5% of the stent group were event-free survivors (log-rank test $P < 0.001$), and 87.2% in the surgical cohort and 79.6% in the stent group were angina-free survivors ($P = 0.001$). In the diabetes subgroup, 82.3% of the surgical group and 56.3% of the stent group were free from any events after 2 years (log-rank test $P < 0.001$).**

INTERPRETATION. The difference in outcome between surgery and stenting observed at 1 year in patients with multivessel disease remained essentially unchanged at 2 years. Stenting was associated with a greater need for repeat revascularization. In view of the relatively greater difference in outcome in patients with diabetes, surgery clearly seems to be the preferable form of treatment for these patients.

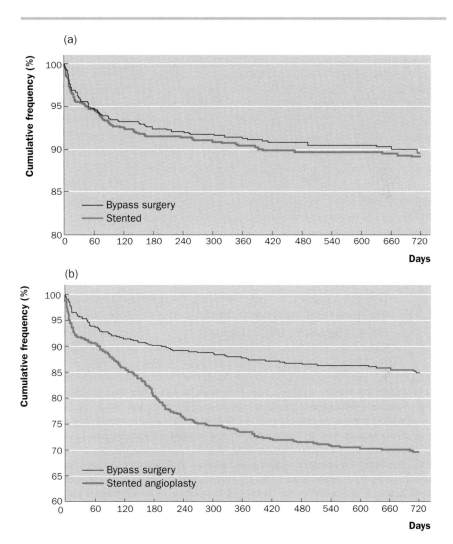

Fig. 4.2 Kaplan–Meier event-free survival curves for (a) death, myocardial infarction or cerebrovascular events for stent group versus surgical group ($P = 0.71$) and (b) death, cerebrovascular events, myocardial infarction or any repeated revascularization stent group versus surgical group ($P = 0.0001$). Source: Unger *et al.* (2003).

Comment

These 2-year follow-up data from the ARTS study reveal similar findings to the original report with no difference in the event-free survival curves for death, MI or stroke between the PCI and surgical groups. There was, however, a divergence of the curves in favour of surgery when freedom from repeat revascularization was included in the composite outcome measure (Fig. 4.2). Furthermore, only 13% of surgical patients had recurrent angina at follow-up compared with 20% in the PCI group.

Results in the PCI group were much improved compared with historical controls from the balloon angioplasty era. There was a reduced need for repeat revascularization and a marked reduction in the need for urgent surgical revascularization for failed PCI (0.5%). This reflects the impact of routine stent implantation. Patient recruitment was completed in June 1998 and there have been important developments in both PCI and surgical approaches over the last 5 years. Very few surgical patients in ARTS (or SoS) were managed as off-pump cases (without cardiopulmonary bypass) – this would be routine in the contemporary management of these low-risk cases. A greater proportion of cases may now involve total arterial revascularization. For PCI patients antiplatelet therapy has improved with general use of clopidogrel and more widespread use of the potent antiplatelet glycoprotein (Gp) IIb/IIIa agents. Drug eluting stent technology holds great promise for minimizing the impact of vessel restenosis.

Bypass surgery versus stenting for the treatment of multivessel disease in patients with unstable angina compared with stable angina.

P J de Feyter, P W Serruys, F Unger, *et al. Circulation* 2002; **105**: 2367–72.

B A C K G R O U N D . Earlier reports have shown that the outcome of balloon angioplasty or bypass surgery in unstable angina is less favourable than in stable angina. Recent improvements in percutaneous treatment (stent implantation) and bypass surgery (arterial grafts) warrant re-evaluation of the relative merits of either technique in the treatment of unstable angina. Seven hundred and fifty-five patients with stable angina were randomly assigned to coronary stenting ($n = 374$) or bypass surgery ($n = 381$), and 450 patients with unstable angina were randomly assigned to coronary stenting ($n = 226$) or bypass surgery ($n = 224$). All patients had multivessel disease considered to be equally treatable using either technique. Freedom from major adverse events, including death, MI and cerebrovascular events, at 1 year was not different in unstable patients (91.2 vs 88.9%) and stable patients (90.4 vs 92.6%) treated, respectively, with coronary stenting or bypass surgery. Freedom from repeat revascularization at 1 year was similar in unstable and stable angina treated with stenting (79.2 vs 78.9%) or bypass surgery (96.3 vs 96%) but was significantly higher in both unstable and stable patients treated with stenting (16.8 vs 16.9%) compared with bypass surgery (3.6 vs 3.5%). Neither the difference in costs between stented or bypassed stable or unstable angina ($2594 vs $3627) nor the cost-effectiveness was significantly different at 1 year.

INTERPRETATION. There was no difference in rates of death, MI and cerebrovascular event at 1 year in patients with unstable angina and multivessel disease treated with either stented angioplasty or bypass surgery compared with patients with stable angina. The rate of repeat revascularization of both unstable and stable angina was significantly higher in patients with stents.

Comment

These data suggest that there is not a marked increase in adverse event rates in patients presenting with unstable angina. This is encouraging considering that the study was conducted before the widespread introduction of platelet Gp IIb/IIIa receptor blockade. Although this was a pre-specified subgroup analysis with a sizeable proportion of unstable patients (more than one-third of the total population) there may be problems with external validity, limiting generalization to routine practice. Patients were excluded if the ejection fraction was <30% or left main stem disease was present. The angiographic findings were reviewed by an interventional cardiologist and surgeon who had to declare suitability for both PCI and surgical revascularization. This, with issues of patient preference and refusal to consent to randomization, meant that only a small proportion of patients screened were randomized. This has been a consistent problem in the PCI versus CABG trials.

Results from the Angina With Extremely Serious Operative Mortality Evaluation (AWESOME) trial were first published in 2001 |5|. This study of PCI versus CABG differed from other contemporary trials in that it sought to recruit patients at high risk for surgical revascularization. The following two papers present results of important sub-studies from this venture.

Percutaneous coronary intervention versus repeat bypass surgery for patients with medically refractory myocardial ischemia: AWESOME randomized trial and registry experience with post-CABG patients.

D A Morrison, G Sethi, J Sacks, *et al. J Am Coll Cardiol* 2002; **40**: 1951–4.

This report compares long-term PCI and CABG survival among post-CABG patients included in the Angina With Extremely Serious Operative Mortality Evaluation (AWESOME) randomized trial and prospective registry.

BACKGROUND. Repeat CABG surgery is associated with a higher risk of mortality than first-time CABG. The AWESOME is the first randomized trial comparing CABG with PCI to include post-CABG patients. Over a 5-year period (1995–2000), patients at 16 hospitals were screened to identify a cohort of 2431 individuals who had medically refractory myocardial ischaemia and at least one of five high-risk factors. There were 454 patients in the randomized trial, of whom 142 had prior CABG. In the physician-directed registry of 1650 patients, 719 had prior CABG. Of the 327 patient-choice registry patients, 119 had at least one prior CABG. The CABG and PCI survivals for the three groups were compared using Kaplan–Meier curves and log-rank

tests. The CABG and PCI 3-year survival rates were 73 and 76%, respectively for the 142 randomized patients (75 and 67 patients) (log-rank non-significant). In the physician-directed registry, 155 patients were assigned to re-operation and 357 to PCI (207 received medical therapy); 36-month survivals were 71 and 77%, respectively (log-rank non-significant). In the patient-choice registry, 32 patients chose re-operation and 74 chose PCI (13 received medical therapy); 36-month survivals were 65 and 86% respectively (log-rank test $P = 0.01$).

INTERPRETATION. PCI is preferable to CABG for many post-CABG patients.

Comment

In contrast to other studies, the AWESOME trial examined the outcome of patients with medically refractory unstable ischaemia who were deemed to be at high risk of an adverse outcome (based on at least one of the following factors: age >70 years, ejection fraction <35%, previous cardiac surgery, pre-procedure intra-aortic balloon pump and MI in the preceding week). Prior CABG had been an exclusion criterion in previous trials but was the focus of this subgroup analysis.

Table 4.2 CABG and PCI outcomes of patients with prior CABG

Outcomes	Assigned revascularization					
	Randomized		Physician-directed		Patient-choice	
	CABG ($n = 75$)	PCI ($n = 67$)	CABG ($n = 155$)	PCI ($n = 357$)	CABG ($n = 32$)	PCI ($n = 74$)
Revascularized as assigned	96%	100%	92%	96%	94%	97%
Cross-over	10%	2%	2%	2%	3%	3%
In-hospital deaths	6	0	13	2†	5	0†
Short-term survival						
1-month	91%	99%	92%	97%	78%	100%
6-month	85%	92%	83%	92%	75%	97%
12-month	81%	89%	79%	88%	72%	95%
36-month survival						
Survival	73%	76%	71%	77%	65%	86%†
Survival free of unstable angina	65%	48%	61%	43%*	62%	43%
Survival free of repeat revascularizations	65%	55%	60%	50%*	66%	56%
Survival free of unstable angina or repeat revascularization	49%	32%	58%	38%*	59%	35%

* Statistically significant difference between CABG and PCI outcomes, $P <0.05$.
† Statistically significant difference between CABG and PCI outcomes, $P <0.01$.
Source: Morrison *et al.* (2002).

In the randomized group, statistical power is limited by small patient numbers. Consent to randomization by patient and cardiologist proved difficult as evidenced by the relative sizes of the randomized trial and registry study. The survival and clinical event rates at 3 years were comparable for PCI and CABG. Survival at all stages of follow-up favoured PCI, whereas survival free of repeat revascularization or recurrent unstable angina favoured CABG. No differences reached conventional levels of statistical significance (Table 4.2).

It is interesting to note the influence of physician and patient choice on treatment allocation. In the registry group PCI procedures outnumbered CABG by 2 to 1.

Percutaneous coronary intervention versus coronary bypass graft surgery for diabetic patients with unstable angina and risk factors for adverse outcomes with bypass: outcome of diabetic patients in the AWESOME randomized trial and registry.

S P Sedlis, D A Morrison, J D Lorin, *et al. J Am Coll Cardiol* 2002; **40**: 1555–66.

B A C K G R O U N D . **This study compared survival after PCI with survival after CABG among diabetics in the Veterans Affairs AWESOME study randomized trial and registry of high-risk patients. Previous studies indicate that CABG may be superior to PCI for diabetics, but no comparisons have been made for diabetics at high risk for surgery. Over five years (1995–2000), 2431 patients with medically refractory myocardial ischaemia and at least one of five risk factors (prior CABG, MI within 7 days, left ventricular ejection fraction <0.35, age >70 years, or an intra-aortic balloon being required to stabilize) were identified. A total of 781 were acceptable for CABG and PCI, and 454 consented to be randomized. The 1650 patients not acceptable for either CABG or PCI constitute the physician-directed registry, and the 327 who were acceptable but refused to be randomized constitute the patient-choice registry. Diabetes prevalence was 32% ($n = 144$) among randomized patients, 27% ($n = 89$) in the patient-choice registry and 32% ($n = 525$) in the physician-directed registry. The CABG and PCI survival rates were compared using Kaplan–Meier curves and log-rank tests. The respective CABG and PCI 36-month survival rates for diabetic patients were 72 and 81% for randomized patients, 85 and 89% for patient-choice registry patients, and 73 and 71% for the physician-directed registry patients. None of the differences was statistically significant.**

I N T E R P R E T A T I O N . We conclude that PCI is a relatively safe alternative to CABG for diabetic patients with medically refractory unstable angina who are at high risk for CABG.

Comment

Studies from the balloon angioplasty era have demonstrated a survival advantage with CABG compared with PCI in diabetic patients – a finding that has influenced clinical practice. These findings indicate a more favourable outcome with PCI in a high-risk group of diabetic patients. For randomized patients in-hospital mortality, 3-year mortality and freedom from revascularization and unstable angina at follow-up were similar for the PCI and CABG groups. The registry data did suggest that there may be a reduction in repeat revascularization and unstable angina with CABG compared with PCI. Again there was difficulty in convincing physicians and patients to permit random allocation in this high-risk population with the majority of patients being allocated treatment based on physician advice or patient choice.

Advocates of PCI may note that procedures in the AWESOME trial do not match current practice norms. In this trial, the stent implantation rate increased from 26% in 1995 to 88% in 1999/2000 but the mean rate was only 54%. Similarly, although the use of Gp IIb/IIIa receptor blockade increased from 1 to 51% over the same period the mean use was only 11%. Similar arguments may apply in the surgical patients with reduced use of arterial conduits and very few off-pump procedures.

It has long been recognized that obstructive coronary disease affecting the proximal portion of the left anterior descending coronary artery (PLAD) has special prognostic significance. This has been established in simple observational studies and in other ventures assessing the prognostic impact of surgical revascularization.

In a meta-analysis examining the results of the first generation balloon angioplasty versus bypass surgery trials, it was identified that initial surgical revascularization appeared particularly effective in patients manifesting single vessel disease with involvement of the PLAD |6|. The results of balloon angioplasty in this group were particularly disappointing, not only in terms of the need for repeat revascularization, but also mortality and subsequent MI. Complex lesions in this territory represent a significant angioplasty challenge particularly if they involve the origin of substantial diagonal or septal branches.

A number of studies, published this year compared surgical- and stent-based PCI strategies for revascularization of this pattern of single vessel disease. Surgical procedures were performed off-pump and, in the main, through limited incisions – so-called minimally invasive surgery.

A prospective randomized trial comparing stenting with off-pump coronary surgery for high-grade stenosis in the proximal left anterior descending coronary artery: three-year follow-up.

D J Drenth, N J Veeger, J B Winter, *et al. J Am Coll Cardiol* 2002; **40**: 1955–60.

BACKGROUND. PCI and off-pump CABG (surgery) are used to treat single-vessel disease of a high-grade stenosis of the PLAD. Mid-term results of both treatments are compared in this prospective randomized study. In a single-centre prospective trial,

102 patients with a high-grade stenosis of the PLAD (American College of Cardiology/American Heart Association classification type B2 or C) were randomly allocated to undergo PCI ($n = 51$) or surgery ($n = 51$). Primary composite end-point was freedom from major adverse cardiac and cerebrovascular events (MACCE) at follow-up, including death, MI, cerebrovascular accident and repeat target vessel revascularization (TVR). Secondary end-points were angina pectoris class and need for anti-anginal medication at follow-up. Analysis was by intention-to-treat (ITT) and received treatment (RT). Mean follow-up time was 3 years (90% midrange, 2–4 years). Incidence of MACCE was 23.5% after PCI and 9.8% after surgery; $P = 0.07$ ITT (24.1 vs 8.3%; $P = 0.04$ RT). After surgery a significantly lower angina pectoris class ($P = 0.02$) and need for anti-anginal medication ($P = 0.01$) was found compared with PCI. Target vessel revascularization was 15.7% after PCI and 4.1% after surgery ($P = 0.09$).

INTERPRETATION. At 3-year follow-up (range, 2–4 years), a trend in favour of surgery is observed in regard to MACCE-free survival with a significantly lower angina pectoris status and significantly lower need for anti-anginal medication.

Comment

This study compares coronary artery stenting with minimally invasive off-pump coronary surgery. As might be expected with a single-centre venture, sample size is relatively small ($n = 102$). This limits the statistical power to detect meaningful

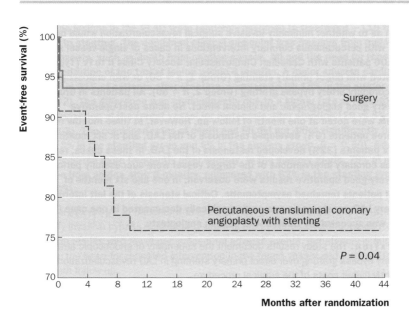

Fig. 4.3 Major adverse cardiac and cerebrovascular events by received treatment analysis. Source: Drenth et al. (2002).

Table 4.3 Major adverse cardiac events during six months of follow-up

Event	Stenting group (n = 108)	Surgery group (n = 108)	P value	Relative risk (95% CI)*
	no. (%)			
Death from cardiac causes	0	2 (2)	0.99	
Acute myocardial infarction	3 (3)	5 (5)	0.68	1.77 (0.41–7.58)
<30 days	2 (2)	4 (4)		
30 days–6 mo	1 (1)	1 (1)		
Acute myocardial infarction or death from cardiac causes	3 (3)	7 (6)	0.50	2.33 (0.34–43.73)
Revascularization of the target vessel	31 (29)	9 (8)	0.003	0.29 (0.09–0.65)
<30 days	2 (2)	4 (4)		
30 days–6 mo	29 (27)	5 (5)		
Any major adverse cardiac event	34 (31)	16 (15)	0.02	0.47 (0.21–0.89)

* CI denotes confidence interval.
Source: Diegeler *et al.* (2002).

revascularization. The difference in this composite outcome measure is driven by a higher rate of repeat revascularization procedures in patients managed initially with stenting (29 vs 8%). The incidence of cardiovascular death or non-fatal MI at 6 months is higher in the surgical group (6 vs 3%). Because of the limited sample size this difference does not achieve conventional levels of statistical significance (see Table 4.3).

Angiographic follow-up again confirmed the essentially universal patency of the bypass graft conduits. This is reflected in the observation that a greater proportion of surgically managed patients are free of angina at follow-up.

Data from this and the papers described above would suggest that newer techniques of minimally invasive surgery appear safe and efficacious. The results appear comparable with those that might be expected with a traditional surgical approach. Clearly, this is an important area and further trials are expected.

Comparative studies of surgery and angioplasty tend to focus on the major adverse cardiac events. It is an interesting observation from the SoS trial that the total number of post-procedural hospital admissions was greater in the surgical group. This was related to a number of key diagnoses including transient atrial arrhythmia, wound infections and pleural effusions. A complete assessment of the procedural morbidity, impact on the patient and implications for cost would demand a more complete description of these outcome measures.

The following two papers report early experience with hybrid revascularization. This approach recognizes the potential value of surgical revascularization of the LAD (as described above), performed off-pump and through minimal incisions. Further revascularization to lesions in other coronary vessels is then performed using PCI techniques.

Hybrid robotic coronary artery surgery and angioplasty in multivessel coronary artery disease.

K D Stahl, W D Boyd, T A Vassiliades, H L Karamanoukian. *Ann Thorac Surg* 2002; **74**: S1358–62.

BACKGROUND. Complete surgical revascularization that includes left internal thoracic artery grafting to the LAD remains the gold standard of treatment for coronary artery disease. Not all patients are good candidates for sternotomy. Therefore, the authors sought to identify a strategy that would combine the long-term advantages of internal thoracic artery grafting to lessen surgical trauma while still allowing complete revascularization. A total of 54 consecutive patients from four institutions underwent hybrid revascularization combining surgery and angioplasty. All internal thoracic artery grafts were harvested endoscopically with robotic assistance using either the Aesop or Zeus system, and all anastomoses were constructed manually through a 4–6-cm anterior thoracotomy incision. Angioplasty was carried out to achieve total revascularization to ungrafted vessels. There were no early or late deaths, MI, strokes or wound infections. Of the patients, 37 (69%) were extubated in the operating theatre. Length of stay in the intensive care unit averaged 24.4 h and hospital stay averaged 3.45 days. In all, 16 patients (29.6%) required transfusion of packed red blood cells. Late complications included one patient with stent occlusion at 3 months and two patients with in-stent restenosis. Three patients were treated for post peri-cardiotomy syndrome. Mean follow-up was 11.7 months. Event-free survival was 87.1% and freedom from recurrent angina 98.3%.

INTERPRETATION. Hybrid endoscopic atraumatic internal thoracic artery to anterior descending coronary artery graft surgery combined with angioplasty is a reasonable revascularization strategy in multiple vessel coronary artery disease in selected patients. Longer follow-up and more patient data in a randomized study are needed to determine the patient cohort most likely to benefit from this approach.

Comment

This early report describes the results of a relatively small series of patients (54 consecutive procedures) performed at four institutions. The strategy under examination involves surgical revascularization of the LAD, performed through minimal incisions with endoscopic techniques and robotic assistance, with PCI to other vessel territories. Interestingly, there was no protocol as to the order in which revascularization procedures were performed. In the early phase of the experience, the authors observe that surgical procedure was performed first, in order that the integrity and patency of the anastomosis could be examined at a subsequent coronary intervention. As experience developed PCI was performed as the initial manoeuvre in some patients. This latter approach would offer the potential for a more expanded surgical approach in the event of acute complications or a failure to achieve adequate revascularization at the time of PCI.

Outcomes in this group were favourable. Major adverse cardiac events were restricted to the development of occlusion or restenosis at stent implantation sites.

The authors present extremely encouraging data on requirements for intensive nursing care and hospital stay. These components of resource utilization have traditionally ensured that the in-hospital costs of surgical revascularization were higher than that for comparable PCI revascularization.

Coronary hybrid revascularization from January 1997 to January 2001: a clinical follow-up.

F C Riess, R Bader, P Kremer, *et al. Ann Thorac Surg* 2002; **73**: 1849–55.

BACKGROUND. Hybrid revascularization (HyR), combining minimally invasive left internal mammary artery (LIMA) bypass grafting to the LAD and catheter interventional treatment of the remaining coronary lesions, avoids the disadvantages associated with cardiopulmonary bypass (CPB). We investigated the clinical follow-up of 57 patients with multivessel disease undergoing this procedure in the last 4 years. Between January 1997 and January 2001, 57 consecutive patients (41 men and 16 women, aged 65.7 ± 7.9 years) with coronary artery disease (two-vessel, $n = 34$; three-vessel, $n = 23$) were treated with off-pump LIMA-to-LAD bypass combined with balloon angioplasty and stenting of the remaining significantly obstructed ($>50\%$) coronary vessels. Clinical follow-up data included an early post-operative and a 6-month control angiography and a patient interview in January 2001. All patients underwent LIMA-to-LAD bypass grafting and balloon angioplasty in 72 coronary lesions without procedural-related complications. However, one early LIMA bypass occlusion was documented during coronary angiography. Post-operatively, no deterioration of pre-existent organ dysfunction was observed in any patient. The mean follow-up was 100.7 ± 37.9 weeks in 55 of 57 patients (97%). Control angiography 6 months after HyR ($n = 34$) revealed a patent LIMA bypass in 33 patients and 8 in-stent restenoses ($>50\%$) in the coronary arteries that were treated interventionally by re-PTCA ($n = 6$) or by conventional CABG ($n = 1$). In one patient medical treatment resulted in a significant reduction of angina so no further intervention was considered necessary. After HyR one patient died 18 months later of an intracerebral haemorrhage. All other patients are alive and doing well.

INTERPRETATION. The results indicate that in selected patients with multivessel disease, including left main stem stenosis, HyR is an effective and secure procedure with excellent early and good mid-term results. In particular, elderly patients with severe concomitant diseases appear to benefit from this approach by avoiding CPB.

Comment

This paper reports a single-centre series of hybrid revascularization procedures using a minimally invasive surgical anastomosis of the left internal mammary to the LAD with subsequent PCI procedures performed a median of 5 days following surgical intervention.

As in the previous study, surgery was scheduled before angioplasty. This again may have been driven by a desire to inspect the nature and quality of the surgical anastomosis during this experimental phase. Clearly further work is required to decide the optimum order of intervention. The advantages of an 'angioplasty first' strategy (described above) must be balanced against the fact that successful surgical revascularization would provide some measure of protection for a subsequent angioplasty intervention. Modern interventional techniques involve the administration of powerful antiplatelet agents. This may, of course, influence decisions about scheduling and the interval between procedures.

The authors comment that their initial enthusiasm for hybrid procedures has diminished somewhat as their experience with complete off pump surgical revascularization has increased. The principal attraction of the hybrid concept is to allow performance of surgical revascularization of the LAD using minimal incisions, reducing operative times and surgical morbidity. Revascularization to other lesions is then provided with percutaneous techniques. Clearly, this represents an alternative to complete off-pump surgical revascularization through a traditional incision. As such it may be an appropriate option for patients with high surgical risk or important co-morbidity. It may also have a role in the development of newer surgical anastomotic techniques and robotic tools. The advent of drug-eluting stents will address the principal limitation of PCI revascularization observed in these hybrid series.

Conclusion

Although randomized control trial methodology demands an adversarial approach, most clinicians recognize that techniques of surgical and PCI revascularization are complimentary. It is usually possible to identify, for each patient, a preferred strategy with consideration of the clinical presentation, angiographic findings and the risk factor and co-morbidity profile. Patient preference is another key element. The final decision should reflect the chronic nature of coronary artery disease and the very real possibility that a patient may require a number of different revascularization procedures, perhaps of different types throughout a protracted clinical course.

The advent of drug-eluting stent technology and the potential to abolish or limit coronary restenosis will further enhance the potential of PCI procedures. Nevertheless, interventional cardiologists must continue to respect the clearly demonstrated safety and efficacy of surgical revascularization. For the interventional cardiologist, problems of incomplete revascularization (usually related to a failure to re-canalize occluded vessels), preservation of important side branches and the management of long segment and small vessel disease remain a considerable challenge.

References

1. De Belder M. British cardiac interventional society audit returns 2001. www.bcis.org.uk.

2. American Heart Association. Heart disease and stroke statistic—2003 update. www. americanheart.org.

3. Serruys PW, Unger F, Sousa JE, Jatene A, Bonnier JRM, Schonberger JPAM, *et al.* Comparison of coronary-artery bypass surgery and stenting for the treatment of multivessel disease. *N Engl J Med* 2001; **344**: 1117–24.

4. Rodriguez A, Bernardi V, Navia J, Baldi J, Grinfield L, Martinez J, *et al.* Argentine randomized study: coronary angioplasty with stenting versus coronary artery bypass surgery in patients with multi-vessel disease (ERACI II): 30-day and one-year follow up results. *J Am Coll Cardiol* 2001; **37**(1): 51–8.

5. Morrison DA, Sethi G, Sacks J, Henderson W, Grover F, Sedlis S, Esposito R, Ramanathan K, Weiman D, Saucedo J, Antakli T, Paramesh V, Pett S, Vernon S, Birjiniuk V, Welt F, Krucoff M, Wolfe W, Lucke JC, Mediratta S, Booth D, Barbiere C, Lewis D. Angina With Extremely Serious Operative Mortality Evaluation (AWESOME). Percutaneous coronary intervention versus coronary artery bypass graft surgery for patients with medically refractory myocardial ischemia and risk factors for adverse outcomes with bypass: a multicenter, randomized trial. Investigators of the Department of Veterans Affairs Cooperative Study #385, the Angina With Extremely Serious Operative Mortality Evaluation (AWESOME). *J Am Coll Cardiol* 2001; **38**(1): 143–9.

6. Pocock SJ, Henderson RA, Rickards AF, Hampton JR, King III SB, Hamm CW, *et al.* Meta-analysis of randomized trials comparing coronary angioplasty with bypass surgery. *Lancet* 1995; **346**: 1184–9.

Part II

Technique

Procedural safety, feasibility, clinical outcome and costs

Direct stenting with the Bx VELOCITY trademark balloon-expandable stent mounted on the Raptor rapid exchange delivery system versus pre-dilatation in a European randomized trial: the VELVET trial.

P W Serruys, S IJsselmuiden, B Hout, *et al. Int J Cardiovasc Intervent* 2003; **5**: 17–26.

BACKGROUND. In phase I, 122 patients (mean age = 62.3 ± 10.1 years, 77% male, 11% with diabetes) with angina pectoris or myocardial ischaemia resulting from a single *de novo* 51–95% coronary stenosis underwent direct stenting. The end-points of phase I included angiographic findings and rates of major adverse cardiac events up to 6 months follow-up. In phase II, 401 patients (mean age = 61.3 ± 10.8 years, 79% male, 16% with diabetes) with angina pectoris or documented myocardial ischaemia resulting from single or multiple, *de novo* or restenotic, coronary lesions were randomized between direct stenting and stenting after pre-dilatation.

INTERPRETATION. In phase I the mean diameter stenosis immediately before and after the procedure, and at six months was 61.7 ± 9.4%, 13.5 ± 6.3% and 33.6 ± 16.2%, respectively. The 6-month binary restenosis rate was 11%. The overall rate of major adverse cardiac events (MACE), including two non-cardiac deaths, was 9.8%. In phase II, the success rates of the intended delivery strategies were 87.9 and 97.9% for direct stenting and pre-dilatation, respectively (*P* <0.001), while the procedural success rates were similar (93.9 vs 96.5%). Over a follow-up period of 9 months, MACE rates were 12.0 and 10.9% in patients randomized to direct stenting and pre-dilatation, respectively (non-significant). Analyses of the costs incurred up to nine months in each treatment group revealed a mean saving of €362 per patient in favour of the direct stenting strategy (non-significant).

Comment

Direct stenting was associated with an equivalent procedural success rate, equivalent clinical results up to 9 months of follow-up, and a reduction in procedural and in-hospital costs (*P* <0.0001 and <0.001, respectively), that is no longer significant after 9 months.

Direct coronary stenting without balloon predilation of lesions requiring long stents: immediate and 6-month results of a multicenter prospective registry.

D Boulmier, M Bedossa, P Commeau, *et al. Catheter Cardiovasc Intervent* 2003; **58**: 51–8.

BACKGROUND. This prospective multicentre registry included 128 consecutive patients who underwent the implantation of stents ≥18 mm in length without balloon pre-dilation of *de novo* coronary artery stenoses.

INTERPRETATION. Mean lesion and stent lengths were 20.7 ± 5.4 and 21.4 ± 3.8 mm, respectively. Rates of direct stenting (DS) success, lesion success and primary success were 82, 99 and 97.7%, respectively. At 6 months, rates of MACE and target vessel revascularization (TVR) were 12.5 and 6.3%, respectively. In multivariate analysis, factors predictive of DS failure versus DS success were presence of calcification (78 vs 45%; $P = 0.004$) and reference vessel diameter (2.77 ± 0.4 vs 3.13 ± 0.42 mm; $P = 0.0002$).

Comment

Direct stenting of long lesions with stents ≥18 mm in length can be performed safely and with a high success rate. This strategy is less successful in the treatment of small vessels and in the presence of calcification. This study is particularly meaningful, as it shows the feasibility of direct stenting in the setting of long lesions. More complex lesions were also selected: B2-type lesion 41%, C-type lesion 38%. The authors acknowledged that a direct stenting strategy was less successful in calcified, type C lesions and small vessels. It should be also noted that a direct stenting strategy was attempted in the circumflex artery location in only 18% of the cases. It has been demonstrated that a circumflex location of the lesion is the strongest predictor of failure for direct stenting |4|. This is particularly true in the case of a long lesion.

A randomized comparison of direct stenting versus stenting with pre-dilatation in native coronary artery disease: results from the multicentric Crosscut study.

F Airoldi, C Di Mario, G Gimelli, *et al. J Inv Cardiol* 2003; **15**: 1–5.

BACKGROUND. This study is a randomized prospective multicentre evaluation including 271 patients (140 patients in the DS group and 131 patients in the provisional stenting [PS] group) with one or two *de novo* or restenotic lesions located in native coronary arteries.

INTERPRETATION. Procedural success was 98.9 and 98.7% in the DS and PS groups, respectively ($P = ns$); cross-over to PS was required in 22/166 lesions (13.2%) enrolled in the DS group because of inability to cross the target lesion without pre-dilatation.

Non-significant reductions in procedural time (−10.5%), fluoroscopy time (−4.7%) and amount of contrast (−3.8%) were observed in the DS group in comparison with the PS group. The number of balloons used (−76.6%) and the global cost of the procedure (−18.8%) were significantly lower in the DS group (*P* <0.01 for both comparisons). After 6 months, no differences (*P* = ns) were observed in the restenosis rate between the two groups (22.0% for DS vs 18.1% for PS group) and in the incidence of major adverse clinical events (5.0% for DS vs 3.0% for PS group).

Comment

Direct stenting is safe and feasible for the treatment of lesions in native coronary arteries and results in a significant reduction in procedural costs, mainly due to the lower number of balloon catheters used. Clinical and angiographic results at 6 months are comparable with those obtained following a conventional pre-dilatation stenting strategy.

Direct coronary stenting versus pre-dilatation followed by stent placement.

M Brueck, D Scheinert, A Wortmann, *et al*. *Am J Cardiol* 2002; **90**: 1187–92.

BACKGROUND. Three hundred and thirty-five symptomatic patients with single or multiple coronary lesions (diameter reduction 60 to 95%) of ≤30 mm length and with a vessel diameter of 2.5–4.0 mm were randomized either to direct stenting (group A, *n* = 171) or stenting after pre-dilatation (group B, *n* = 164). Patients with vessels with excessive calcification, severe proximal tortuosity or occlusion were excluded. All patients were asked to return for routine repeat angiography at 6 months, irrespective of symptoms.

INTERPRETATION. The feasibility of direct stenting was 95% in group A, with 5% requiring cross-over to pre-dilatation. Successful stent placement after pre-dilatation was performed in all 164 patients in group B. Direct stenting was associated with a shorter procedural duration (group A 42.1 ± 18.7 min vs group B 51.5 ± 23.8 min, *P* = 0.004), radiation exposure time (group A 10.3 ± 7.7 min vs group B 12.5 ± 6.4 min, *P* = 0.002), amount of contrast dye used (group A 163 ± 69 ml vs group B 197 ± 84 ml, *P* <0.0001), and lower procedural costs (group A 845 ± 167 vs group B 1064 ± 175, *P* <0.0001). Immediate angiographic results and in-hospital clinical outcomes (death, Q-wave myocardial infarction, repeat revascularization) were not significantly different between both strategies. However, at 6-month follow-up, direct stenting was associated with a lower angiographic restenosis (group A 20% vs group B 31%, *P* = 0.048) and target lesion revascularization rates (group A 18% vs group B 28%, *P* = 0.03).

Comment

This study demonstrates the feasibility, safety and outcomes of direct stenting in eligible coronary lesions. In appropriately selected cases, direct stenting has a lower rate of angiographic restenosis up to 6 months after the procedure, resulting in fewer coronary reinterventions compared with the conventional strategy of stenting with prior dilatation. It is likely that this observation results from chance as the study would appear to be underpowered to detect significant differences in categorical restenosis rates.

Clinical and angiographic outcome after conventional angioplasty with optional stent implantation compared with direct stenting without pre-dilatation.
S Miketic, J Carlsson, U Tebbe. *Heart* 2002; **88**: 622–6.

BACKGROUND. Patients undergoing coronary intervention for symptomatic coronary artery disease were randomly assigned to conventional angioplasty with optional stenting (provisional stenting) or to direct stent implantation without pre-dilatation. The post-stent treatment consisted of antiplatelet therapy. Follow-up angiography was performed 6 months after the initial procedure.

INTERPRETATION. Between December 1998 and August 1999, 181 of 190 eligible patients were randomly assigned to either provisional stenting ($n = 92$) or direct stenting ($n = 89$). The procedural success was similar in both groups (87 [97.8%] in the optional vs 87 [94.6%] in direct stenting group, $P = 0.88$). There were five cases of cross-over from the direct stenting to the provisional stenting group. Six patients experienced a Q-wave myocardial infarction without further complications (4 in the optional vs 2 in the direct stenting group, $P = 0.36$). One patient in whom coronary angioplasty failed underwent elective bypass surgery. No patients required urgent bypass surgery and no patients died. The reduction in late luminal loss (mean [SD] 1.19 [0.87] mm in the provisional vs 0.62 [0.69] mm in the direct stenting group, $P = 0.004$) led to a significant improvement in minimal luminal diameter at follow-up (1.87 [0.93] mm in the provisional vs 2.56 [0.86] mm in the direct stenting group, $P = 0.002$), resulting in a significant reduction in restenosis rate, defined as >50% diameter stenosis at follow up 6.5 (2.1) months after the initial procedure: 28 (30.4%) in the provisional versus 14 (15.7%) in the direct stenting group ($P = 0.019$).

Comment

Direct stent implantation without pre-dilatation significantly reduces late luminal loss, resulting in a larger minimal luminal diameter and reduced restenosis rates compared with provisional stenting. According to this strategy, stent implantation is needed only when the immediate result after plain balloon angioplasty is poor or when the risk of restenosis following balloon angioplasty is high. In contrast, with direct stenting, all technically eligible stenoses receive a stent, by primary intention. The issue is how one determines the quality of the result of balloon angioplasty. Intravascular ultrasound (IVUS) and Doppler flow measurements have been proposed to identify patients who would be unlikely to benefit from stent implantation after successful balloon angioplasty. Balloon-treated vessels that meet the quantitative coronary angioplasty (QCA), IVUS or Doppler criteria of an 'optimal stent-like' result, range from 22 to 52% of all attempted cases and were shown to have very low restenosis rates. The avoidance of stent implantation in this subset of patients might reduce procedural costs without compromising the clinical outcome. However, the DEBATE II (Doppler Endpoints Balloon Angioplasty Trial in Europe) trial |5| demonstrated no significant difference in outcome between the 'per principle' and provisional stenting approach, but the costs of the latter strategy at 1 year were significantly higher. Furthermore, in the DEBATE II study, stent implantation, despite achievement of a 'stent-like' result following balloon dilatation, incrementally ($P = 0.07$) reduced the event rate at 1 year from 16 to 6.5%. The OPUS-TIMI trial |6| showed a significantly higher MACE rate (death, myocardial infarction [MI] and target lesion revascularization) in the provisional stenting group than in the elective stenting group, demonstrating that angiography alone is not sensitive enough to identify patients who do not require stent implantation. Thus it appears that the clinical applicability of the provisional stenting strategy is limited because its application requires detailed physiological and morphological (IVUS) assessment of the angioplasty result, which will jeopardize potential savings. A word of caution applies to the case of small vessels and long lesions. Clinical data have clearly demonstrated increasing restenosis rates with decreasing vessel size. However, the results of trials comparing stent implantation and balloon-percutaneous transluminal coronary angioplasty (PTCA) in small vessels have demonstrated equivalent results in terms of long-term outcome. In long lesions, procedural success rate was not different between stent implantation and balloon-PTCA. An initially larger minimal lumen diameter, observed with stent implantation, was associated with reduced angiographic restenosis at 9 months. However, no differences in freedom from MACE were observed between the two strategies. In the setting of small vessels and long lesions, a strategy of provisional stenting would thus be advisable.

Is direct coronary stenting the best strategy for long-term outcome? Results of the multicentric randomized benefit evaluation of direct coronary stenting (BET) study.

M Elbaz, E El Mokhtar, K Khalife, *et al. Am Heart J* 2002; **144**: E7.

BACKGROUND. Between January and September 1999, 338 patients were randomly assigned to either direct stent implantation (DS+, *n* = 173) or standard stent implantation with balloon pre-dilatation (DS–, *n* = 165). Clinical follow-up was performed.

INTERPRETATION. Baseline characteristics were similar in the two groups. Procedural success was achieved in 98.3% of patients assigned to DS+ and 97.5% in patients assigned to DS– (ns). Clinical follow-up was obtained in 99% of patients (mean 16.4 ± 4.6 months). MACE – defined as whichever of the following occurred first; cardiac death, MI, unstable angina, new revascularization were observed at a higher rate in the DS+ group than in the DS– group, but this difference was not significant (11.3 vs 18.2%, P = ns). The difference in target lesion revascularization (TLR) rate in the DS+ (7%) and DS– (5.2%) groups was also not significant. Multivariate analysis showed that direct stenting had no influence on long-term MACE rate. Independent relationships were found between long-term MACE rate and final minimal lumen diameter <2.48 mm (relative risk [RR] 0.449, confidence interval [CI] 0.239–0.845, P = 0.013), prior MI (RR 2.028, CI 1.114–3.69, P = 0.02), and hypertension (RR 1.859, CI 1.022–3.383, P = 0.042).

Comment

The influence of direct stenting on the long-term need for new TLR does not differ from that of stenting that follows balloon pre-dilatation.

Direct coronary stenting versus stenting with balloon pre-dilation: immediate and follow-up results of a multicentre, prospective, randomized study; the DISCO (DIrect Stenting of COronary Arteries) trial.

L Martinez-Elbal, J M Ruiz-Nodar, J Zueco, *et al. Eur Heart J* 2002; **23**: 633–40.

BACKGROUND. In this study, 416 patients were randomized (446 lesions) to direct stent implantation or stent implantation following balloon pre-dilation. Patients >75 years old, with heavily calcified lesions, bifurcations, total occlusions, left main lesions and very tortuous vessels were excluded.

INTERPRETATION. Direct stenting was successful in 217/224 lesions (96.8%). No single loss or embolization of the stent occurred. All stents in the group with pre-dilation were effectively deployed. The immediate post-procedure angiographic results were similar with both techniques. Fluoroscopy and procedural time were significantly lower in direct stenting (6.4 ± 0.3 and 21 ± 0.9 min) than in pre-dilated stenting (9.1 ± 0.4 and 27.5 ± 1.1 min) (P >0.001). MACE during hospitalization were one in direct and four in pre-dilated stenting (P = 0.05), but there were no significant differences at 1-, 6- and 12-month follow-up between the two groups. Angiographic re-evaluation at 6 months was performed in 94% of the cases. Restenosis rate was 16.5% in direct stenting and 14.3% in pre-dilatation stenting (P = ns).

Comment

Direct stenting is as safe as pre-dilatation stenting in selected coronary lesions. Acute angiographic results are similar but procedural costs, duration of the procedure and radiation exposure are lower in direct stenting. Overall success rate, mid-term clinical outcome and restenosis rates are similar with both techniques (see Table 5.1).

Table 5.1 Clinical outcome results of the DISCO trial: no difference between direct stenting and pre-dilatation stenting

	DS	PS	P
6 month clinical follow-up	**n = 224**	**n = 222**	
MI	2 (0.9%)	6 (2.7%)	0.3
Death	1 (0.5%)	2 (1%)	0.55
PTCA	25 (11.9%)	26 (11.7%)	0.93
CABG	1 (0.5%)	1 (0.5%)	0.94
MACE	28 (13.3%)	32 (15.5%)	0.52
12 month clinical follow-up	**n = 194**	**n = 188**	
MI	3 (1.5%)	7 (3.7%)	0.18
Death	1 (0.5%)	2 (1%)	0.55
PTCA	30 (15.5%)	29 (15.4%)	0.93
CABG	1 (0.5%)	2 (1%)	0.54
MACE	33 (15.2%)	35 (16.9%)	0.89

DS = direct stenting; PS = pre-dilatation stenting; MI = myocardial infarction; PTCA = percutaneous transluminal coronary angioplasty; CABG = coronary artery bypass graft surgery; MACE = major adverse cardiovascular events.
Source: Martinez-Elbal *et al.* (2002).

Intracoronary stenting and angiographic results: restenosis after direct stenting versus stenting with pre-dilatation (ISAR-DIRECT) trial.

J Mehilli, A Kastrati, J Dirschinger, *et al. Circulation* 2002; **II-391**: 1944.

BACKGROUND. This trial included 910 patients with stable or unstable angina and lesions in native vessels (total occlusions were excluded): 456 were randomly assigned to direct stenting (DS) and 454 to pre-dilatated stenting (SP). The protocol included a follow-up angiography at 6 months. Angiographic restenosis (>50% diameter stenosis) was the primary end-point). Patients were also monitored for death, MI and TVR over 1 year after randomization.

INTERPRETATION. DS was not superior to PS with respect to angiographic and clinical outcomes. On the contrary, there was a trend for a higher risk for restenosis (RR, 1.1 [0.8–1.5]), TVR (RR, 1.2 [0.8–1.6]) and death or MI (RR, 1.3 [0.8–2.0]) in the DS group (see Fig. 5.1).

Comment

These data do not support a role of direct stenting for the prevention of in-stent restenosis in clinical practice. This is just another study pointing in the same direction.

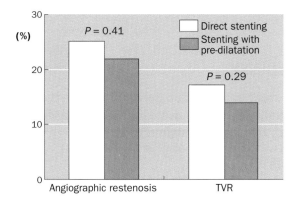

Fig. 5.1 Angiographic and clinical outcome of the ISAR-DIRECT trial: no difference between direct stenting and stenting with pre-dilatation. TVR = target vessel revascularization. Source: Mehilli *et al.* (2002).

Reduction of restenosis rate for direct stenting with intracoronary ultrasound guidance; results from the prospective, randomized trial.

R Gil, T Pawlowski, K Zmudka, *et al. Eur Heart J* 2002; **310**: 1661.

BACKGROUND. **This study compared analysis of early and late results of DS guided using QCA and intracoronary ultrasound (ICUS). The study population consisted of 120 patients divided into two groups according to the type of stent implantation guidance. There were 62 patients in the DS-QCA group (group 1) and 58 patients in the DS-ICUS group (group 2). In group 1 the stent was sized according to QCA vessel reference diameter (RD), whereas in group 2 media-to-media diameter measured using ICUS was used for that reason. Stent length was chosen in accordance with QCA (group 1) and with ICUS (group 2) measurements. MACE and TLR were observed during follow-up. Coronary angiography for restenosis detection between 6–9 months was planned.**

INTERPRETATION. There was 100% procedural success and no early (30 days) complications. There were no differences in procedural variables (maximum inflation pressure and time) between the two groups. Mean stent size used for DS was significantly bigger in group 2 than in group 1 (3.8 ± 0.55 vs 3.41 ± 0.42 mm, $P < 0.001$). The need for stent redilatation was 33% in group 1 and 39% in group 2 (P = ns). QCA results did not differ between groups except for minimal lumen diameter obtained after the procedure (2.98 ± 0.62 vs 3.35 ± 0.56 mm, respectively group 1 vs group 2, $P < 0.05$). The evidence of MACE at 6-month follow-up was 18.4 and 10.4% for groups 1 and 2 respectively (P = ns). The control angiography revealed in-stent restenosis in 23.7% of group 1 and 9.3% of group 2 patients ($P < 0.05$).

Comment

ICUS-guided DS is associated with use of bigger stents which provides a better clinical outcome and lower restenosis rate.

Direct coronary stent implantation does not reduce the incidence of in-stent restenosis or major adverse cardiac events; six-month results of a randomized trial.

A J IJsselmuiden, P W Serruys, A Scholte, *et al. Eur Heart J* 2003; **24**: 421–9.

BACKGROUND. Patients ($n = 400$) with coronary stenoses in a single native vessel were randomly allocated to direct stenting or stenting after pre-dilatation. A major adverse cardiac and cerebrovascular event (MACCE) was defined as death, MI, stent thrombosis, target restenosis, repeat target- and non-target vessel-related PCI, TLR, coronary artery bypass surgery and stroke.

INTERPRETATION. Stents were successfully implanted in 98.3% of patients randomized to direct stenting compared with 97.8% randomized to stenting preceded by pre-dilatation. The primary success rate of direct stenting was 88.3%, compared with 97.8% for stenting preceded by balloon dilatation ($P = 0.01$). The angiographic follow-up at 6 months included 333 of the 400 patients (83%). The binary in-stent restenosis rate was 23.1% of 163 patients randomized to direct stenting and 18.8% of 166 patients randomized to balloon pre-dilatation ($P = 0.32$). By 185 ± 25 days, MACCE had occurred in 31 of 200 (15.5%) patients randomized to direct stenting, and 33 of 200 (16.5%) randomized to pre-dilatation ($P = 0.89$). At 6 months, costs associated with the direct stenting strategy (€3222/patient) were similar to those associated with pre-dilatation (€3428/patient, $P = 0.43$). However, procedural costs were significantly lower. It is noteworthy that, on multivariate analysis, a baseline C-reactive protein (CRP) level >10 mg/l was a predictor of restenosis (odds ratio: 2.10, $P = 0.025$) as well as of MACCE (odds ratio: 1.94, $P = 0.045$).

Comment

Compared with stenting preceded by balloon pre-dilatation, direct stenting is associated with similar 6-month restenosis and MACCE rates. Procedural, but not overall 6-month, costs are reduced by direct stenting. An increased baseline CRP level is an independent predictor of adverse long-term outcome after coronary stent implantation.

Mechanisms of stent expansion with direct stenting

Is coronary stent deployment and remodeling affected by pre-dilatation? An intravascular ultrasound randomized study; stenting with or without pre-dilatation: an IVUS study.

J Boschat, H Le Breton, P Commeau, *et al*. and the Stent WIthout BAlloon Pre-dilatation (SWIBAP) Study Group. *Int J Cardiovasc Imaging* 2002; **18**: 399–404.

BACKGROUND. In this IVUS randomized trial, a strategy of DS without pre-dilatation (*n* = 30) was compared with a strategy of conventional stenting with pre-dilatation (SWP) (*n* = 30) in patients with suitable type A or B non-calcified lesions in native vessels ≥3 mm. Optimal deployment was achieved using angiographic criteria without interactive IVUS. The goal of the study was to determine whether stent expansion and coronary remodelling were similar.

INTERPRETATION. Maximal pressure inflation was comparable in the two groups (11.4 ± 2.2 vs 11.8 ± 1.9 atm; ns). Stent deployment was obtained in all patients with complete apposition to the vessel wall. DS and SWP resulted in comparable lumen enlargement (5.4 ± 2.5 vs 5.5 ± 2.1 mm^2) with an identical mechanism: 66% of lumen enlargement was due to increased enlarged elastic membrane (EEM) cross-sectional area (CSA) (delta = 3.7 ± 2.1 mm^2 and 2.4 ± 6.8 mm^2, respectively, *P* <0.49) and 34% was due to a reduced plaque + media (P+M)-CSA (delta = 0.02 ± 6.9 mm^2 and 1.2 ± 6.3 mm^2, respectively, *P* <0.50).

Comment

At the same maximal inflation pressure the mechanisms of stent expansion are similar in both DS and SWP groups. In this study, the IVUS data clearly showed under-expansion of stents in both groups in comparison with previously published CSA values (minimum stent CSA of 7.5 mm^2).

Mechanism of lumen enlargement with direct stenting versus pre-dilatation stenting: influence of remodelling and plaque characteristics assessed by volumetric intracoronary ultrasound.

G Finet, N J Weissman, G S Mintz, *et al. Heart* 2003; **89**: 84–90.

BACKGROUND. To compare the effects of arterial remodelling and plaque characteristics on the mechanisms of direct stenting and pre-dilatation stenting. Pre- and post-interventional volumetric IVUS was undertaken in 30 patients with direct stenting and 30 with pre-dilatation stenting of non-calcified native coronary lesions, using the same stent design and stent length. Lumen, vessel (EEM), and plaque (P+M) volumes were calculated. Remodelling was determined by comparing the EEM area at the centre of the lesion with the EEM areas at proximal and distal reference sites. Plaque eccentricity was defined as the thinnest plaque diameter to the thickest plaque diameter ratio. Plaque composition was characterized as soft, mixed or dense.

INTERPRETATION. All volumetric IVUS changes were similar in the two groups. Pre-intervention remodelling remained uninfluenced after direct stenting, but was neutralized after pre-dilatation stenting. Eccentric lesions responded to intervention by a greater luminal gain owing to greater vessel expansion in direct stenting. Plaque composition influenced luminal gain in direct stenting, the gain being greatest in the softest plaques; in pre-dilatation stenting, luminal gain was equivalent but vessel expansion was greater for 'dense' plaque and plaque reduction greater for 'soft' plaque.

Comment

In non-calcified lesions, the mechanisms of lumen enlargement after direct or pre-dilatation stenting are significantly influenced by atherosclerotic remodelling, plaque eccentricity and plaque composition.

Coronary and myocardial procedural injury

Side-branch occlusion after coronary stenting with or without balloon pre-dilation: direct versus conventional stenting.

T Timurkaynak, H Ciftci, M Ozdemir, *et al. J Invasive Cardiol* 2002; **14**: 497–501.

BACKGROUND. This study evaluates side branches occlusion (SBO) >1 mm in diameter after DS and compares it with conventional stenting (CS) with balloon pre-dilation.

INTERPRETATION. The study population consisted of 151 patients (88 underwent DS, 63 underwent CS) with 185 side branches jailed by the stent (110 in DS group, 75 in CS group). SBO was observed in 20 of 110 patients in the DS group (18.2%) and 18 of 75 patients in the CS group (24%). Although the incidence of SBO was higher in the CS group than the DS group (24 vs 18.2%, respectively), these values did not reach statistical significance ($P > 0.05$). Most of the SBOs were observed in cases with type D side branch morphology ($P < 0.001$) and in cases with side branch ostial diameter stenosis 50% ($P = 0.019$). None of the other clinical and angiographic variables predicted the SBO.

Comment

Direct stenting does not bear a higher risk of side branch occlusion than conventional stenting.

Randomized comparison of direct stenting and stenting after pre-dilatation in acute myocardial infarction; in-hospital results of DIRAMI trial.

M Gasior, M Gierlotka, A Lekston, *et al. Eur Heart J* 2002; **390**: 2060.

BACKGROUND. The aim of this study was to evaluate feasibility, safety and effectiveness of direct stenting in AMI. Consecutive patients with AMI were randomized before angiography to DS or stenting after balloon pre-dilatation (PS). Exclusion criteria were pulmonary oedema and cardiogenic shock. After coronary angiography, patients were excluded if the operator decided not to perform angioplasty or stenting. Thrombolysis in myocardial infarction (TIMI) flow grades 0 or 1 were not considered a contraindication for DS.

INTERPRETATION. One-year clinical and angiographic follow-up is pending. Analysis was performed on an intention to treat basis. Between November 2000 and September 2001, a total of 248 patients were randomized: 125 to DS and 123 to PS. After coronary angiography 31 patients were further excluded. Final study groups comprised 110 and 107 patients in the DS and PS groups, respectively. Cross-over to pre-dilatation occurred in 13 (11.8%) in DS group (inability to cross the lesion with a stent, 7; uncertain guidewire placement, 4; lesion type, 2). Except for in two patients (one per group), the stents were implanted successfully (see Table 5.2).

Comment

Direct stenting during angioplasty for AMI is feasible, safe and effective in a majority of patients/lesions that are suitable for stent implantation.

Table 5.2 Procedural results in the DIRAMI trial

	DS (*n* = 110)	PS (*n* = 107)	*P*
TIMI flow grade 3 (%)	95.4	93.5	0.52
TMP grade 2 or 3 (%)	81.3	76.2	0.41
MLD, mm (SD)	2.66 (0.41)	2.70 (0.52)	0.46
Additional stent(s) (%)	12.7	14.9	0.63
Side branch occlusion (%)	2.7	3.7	0.72
Fluoroscopy time, min (SD)	12.2 (7.5)	14.9 (7.7)	0.011
Procedure time, min (SD)	59 (22)	72 (31)	0.0006
Reocclusion or reinfarction (%)	1.8	2.8	0.68
Death (%)	0	1.9	0.24

TMP, TIMI myocardial perfusion; grade was accessible in 83% of patients in the DS group and 78% of patients in the PS group. MLD, mean lumen diameter.
Source: Gasior *et al*. 2002.

Direct stenting may limit myocardial injury during percutaneous coronary intervention.

T Nageh, M R Thomas, R A Sherwood, B M Harris, D E Jewitt, R J Wainwright. *J Invasive Cardiol* 2003; **15**: 115–18.

BACKGROUND. **Direct stenting may limit distal embolization of atherosclerotic plaque and consequently reduce myocardial cell injury following PCI, which may have important prognostic implications. Cardiac troponin I (cTnI) release was assessed in the 24 h following direct coronary stenting as compared with stenting with balloon pre-dilatation (PD) in a total of 311 patients and 440 vessels/lesions (vessel to lesion ratio = 1:1) (DS: n = 107 patients and 149 vessels/lesions; PD: n = 204 patients and 291 vessels/lesions).**

INTERPRETATION. The two groups were well matched except for a greater proportion of diabetic patients in the PD group (21%) compared with the DS group (11%) ($P <0.05$). There were no significant differences in the distribution of target lesion site or angiographic complexity between the two groups. Primary angiographic success was achieved in 97% of vessels in the DS group and 98% of vessels in the PD group (P = ns). DS failed in 7/114 patients (6%) deemed suitable for DS by the operator, but all stents were subsequently successfully deployed following balloon pre-dilatation. Abciximab (ReoPro) was used in 11 patients (10%) in the DS group and 24 patients (12%) in the PD group (P = 0.68). The post-procedural median (IQR) peak cTnI concentrations were 0.2 ± 0.1 g/l in the DS group and 0.5 ± 0.3 g/l in the PD group (P = 0.02). Post-procedural cTnI concentrations were >0.2 g/l in 11 patients (10%) in the DS group and in 53 patients (26%) in the PD group (x^2 = 58.6; $P <0.0001$). The rate of major adverse cardiac events at 6–18-month follow-up was 8% in the DS group and 15% in the PD group (x^2 = 38.5; P = 0.02).

Comment

Direct stenting without balloon pre-dilatation is associated with lower post-procedural cTnI concentrations and lower incidence of major adverse events compared to traditional stenting with pre-dilatation.

Effect of direct stent implantation on minor myocardial injury.

Y Atmaca, F Ertas, S Gulec, I Dincer, D Oral. *J Invasive Cardiol* 2002; **14**: 443–6.

BACKGROUND. **This non-randomized study evaluated the incidence of minor myocardial injury (MMI) in prospectively selected patients with simple lesion morphology and class II stable angina undergoing stenting with or without pre-dilatation. A total of 154 patients were divided into two arms based on the stenting technique used: direct stenting without pre-dilatation (group I; n = 78) and stenting with pre-dilatation (group**

II; *n* = 76). **Cardiac troponin T (cTnT) was measured immediately before, at 12 h and 24 h post procedure. The primary end-point was the MMI in-hospital. The secondary end-point of the study was the major clinical event (MCE) rate in-hospital and up to 6 months.**

INTERPRETATION. The frequency increase in group I was found to be significantly lower compared with group II (5.1 vs 21%, respectively; $P < 0.007$), as was the amount of cTnT release (0.28 ± 0.04 vs 0.51 ± 0.12 ng/ml at 12 h, $P < 0.001$; 0.28 ± 0.06 vs 0.51 ± 0.10 ng/ml at 24 h, $P < 0.0004$). No MCE was seen during the in-hospital period in both groups. Furthermore, no significant differences were found between the two groups with respect to MCE (12.8 vs 18.4%, respectively; $P > 0.05$) at 6 months. The balloon inflation time (BIT) was significantly longer in patients with abnormal cTnT level than in those with normal cTnT level in group II (120.3 ± 4.7 vs 118.2 ± 1.3 s; $P < 0.002$) but there was no statistical difference in group I (32.4 ± 2.1 vs 30.6 ± 2.4 s; $P > 0.05$). Furthermore, there was no statistical difference with respect to the number of balloon inflations in patients with normal and abnormal cTnT levels in either group (1.2 ± 0.2 vs 1.3 ± 0.4 inflations in group I, $P > 0.05$; 3.2 ± 0.9 vs 3.0 ± 1.4 inflations in group II, $P > 0.05$).

Comment

This study showed that MMI probably occurs less frequently after direct stenting than with pre-dilatation stenting.

Conventional versus direct stenting in AMI: effect on immediate coronary blood flow.

T Timurkaynak, M Ozdemir, A Cengel, *et al. J Invasive Cardiol* 2002; **14**: 372–7.

BACKGROUND. **The aim of this study was to evaluate the impact of direct stenting on the angiographic results and compare it to conventional stenting performed in the setting of AMI. Forty-four patients underwent stenting in the setting of AMI (29 primary and 15 rescue angioplasty). Patients were divided into two groups; group A consisted of patients who had undergone conventional stenting (23 patients) and group B those who had undergone direct stenting (21 patients). Angiographic success was defined as TIMI flow grade 2.**

INTERPRETATION. The baseline TIMI 0–1 flow was higher in group A than group B (74 vs 24%; $P < 0.05$). TIMI flow rates before stenting (after balloon pre-dilation in group A and after guidewire crossing in group B) and angiographic success (TIMI flow 2) after stenting were similar in both groups ($P > 0.05$). However, the final TIMI 3 flow were significantly better in group B after stenting (65 vs 95%; $P < 0.05$). Although there was no 'no reflow' in group B, three patients in group A had 'no reflow' after balloon pre-dilatation of lesions with baseline TIMI 2 flow. There was a statistical tendency to a higher TIMI 3 flow in patients treated with direct stenting in the setting of AMI.

Comment

Direct stenting strategy in thrombus-containing lesions seems to be a safe and feasible approach that may in addition be associated with reduced incidence of 'no reflow'.

Could direct stenting reduce no-reflow in acute coronary syndromes? A randomized pilot study.

R Sabatier, M Hamon, Q M Zhao, *et al. Am Heart J* 2002; **143**: 1027–32.

BACKGROUND. This randomized pilot study was designed to compare the incidence of no-reflow after direct stenting or conventional stenting after balloon pre-dilation in acute coronary syndrome-related lesions. Between December 1998 and October 1999, 130 patients with acute coronary syndromes were included in this study and randomized into two groups. In group A (*n* = 65), direct stent implantation was performed without balloon pre-dilation. In group B (*n* = 65), conventional balloon pre-dilation was carried out before stent implantation.

INTERPRETATION. Baseline clinical and angiographic characteristics before the procedure were similar in the two groups. No-reflow was observed in 7.7% after direct stenting and in 6.1% after conventional stent implantation (*P* = ns). The immediate clinical success rate

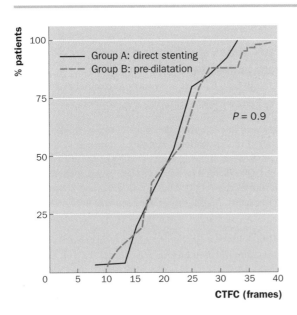

Fig. 5.2 Distribution of corrected TIMI frame count (CTFC) in study population. Source: Sabatier *et al.* (2002).

was similar in the two groups. Among the procedural data, only duration of the procedure (shorter in the direct stenting group), the number of balloons used and the quantity of contrast agent (lower in the direct stenting group) were significantly different between the two groups ($P < 0.05$). The 6-month clinical outcome was similar in the two groups (see Fig. 5.2).

Comment

This randomized study confirms the feasibility and the safety of direct coronary stenting in highly selected acute coronary syndrome-related lesions. The major impact of this strategy is the improvement of the cost–benefit ratio, with no major influence on the acute complications and especially on the occurrence of no-reflow in this high-risk population.

Conclusion

The strategy of direct stenting was introduced because it was thought that this approach would reduce procedural duration and costs.

Several reports indicated that indeed direct coronary stenting in patients with stable angina was feasible, safe and associated with a short- and long-term clinical outcome and six-month restenosis rate not different from a strategy of pre-dilatation followed by stent implantation.

Direct stenting in patients with acute coronary syndrome is also feasible and safe and a few studies even suggested that direct stenting is associated with a lower incidence of MACE, lower post-procedural troponin levels and lesser occurrence of no-reflow.

There was concern that direct stenting might be associated with a higher incidence of stent under-expansion compared to a pre-dilatation strategy with stenting, but data from two studies suggested that this was not the case.

Although direct stenting may be feasible in the majority of cases, it may be difficult in calcified lesions or vessels with severe tortuosity and in general less easy in lesions located in the left coronary circumflex artery.

It may be concluded that direct coronary stenting is feasible and safe and associated with a shorter procedural duration and lower cost mainly due to the lesser use of balloons. The in-hospital outcome is similar, or possibly slightly better, than compared to a strategy of pre-dilatation and stent-implantation, but the restenosis at six months is not different from a strategy of pre-dilatation and stenting. Lastly, prior dilatation has been recommended so far with the use of most drug-eluting stents. How the widespread usage of currently available and future drug-eluting stents will influence the practice of direct stenting remains to be seen.

References

1. Carrié D, Khalifé K, Citron B, *et al.* Comparison of direct coronary stenting with and without balloon pre-dilatation in patients with stable angina pectoris. BET (Benefit Evaluation of Direct Coronary Stenting) Study Group. *Am J Cardiol* 2001; **87**: 693–8.

2. Baim D, Flatley M, Caputo R. Comparison of pre-dilatation vs direct stenting in coronary treatment using the Medtronic AVE S670 Coronary Stent System (the PREDICT trial). *Am J Cardiol* 2001; **88**: 1364–9.

3. Martinez-Elbal L, Ruiz-Nodar JM, Zueco J, *et al.* Direct coronary stenting versus stenting with balloon pre-dilatation: immediate and follow-up results of a multi-centre, prospective, randomized study. The DISCO trial. DIrect Stenting of COronary Arteries. *Eur Heart J* 2002; **23**(8): 633–40.

4. Chevalier B, Guyon P, Roger T, *et al.* Comparison of three coronary stenting techniques in acute myocardial infarction angioplasty. *Eur Heart J* 2000; **21**: 644, P3533.

5. Albertal M, Voskuil M, Piek JJ, *et al.* Coronary flow reserve after percutaneous intervention is predictive of peri-procedural outcome. *Circulation* 2002; **105**: 1573–8.

6. Cannon CP, McCabe CH, Wilcox RG, *et al.* Oral glycoprotein IIb/IIIa inhibition with orbofiban in patients with unstable coronary syndromes (OPUS-TIMI 16) trial. *Circulation* 2000; **102**: 149–56.

6

Pressure and flow measurements in percutaneous coronary intervention

Introduction

In the last decade, quantification of the effects of an epicardial stenosis on distal coronary perfusion pressure and on regional blood flow in the myocardium supplied by the stenosed vessel has come into widespread use in the catheterization laboratory. Thanks to the development and validation of minaturized angioplasty guidewires with flow or pressure sensors at the tip, such information can be used to assess the need for percutaneous intervention, to physiologically guide the procedure and to assess the results. A brief overview of flow and pressure measurements is presented below, addressing the relative advantages and limitations of flow and pressure measurements, and alluding to some of the areas of uncertainty that are covered by the papers reviewed in this chapter.

Coronary flow reserve

When an epicardial lesion is severe enough to produce an increased resistance to flow, the resistance in the microcirculatory bed distal to the stenosis decreases to maintain blood flow, in the myocardium subtended by the vessel, at a level appropriate for myocardial oxygen utilization. If the stenosis is moderately severe, resting flow is usually maintained and the impediment to flow only becomes apparent when myocardial oxygen utilization increases. If we consider the simplest scenario, that of a patient with a moderately severe single lesion in one coronary artery, this is usually manifested clinically as effort-induced stable angina.

In patients undergoing catheterization with risk factors for coronary disease but who were found to have angiographically normal coronary arteries – the absolute coronary flow reserve (CFR), defined as the ratio of hyperaemic to basal mean flow with the Flow wire, was found to be 2.7 ($\pm$ 0.6) with little (<15%) regional variation |1|. Maximal hyperaemia in the catheterization laboratory is achieved with pharmacological stimuli such as papaverine, ADP or ATP, exclusively by the intracoronary route for papaverine, or by the intracoronary or intravenous route for the others.

In the presence of a physiologically significant epicardial lesion, the distal microvascular bed is already dilated at rest and thus the relative increase in flow induced by hyperaemic stimuli is reduced proportionately. However, the use of CFR to assess the physiological significance of an epicardial lesion is subject to several limitations. As CFR is a ratio, its value is influenced by changes in basal flow. Thus, changes in heart rate and blood pressure can affect CFR by altering basal flow. Interpretation of CFR is also complicated by the fact that CFR measures the sum of resistance to flow in both the epicardial and microcirculation. Therefore, the presence of left ventricular hypertrophy, diabetes mellitus or of a myocardial infarction (MI) in the myocardium supplied by the target vessel, all of which decrease CFR by their effects on the microcirculation, also confounds interpretation of the relative contribution of an epicardial lesion to CFR. In order to overcome these limitations, the concept of rCFR defined as the CFR in the target vessel divided by the CFR in a reference vessel ($CFR_{Target}/CFR_{Reference}$) was introduced. A normal value (>0.8) of rCFR excludes a physiologically significant epicardial stenosis |2,3|. Of course, in patients with triple-vessel disease no suitable reference vessel exists. Finally, the concept of rCFR assumes that microvascular disease, if present, is distributed homogenously throughout the myocardium; thus it cannot be used in patients with MI or other causes of regional microvascular dysfunction.

Pressure measurements

A physiologically significant stenosis also results in a decrease in distal pressure. There is thus a difference in pressure between the reference pressure in the aorta and the pressure distal to the epicardial lesion. By analogy with the arguments presented previously for flow, the pioneering work of Pijls *et al.* showed that the physiological significance of a stenosis was best demonstrated by the pressure gradient during hyperaemia |4–6|. This group introduced the concept of myocardial fractional flow reserve (FFR). This is the ratio of distal coronary pressure to aortic pressure during maximal hyperaemia and it has been shown to reflect myocardial perfusion (both antegrade and from collateral flow). In contrast to CFR, FFR is independent of haemodynamic conditions (blood pressure and heart rate) and relatively independent of the state of the microcirculation. A normal FFR is 1.0 and any decrease reflects the effect of epicardial obstruction. An FFR <0.75 has been shown to be a reliable indicator of an epicardial lesion that can cause myocardial ischaemia in patients with single-vessel disease and normal left ventricular function.

As for CFR, FFR may be difficult to interpret in some situations. The definition of FFR assumes that maximal dilation of the microcirculation has been obtained with the drug used. The use of different agents at different doses means that this may not always be the case. One of the papers discussed in this chapter addresses the effect of the dose and route of administration of commonly used drugs on measured FFR. In a vessel that was the site of a recent or remote MI, FFR may be difficult to interpret. If there is little viable myocardium in the area subtended by a stenosis, a lesion with an FFR <0.75 may still provide adequate perfusion at hyperaemia for the remaining viable myocardium. The role of FFR in patients with recent MI and in selected patients with unstable angina is also investigated by papers reviewed in this chapter. FFR measurements must, of course, be interpreted taking into account the clinical presentation. Episodic variations in vasomotor tone such as intermittent constriction of the epicardial vessels (variant angina) or of the epicardial vessels ± the microcirculation (effort angina with a variable threshold) may contribute to the pathophysiology of myocardial ischaemia. In such patients, FFR can assess the potential of the epicardial lesion to cause ischaemia after conventional hyperaemic stimuli but does not exclude that the lesion may be responsible for symptomatic myocardial ischaemia. Conceptually, the presence of an FFR >0.75 suggests that intervention at the epicardial lesion would not improve myocardial perfusion or prognosis. However, there is discordance in the results of FFR and CFR in some patients that might be overcome by using both FFR and CFR to assess the functional implications of a stenosis. Finally, an inherent limitation of FFR relates to the fact that prognosis both to the potential of an epicardial lesion to cause ischaemia and to its potential to cause ischaemic events such as sudden death, or acute MI. This cannot be predicted by FFR or by any other currently validated modality. This is particularly relevant in the context of lesion evaluation after acute MI or in patients with unstable angina.

Pressure and flow measurements at intermediate lesions in diverse clinical contexts

The first two papers reviewed concern the use of FFR at isolated moderate coronary lesions in stable patients or in patients with recent unstable angina/non-ST segment elevation MI. The third examines the validity of FFR in patients with prior acute ST-segment elevation MI, and the fourth looks at the use of CFR as a potential surrogate for non-invasive testing in patients with multivessel disease.

Fractional flow reserve to determine the appropriateness of angioplasty in moderate coronary stenosis. A randomized trial.

G J W Bech, B De Bruyne, N H J Pijls, *et al. Circulation* 2001; **103**: 2928–34.

BACKGROUND. Percutaneous intervention at a coronary stenosis without documented ischaemia at non-invasive stress testing is often performed, but its benefit is unproven. Coronary pressure-derived FFR is a reliable substitute for non-invasive stress testing with a value of <0.75 identifying haemodynamically significant stenoses. FFR was measured in 325 patients for whom percutaneous transluminal coronary angioplasty (PTCA) was planned and who did not have documented ischaemia. If FFR was >0.75, patients were randomly assigned to deferral (*n* = 91) or percutaneous coronary intervention (PCI, *n* = 90). If FFR was <0.75, PCI was performed as planned (reference group; *n* = 144). Clinical follow-up was obtained at 1, 3, 6, 12 and 24 months. Event-free survival was similar between the deferred and PCI groups (92 vs 89% at 12 months and 89 vs 83% at 24 months), but was significantly lower in the reference group (80% at 12 months and 78% at 24 months). In addition, the percentage of patients free from angina was similar between the deferral and performance groups

(49 vs 50% at 12 months and 70 vs 51% at 24 months), but was significantly higher in the reference group (67% at 12 months and 80% at 24 months).

INTERPRETATION. It is not uncommon that patients with coronary lesions, that have not been documented on non-invasive testing to be responsible for ischaemia, undergo PCI. This paper demonstrates that coronary pressure-derived FFR identifies those who will benefit from PCI.

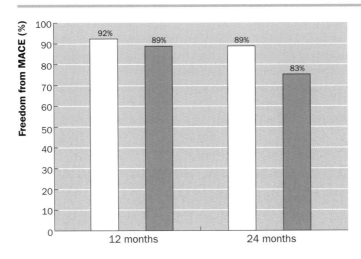

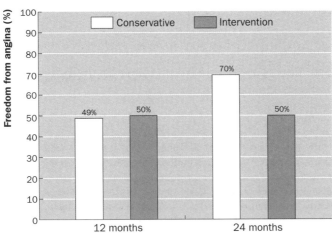

Fig. 6.1 Clinical outcome one and two years after randomization to percutaneous intervention or conservative therapy at lesions with a FFR >0.75. Percentages of patients who were free from MACE are shown in the top panel with the corresponding percentages of patients who were free from angina in the bottom panel. There were no significant differences between groups. Source: Bech *et al.* (2001).

Comment

For a variety of reasons, many patients undergo PCI at lesions that are judged angiographically significant but whose potential to cause ischaemia has not been shown objectively. This study found that half of the stenoses in these patients, who had predominantly single-vessel disease, were haemodynamically not significant. Situations that mimic this scenario in somewhat different clinical contexts are frequently encountered by interventional cardiologists. In patients presenting with stable angina who have multivessel disease, several lesions are dilated during the same procedure to achieve 'complete' revascularization. In some, but not all, cases this also reflects genuine doubt as to the true culprit lesion. Another common situation is the patient after an acute MI or with unstable angina in whom, after initial treatment of the 'culprit lesion' a staged procedure is planned to treat the remaining lesions that are judged to be significant on angiography. This study does not specifically address these situations. However, it was a landmark study as it provides convincing evidence that in patients in whom non-invasive testing was not performed or was inconclusive, deferral of intervention is justified if FFR measurements show that the lesion is haemodynamically not significant. The proportion of patients who were free from major adverse cardiac events did not differ significantly between the deferral and intervention groups up to two years. It is noteworthy, however, that the majority of these events were further revascularizations. In addition, the proportion of patients who were free from angina did not differ between groups (Fig. 6.1).

Use of fractional flow reserve versus stress perfusion scintigraphy after unstable angina. Effect on duration of hospitalization, cost, procedural characteristics, and clinical outcome.

M A Leesar, T Abdul-Baki, N I Akkus, *et al. J Am Coll Cardiol* 2003; **41**: 1115–21.

BACKGROUND. FFR, an invasive index of stenosis severity, is a reliable surrogate for stress perfusion scintigraphy (SPS) in patients with normal left ventricular function. An FFR ≥0.75 can distinguish patients after MI with a positive SPS from those with a negative SPS. However, the use of FFR has not been investigated after unstable angina/non-ST-segment elevation myocardial infarction (UA/NSTEMI). This study sought to determine the value of FFR compared with SPS in patients with recent UA/NSTEMI. Seventy such patients with an intermediate single-vessel stenosis were randomized to either SPS (*n* = 35) or FFR (*n* = 35). Patients in the SPS group were discharged if the SPS revealed no ischaemia, whereas those in the FFR group were discharged if the FFR was ≥0.75. Patients with a positive SPS and those with an FFR <0.75 underwent percutaneous angioplasty. The use of FFR markedly reduced the duration and cost of hospitalization compared with SPS (11 ± 2 h vs 49 ± 5 h [−77%], *P* <0.001; and US$1329 ± 44 vs 2113 ± 120, respectively, *P* <0.05). There were no significant differences in procedure time, radiation exposure time, or event rates during follow-up, including death, MI or revascularization.

Prognostic value of coronary blood flow velocity and myocardial perfusion in intermediate coronary narrowings and multivessel disease.

S A J Chamuleau, R A Tio, C C de Cock, *et al.*, on behalf of the Intermediate Lesions: Intracoronary Flow Assessment versus ^{99m}Tc-MIBI SPECT (ILIAS) Investigators. *J Am Coll Cardiol* 2002; **39**: 852–8.

B A C K G R O U N D . **This study aimed to investigate the roles of intracoronary derived coronary flow velocity reserve (CFVR) and myocardial perfusion scintigraphy (SPECT) for management of an intermediate lesion in patients with multivessel coronary artery disease. SPECT was performed in 191 patients with stable angina and multivessel disease and scheduled for angioplasty (PCI) of a severe coronary narrowing. CFVR was determined selectively distal to an intermediate lesion in another artery using a Doppler guidewire. PCI of the intermediate lesion was deferred when SPECT was negative or CFR ≥2.0. Patients were followed for 1 year to document major cardiac events (death, infarction, revascularization), related to the intermediate lesion. Reversible perfusion defects were documented in the area of the intermediate lesion in 30 (16%) patients; CFVR was positive in 46 (24%) patients. PCI of the intermediate lesion was deferred in 182 patients. During follow-up, 19 events occurred – 3 MI and 16 revascularizations. CFVR was a more accurate predictor of cardiac events than was SPECT; relative risk: CFVR 3.9 (1.7–9.1), P <0.05; SPECT 0.5 (0.1–3.2), P = ns. Multivariate analysis revealed CFR as the only significant predictor for cardiac events.**

I N T E R P R E T A T I O N . Deferral of PCI of intermediate lesions in multivessel disease, when CFVR ≥2.0 is associated with an event rate of 6% per year. The authors suggest that selective evaluation of coronary lesion severity with CFVR during cardiac catheterization allows a more accurate risk stratification than does SPECT in patients with multivessel disease (Fig. 6.2).

Comment

Although CFVR is a useful measure of the potential of individual stenoses to cause ischaemia, this does not imply that it can be used as a replacement for the currently accepted diagnostic approach in multivessel disease, as the authors suggest. Exercise testing and stress imaging with nuclear or echocardiographic techniques provide an assessment of the cumulative physiological impact of all significant and non-significant lesions and provide important prognostic information that is additional to that obtained by invasive evaluation. Furthermore, the majority of events in the trial were elective revascularizations |**8–10**|. The study was not powered to detect a significant difference in the more clinically relevant 'hard' end-points of death or MI. The only conclusion to be drawn from this study is that CFVR is a useful tool in the interventional laboratory. However, it was never intended to be used as an index of future cardiac risk and this study provides no evidence that would prompt a re-evaluation of current clinical and non-invasive attitudes to risk stratification in patients with multivessel disease |**11**|.

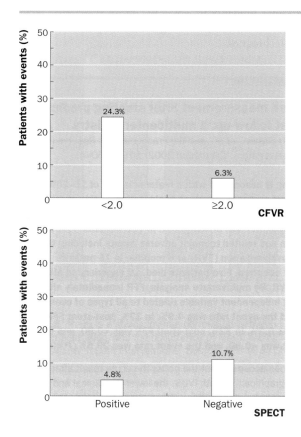

Fig. 6.2 MACE related to the intermediate lesion in patients in whom PCI was deferred as a function of the results of CFVR (top panel) and SPECT (bottom panel) at baseline. The cut-off value for CFVR was 2.0. A positive SPECT was defined as a reversible perfusion defect in the region of interest. The vast majority of MACE were elective repeat PCIs. The high rate of MACE in patients with a negative SPECT is unexpected and in conflict with the results of previous studies. Source: Chamuleau *et al.* (2002).

Pressure measurements and stent implantation

The following two papers concern the use of FFR in the context of coronary stent implantation. The first paper is a multicentre registry study on the potential role of FFR after angiographically satisfactory stent implantation as a predictor of adverse clinical events during the 6 months after the procedure. The second directly compares traditional intravenous ultrasound (IVUS) criteria with FFR after stent implantation. As discussed in the comments section, it is unfortunate that neither

higher doses (>30 μg) of intracoronary adenosine, suggesting that FFR might be overestimated in the other group.

INTERPRETATION. A fractional flow reserve <0.96 after stent deployment, predicts a suboptimal result based on validated IVUS criteria; however, an FFR ≥0.96 does not reliably predict an optimal stent result. Higher doses of intracoronary adenosine than previously used to measure FFR improve these results.

Comment

This study directly compared FFR after stent deployment with standard IVUS criteria for optimal stent deployment. Although an FFR <0.96 was predictive of a suboptimal result on IVUS, an FFR >0.96 did not reliably predict an optimal result as defined by IVUS. There were several potential reasons why FFR did not correlate better with IVUS criteria. First, the hyperaemic stimulus may have been insufficient in some patients. Intracoronary adenosine at doses of 15–20 μg was recommended and thus full hyperaemia may not always have been obtained for the FFR measurements. This hypothesis is supported by the fact that when higher doses (30–40 μg) were used the correlation with IVUS was significantly improved. Second, FFR is influenced by the presence of other evident or occult lesions in the treated vessel and systematic measurements just distal to the stent were not performed to identify this potential confounding factor. Third, FFR measures functional severity and thus may not be sensitive to subtle changes in stent expansion. The authors state that the practical clinical implications of the study are clear in that FFR provides a convenient method to identify most cases in which the stent is significantly under-expanded despite a reasonable angiographic appearance. However, as they acknowledge in the limitations of the study IVUS only provides anatomic information, whereas FFR provides a functional assessment. Of course both IVUS and FFR can provide additional information regarding the rest of the vessel that was not incorporated in this study. As for the previous article, these observations need to be reconsidered in the era of drug-eluting stents. It is possible that a physiologically guided approach, after FFR pullback of the entire vessel may be appropriate in patients with diffuse disease or multiple lesions. This could be used to stent the entire 'physiologically' relevant segment with a repeat pullback after stenting to identify a residual gradient within the stent. More focal lesions might be treated with angiographic guidance alone.

Pressure measurements and diffuse epicardial atherosclerosis

The following paper was designed to test a novel hypothesis. The authors postulated that in patients with diffuse epicardial atherosclerosis but without focal angiographic stenoses, myocardial ischaemia might result from a flow-limiting decrease in pressure along the epicardial vessels.

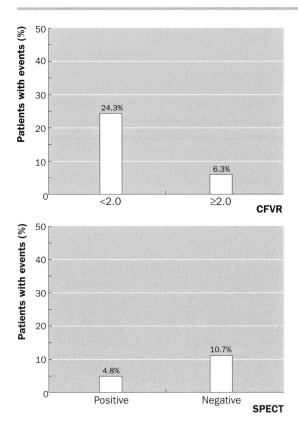

Fig. 6.2 MACE related to the intermediate lesion in patients in whom PCI was deferred as a function of the results of CFVR (top panel) and SPECT (bottom panel) at baseline. The cut-off value for CFVR was 2.0. A positive SPECT was defined as a reversible perfusion defect in the region of interest. The vast majority of MACE were elective repeat PCIs. The high rate of MACE in patients with a negative SPECT is unexpected and in conflict with the results of previous studies. Source: Chamuleau *et al.* (2002).

Pressure measurements and stent implantation

The following two papers concern the use of FFR in the context of coronary stent implantation. The first paper is a multicentre registry study on the potential role of FFR after angiographically satisfactory stent implantation as a predictor of adverse clinical events during the 6 months after the procedure. The second directly compares traditional intravenous ultrasound (IVUS) criteria with FFR after stent implantation. As discussed in the comments section, it is unfortunate that neither paper took full advantage of either modality to assess the entire vessel after stent implantation. This would have provided additional insights into the potential advantages and limitations of the two techniques.

Coronary pressure measurement after stenting predicts adverse events at follow-up: a multicenter registry.

N H J Pijls, V Klauss, U Siebert, *et al.*, and the Fractional Flow Reserve (FFR) Post-Stent Registry Investigators. *Circulation* 2002; **105**: 2950–4.

BACKGROUND. **Coronary stenting is associated with a restenosis rate of 15–20% at 6-month follow-up, despite optimum angiographic stent implantation. In this multicentre registry, the relation between optimum physiological stent implantation as assessed by post-stent FFR and outcome at 6 months was investigated. In 750 patients, FFR was measured after stent implantation and related to major adverse events including the need for repeat target vessel revascularization (TVR) at 6 months. In 76 patients (10.2%), at least 1 adverse event occurred. Five patients died, 19 experienced MI, and 52 underwent at least 1 repeat TVR. By multivariate analysis, FFR immediately after stenting was the most significant independent variable related to all types of events. In 36%, FFR normalized (>0.95), and the event rate was 4.9%. In 32%, post-stent FFR was 0.90–0.95, and the event rate was 6.2%. In 32%, post-stent FFR was <0.90, and the event rate was 20.3%. In 6%, FFR was <0.80, and the event rate was 29.5% (*P* <0.001).**

INTERPRETATION. It has long been accepted that the better the acute result after stenting, whether measured angiographically or with IVUS, the lower the clinical and angiographic restenosis rates. This study extends these observations to include the functional outcome, assessed by FFR after stenting, by demonstrating that the post-stent FFR is a strong independent predictor of clinical outcome at 6 months.

Comment

This study convincingly demonstrates that a normalized FFR after stenting is associated with a very low clinical event rate at 6 months; when a lower FFR was obtained, the FFR was inversely correlated with the rate of adverse events (Fig. 6.3). There are several potential explanations for a suboptimal FFR after stent implantation including: (1) inadequate stent deployment or edge dissection that may not be apparent on angiography, and (2) the presence of other lesions or of diffuse disease in the rest of the vessel. The optimal use of FFR in this situation would involve a pullback approach before stent implantation to identify the degree to which the target lesion contributes to the overall pressure gradient in the vessel. A repeat pullback after stent implantation would identify the source of a persistent gradient, where present, and when appropriate, optimization of stent deployment or treatment of additional lesions could be performed. With drug-eluting stents more liberal use of longer stents will be possible. The incremental value of IVUS compared with FFR in this new situation will need re-evaluation.

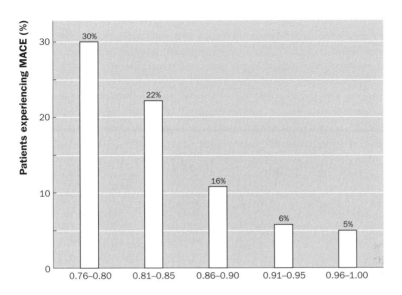

Fig. 6.3 There is a strong inverse correlation between FFR, measured immediately after stent implantation, and the occurrence of MACE during follow-up. The majority of MACE were elective repeat interventions. Source: Pijls *et al.* (2002).

Fractional flow reserve compared with intravascular ultrasound guidance for optimizing stent deployment.

W F Fearon, J Luna, H Samady, *et al. Circulation* 2001; **104**: 1917–22.

B A C K G R O U N D . Determination of FFR has been proposed as a means to assess stent deployment. In this prospective, multicentre trial, the use of FFR to optimize stenting was evaluated by comparing it with standard IVUS criteria. Stable patients ($n = 84$) with isolated coronary lesions underwent coronary stent deployment starting at 10 atm with incremental inflations (2 atm more) until FFR was ≥ 0.94 or 16 atm. IVUS was then performed. FFR was measured after intracoronary adenosine. The diagnostic characteristics of an FFR <0.94 to predict suboptimal stent expansion by IVUS, defined in both absolute and relative terms, were calculated. Over a range of IVUS criteria, the highest sensitivity, specificity and predictive accuracy of FFR were 80, 30 and 42%, respectively. ROC analysis defined an optimal FFR cut-off point at ≥ 0.96; at this threshold, the sensitivity, specificity and predictive accuracy of FFR were 75, 58 and 62%, respectively ($P = 0.03$ for comparison of predictive accuracy, $P = 0.01$ for concordance between FFR and IVUS). The negative predictive value was 88%. Significantly better diagnostic performance was achieved in a subgroup that received

higher doses (>30 μg) of intracoronary adenosine, suggesting that FFR might be overestimated in the other group.

INTERPRETATION. A fractional flow reserve <0.96 after stent deployment, predicts a suboptimal result based on validated IVUS criteria; however, an FFR ≥0.96 does not reliably predict an optimal stent result. Higher doses of intracoronary adenosine than previously used to measure FFR improve these results.

Comment

This study directly compared FFR after stent deployment with standard IVUS criteria for optimal stent deployment. Although an FFR <0.96 was predictive of a suboptimal result on IVUS, an FFR >0.96 did not reliably predict an optimal result as defined by IVUS. There were several potential reasons why FFR did not correlate better with IVUS criteria. First, the hyperaemic stimulus may have been insufficient in some patients. Intracoronary adenosine at doses of 15–20 μg was recommended and thus full hyperaemia may not always have been obtained for the FFR measurements. This hypothesis is supported by the fact that when higher doses (30–40 μg) were used the correlation with IVUS was significantly improved. Second, FFR is influenced by the presence of other evident or occult lesions in the treated vessel and systematic measurements just distal to the stent were not performed to identify this potential confounding factor. Third, FFR measures functional severity and thus may not be sensitive to subtle changes in stent expansion. The authors state that the practical clinical implications of the study are clear in that FFR provides a convenient method to identify most cases in which the stent is significantly under-expanded despite a reasonable angiographic appearance. However, as they acknowledge in the limitations of the study IVUS only provides anatomic information, whereas FFR provides a functional assessment. Of course both IVUS and FFR can provide additional information regarding the rest of the vessel that was not incorporated in this study. As for the previous article, these observations need to be reconsidered in the era of drug-eluting stents. It is possible that a physiologically guided approach, after FFR pullback of the entire vessel may be appropriate in patients with diffuse disease or multiple lesions. This could be used to stent the entire 'physiologically' relevant segment with a repeat pullback after stenting to identify a residual gradient within the stent. More focal lesions might be treated with angiographic guidance alone.

Pressure measurements and diffuse epicardial atherosclerosis

The following paper was designed to test a novel hypothesis. The authors postulated that in patients with diffuse epicardial atherosclerosis but without focal angiographic stenoses, myocardial ischaemia might result from a flow-limiting decrease in pressure along the epicardial vessels.

Abnormal epicardial coronary resistance in patients with diffuse atherosclerosis but 'normal' coronary angiography.

B De Bruyne, F Hersbach, N H J Pijls, *et al. Circulation* 2001; **104**: 2401–6.

BACKGROUND. Coronary arteries without focal stenosis at angiography are generally considered non-flow-limiting. However, atherosclerosis is a diffuse process that often remains invisible at angiography. This study tested the hypothesis that in patients with coronary artery disease, non-stenotic coronary arteries induce a decrease in pressure along their length due to diffuse coronary atherosclerosis. Coronary pressure and FFR, as indices of coronary conductance, were obtained from 37 arteries in 10 individuals without atherosclerosis (group I) and from 106 non-stenotic arteries in 62 patients with arteriographic stenoses in another coronary artery (group II). In group I, the pressure gradient between aorta and distal coronary artery was minimal at rest (1 ± 1 mmHg) and during maximal hyperaemia (3 ± 3 mmHg). Corresponding values were significantly larger in group II (5±4 mmHg and 10±8 mmHg, respectively; both P <0.001). The FFR was near unity (0.97 ± 0.02; range, 0.92–1) in group I, indicating no resistance to flow in truly normal coronary arteries, but it was significantly lower (0.89 ± 0.08; range, 0.69–1) in group II, indicating a higher resistance to flow. In 57% of arteries in group II, FFR was lower than the lowest value in group I. In 8% of arteries in group II, FFR was <0.75, the threshold for inducible ischaemia.

INTERPRETATION. Diffuse coronary atherosclerosis without focal stenosis at angiography causes a graded, continuous pressure fall along arterial length and this resistance to flow may contribute to myocardial ischaemia in such patients. The authors suggest that this observation has consequences for decision-making during PCI.

Comment

Chest pain in patients with angiographically normal coronary arteries is a vexing clinical problem. It may be related to myocardial ischaemia due to microvascular dysfunction, as can occur in patients with hypertension, to coronary artery spasm, to intermittent constriction of the microcirculation, or to other as yet non-elucidated mechanisms. Some patients may be exquisitely sensitive to very minimal degrees of ischaemia that are below the threshold of detection with current methods. Finally, many patients may have a non-cardiac explanation for their symptoms. Whatever the underlying cause, such patients often repeatedly seek medical attention and are difficult to manage. This article suggests a 'novel' mechanism for myocardial ischaemia: an increase in resistance to flow due to diffuse epicardial atherosclerosis. Although the concept is attractive, and the pressure tracings shown demonstrate a continuous pressure gradient from distal to proximal, the accompanying figure suggests that at least some of the patients did not have 'normal' coronary vessels. The angiograms suggest that some patients had multiple discrete lesions that were probably superimposed on diffuse atherosclerosis. In such a situation the contribution of each of these individual lesions to the overall drop in pressure may be difficult to determine as the authors have previously pointed out in patients with serial stenoses in the same vessel. In that situation, each lesion influences the haemodynamic effect of the others that may result in underestimation of the severity of each individual lesion |12|. As pointed out in a subsequent editorial comment, it would have been helpful to perform IVUS to assess the extent and severity of atherosclerosis |13|. However, this would not be without risk in such diffusely diseased vessels. Additional points to consider are also discussed in this editorial such as the fact that microvascular constriction or an inability of the microcirculation to dilate in response to adenosine could have influenced FFR measurements. At present, the concept, although attractive, needs further confirmation. Patients after cardiac transplantation are an obvious group in whom these observations could be further explored.

Achieving maximal vasodilatation. Which drugs and what doses?

There has been controversy regarding the most reliable agent (papaverine, adenosine, ATP), the appropriate doses, and, for adenosine and ADP, the most appropriate route of administration (intracoronary, arm vein or femoral vein). The following paper provides convincing answers to all these questions and the findings are of considerable practical importance.

Intracoronary and intravenous adenosine 5'-triphosphate, adenosine, papaverine, and contrast medium to assess fractional flow reserve in humans.

B De Bruyne, N H J Pijls, E Barbato, *et al. Circulation* 2003; **107**: 1877–83.

B A C K G R O U N D . Inducing both maximal and steady-state coronary hyperaemia is of clinical importance to take full advantage of fractional flow reserve measurements. This study compared different doses and routes of administration of adenosine 5'-triphosphate (ATP), adenosine, contrast medium and papaverine to assess their potential to achieve both maximal and steady-state hyperaemia. In patients with an isolated coronary stenosis ($n = 21$), coronary vasodilation was induced successively by papaverine (20 mg, intracoronary), adenosine (20 and 40 μg, intracoronary), ATP (20 and 40 μg, intracoronary), iohexol (6 ml, intracoronary), adenosine or ATP through an antecubital vein (140 and 180 μg/kg/min), or adenosine or ATP through a femoral vein (140 and 180 μg/kg/min). Because vessel dimensions did not change, the ratio of distal coronary (Pd) to aortic (Pa) pressure was used as an index of myocardial resistance (FFR). FFR was 0.77 ± 0.21 at rest and decreased to 0.61 ± 0.21 after papaverine. FFR decreased to a similar level with all other vasodilators, except with contrast medium (0.68 ± 0.21; $P < 0.01$ vs papaverine). Steady-state hyperaemia could only be obtained by intracoronary papaverine and by intravenous ATP or adenosine. In another 23 patients, an intravenous infusion of ATP was varied from 0 to

280 µg/kg/min. At doses >140 µg/kg/min, there was neither a further decrease in FFR nor a further increase in coronary flow velocities.

INTERPRETATION. Provided sufficient doses are used, ATP, adenosine and papaverine all induce maximal hyperaemia and can be used to assess FFR. However, when assessment of multiple stenoses in the same vessel is indicated, only intracoronary papaverine and intravenous ATP or adenosine induce steady-state hyperaemia that permits a pressure pullback manoeuvre.

Comment

The authors show that appropriate doses of ATP, adenosine and papaverine all induce maximal hyperaemia and can be used to assess FFR. For adenosine and ATP, intracoronary infusion and peripheral infusion were equally effective when FFR measurement was required to assess a discrete lesion (Table 6.1). Furthermore, peripheral infusion in an arm vein was as effective as infusion in the femoral vein. This is an important finding as femoral vein catheterization is a potential source of iatrogenic injury, especially in fully anticoagulated patients. However, when assessment of multiple stenoses in the same vessel is indicated, only intracoronary papaverine and intravenous ATP or adenosine induce steady-state hyperaemia that permits a pressure pullback manoeuvre. The authors suggest that femoral vein infusion may be preferable in patients with borderline FFRs as the response is less variable. The evidence for this assertion is not very convincing but this approach could certainly be adopted as a fallback strategy.

Table 6.1 Mean FFR, time to peak action, and duration of the plateau phase induced by different vasodilatory stimuli

	FFR	Peak action (seconds)	Plateau phase (seconds)
Bolus Intracoronary Injection			
Papaverine 20 mg	0.61 ± 0.20	23 ± 5	22 ± 7
Adenosine 20 µg	0.62 ± 0.20	15 ± 2	7 ± 3
Adenosine 40 µg	0.62 ± 0.19	15 ± 2	5 ± 1
ATP 20 µg	0.62 ± 0.20	14 ± 3	4 ± 1
ATP 40 µg	0.60 ± 0.19	14 ± 3	5 ± 1
Intravenous Infusion			
Adenosine 140 µg kg-1 min-1 (Femoral vein)	0.61 ± 0.19	80 ± 3	
ATP 140 µg kg-1 min-1 (Femoral vein)	0.61 ± 0.19	76 ± 28	
Adenosine 140 µg kg-1 min-1 (Peripheral vein)	0.61 ± 0.19	112 ± 48	
ATP 140 µg kg-1 min-1 (Peripheral vein)	0.61 ± 0.17	104 ± 36	

Values are mean ± SD. ATP = adenosine 5'-triphosphate.
Source: De Bruyne et al. (2003).

Novel approaches to flow and pressure measurements

Both FFR, measured with a PressureWire, and CFR, measured with a Flowire, provide information on coronary physiology and its alterations by diverse pathological conditions. However, FFR measures only the physiological significance of obstruction(s) in the epicardial circulation, whereas CFR assesses the combined effect of both epicardial and microvascular disease but cannot aid in discriminating between them. Although it would thus be useful to have both measurements available, until now, this has required the use of two different consoles and two different wires. The following four papers concern the potential assessment of both epicardial and microcirculatory resistance with the same wire.

Coronary thermodilution takes advantage of the fact that the PressureWire is very sensitive to changes in temperature. Modified software allows the pressure sensor of the wire to act as a distal thermistor, while the shaft of the wire serves as a proximal thermistor. The first two papers that were both co-authored by the groups from Aalst and Eindhoven describe the experimental and clinical validation of the measurement of CFR by thermodilution with the PressureWire. The Stanford group used the experimental validation of the thermodilution method to derive a novel index of microcirculatory resistance (IMR) that might allow an independent assessment of the function of the microcirculation. The third paper describes the experimental validation of this index. The fourth paper describes a novel index to assess the functional severity of a stenosis derived from Doppler flow and pressure measurements obtained sequentially with two different wires. The fifth paper describes a novel approach to CFR in which CFR measurements are derived from the pressures recorded proximal and distal to the stenosis. The final paper describes how the physiological significance of an epicardial lesion might be derived from analysis of the dicrotic notch segment of the arterial pressure waveform by spectral analysis of the high frequency components. The pulse transmission coefficient (PTC) approach has the advantage that it does not require a hyperaemic stimulus.

Coronary thermodilution to assess flow reserve: experimental validation.

B De Bruyne, N H J Pijls, L Smith *et al. Circulation.* 2001; **104**: 2003–6.

B A C K G R O U N D . FFR and CFR are indices of coronary stenosis severity that provide the clinician with complementary information on the contribution of epicardial arteries and the microcirculation to total resistance to myocardial blood flow. At present, FFR and CFR can only be obtained using two separate guidewires. This study tested the validity of the thermodilution principle in assessing CFR with one pressure–temperature sensor-tipped guidewire. In an *in vitro* model, absolute flow was compared with the inverse mean transit time ($1/T_{mn}$) of a thermodilution curve obtained after a bolus injection of 3 ml saline at room temperature. A very close correlation was found between absolute flow and $1/T_{mn}$ when the sensor was placed $\geq$6 cm from the injection site. In six chronically instrumented dogs (60 stenoses; FFR 0.19–0.98), a significant correlation was found between $CFR_{Doppler}$, which was calculated from the ratio of hyperaemic to resting flow velocities, and CFR_{Thermo}, which was calculated from the ratio of resting to hyperaemic T_{mn}.

INTERPRETATION. The results show that using either hand or ECG-triggered injection of 3 ml boluses of saline, the CFR calculated by thermodilution method is closely correlated with absolute coronary flow and coronary flow velocity.

Comment

Based on the indicator dilution theory, which is familiar to cardiologists as the principle used to measure cardiac output using dye dilution or thermodilution, the formula CFR = T_{mn} at rest/T_{mn} at hyperaemia, can be used to calculate CFR using a PressureWire with modified softwire and injections of small amounts of saline (at room temperature). The mathematical derivation of the formula is outlined in the paper. The formula assumes that:

1. The epicardial volume remains constant at rest and at hyperaemia.
2. The injection of saline does not influence coronary flow.
3. The indicator (saline) is adequately mixed with blood before arriving at the distal sensor.
4. The position of the distal sensor remains constant between measurements.

The first condition is satisfied if maximal epicardial dilatation is obtained with nitrates before CFR measurement to counteract the effects of flow-mediated epicardial dilatation. The validity of the other two assumptions is shown by the authors who demonstrate that the volume of saline used (3 ml) does not affect flow and provide evidence that adequate mixing is obtained if the distal sensor is $\geq$6 cm from the injection site.

An advantage of this approach is that it does not require knowledge of either the exact volume or temperature of the injected saline but only precise timing of the start of the injection and the measurement of changes over time in coronary blood temperature by the distal sensor.

The results show that using either hand or ECG-triggered injection of 3 ml boluses of saline, the CFR calculated by thermodilution method is closely correlated with either absolute flow (for the *in vitro* experiments) or with flow velocity (measured simultaneously with a Flowire) for the *in vivo* experiments. In order to reduce the potential for error (especially at low heart rates) the authors suggest that measurements should be performed in triplicate and averaged.

Coronary thermodilution to assess flow reserve: validation in humans.

N H J Pijls, B De Bruyne, L Smith, *et al. Circulation* 2002; **105**: 2482–6.

B A C K G R O U N D . The aim of this study was to investigate the feasibility of simultaneous measurement of FFR and CFR using one pressure–temperature sensor-tipped guide wire with the use of coronary thermodilution and to compare CFR by thermodilution (CFR_{Thermo}) with simultaneously measured Doppler CFR ($CFR_{Doppler}$). In 103 coronary arteries in 50 patients, a pressure–temperature sensor-tipped 0.014-inch floppy guide wire and a 0.014-inch Doppler guide wire were introduced. Both normal vessels and a wide range of stenotic vessels were included. With 3 ml of saline at room temperature used as an indicator, by hand-injection, thermodilution curves in the coronary artery were obtained in triplicate, both at baseline and at intravenous adenosine-induced maximum hyperaemia. After adequate curve-fitting, CFR_{Thermo} was calculated from the ratio of inverse mean transit times and compared with $CFR_{Doppler}$ calculated by velocities at hyperaemia and baseline. Adequate sets of thermodilution curves and corresponding CFR_{Thermo} could be obtained in 87% of the arteries versus 91% for Doppler CFR and 100% for FFR. CFR_{Thermo} correlated fairly well to $CFR_{Doppler}$ ($CFR_{Thermo} = 0.84\ CFR_{Doppler} + 0.17$; $r = 0.80$; $P < 0.001$), although individual differences of >20% between both indexes were seen in a quarter of all arteries.

I N T E R P R E T A T I O N . In conjunction with the experimental validation in the preceding paper, this study shows the feasibility of simultaneous measurement of FFR (by coronary pressure) and CFR (by coronary thermodilution) in humans by a single guide wire in a practical and straightforward way.

Comment

Thermodilution-derived CFR will facilitate the assessment of the relative contribution of epicardial lesions and microvascular resistance in patients. A major advantage of this method of 'simultaneous' assessment of FFR and CFR is that, despite the fact that the two measurements are obtained using a single wire, the measurements are 'independent'. This is not the case with alternative methods to derive CFR from pressure measurements described later in this section. Furthermore, CFR_{Thermo} can be measured in normal vessels and thus the relative CFR (CFR in the diseased vessel/ CFR in the reference normal vessel) can be calculated. This index, which is invaluable in patients with diffuse impairment of microvascular function (hypertension, left ventricular hypertrophy, etc.), cannot be derived from pressure measurements as there is no pressure gradient in a normal vessel.

Novel index for invasively assessing the coronary microcirculation.

W F Fearon, L B Balsam, O Farouque, *et al. Circulation* 2003; **107**: 3129–32.

BACKGROUND. A relatively simple, invasive method for quantitatively assessing the status of the coronary microcirculation independent of the epicardial artery is lacking. By using a coronary pressure guide wire and modified software, it is possible to calculate the mean transit time of room-temperature saline injected down a coronary artery. The inverse of the hyperaemic mean transit time has been shown to correlate with absolute flow. We hypothesize that distal coronary pressure divided by the inverse of the hyperaemic mean transit time provides an IMR that will correlate with true microcirculatory resistance (TMR) defined as the distal left anterior descending (LAD) pressure divided by hyperaemic flow, measured with an external ultrasonic flow probe. A total of 61 measurements were made in 9 Yorkshire swine at baseline and after disruption of the coronary microcirculation, both with and without an epicardial LAD stenosis. The mean IMR (16.9 ± 6.5 U to 25.9 ± 14.4 U, $P = 0.002$) and TMR (0.51 ± 0.14 to 0.79 ± 32 mmHg/ml/min, $P = 0.0001$), as well as the per cent change in IMR ($147 \pm 66\%$) and TMR ($159 \pm 105\%$, $P = $ NS vs IMR per cent change) increased significantly and to a similar degree after disruption of the microcirculation. These changes were independent of the status of the epicardial artery.

INTERPRETATION. There was a significant correlation between mean IMR and TMR values, as well as between the per cent change in IMR and per cent change in TMR.

Comment

The experimental validation of thermodilution showed that absolute coronary blood flow was highly correlated with the inverse of the mean transit time of a saline bolus in a coronary artery. The thermodilution method was then applied to measure CFR as described previously. CFR, by definition, reflects the flow status of both the epicardial vessel and the microcirculation and cannot therefore be used to describe the state of the microcirculation independently.

The distal coronary pressure divided by the absolute coronary flow provides a direct measure of microcirculatory function. The inverse of the hyperaemic mean transit time (measured by thermodilution) can be used as a surrogate for the absolute coronary flow. The authors thus propose a novel index of microcirculatory resistance (IMR) defined as the distal coronary pressure multiplied by the hyperaemic mean transit time that can be obtained using the pressure wire. Because both distal pressure and flow will fall in the presence of an epicardial lesion the IMR, in theory, should not change. At peak hyperaemia, it is assumed that the variability of resting vascular tone and haemodynamics will be eliminated and thus the IMR will reflect minimum microvascular resistance.

In this study, the validity of these assumptions was tested by comparing IMR with the true microvascular resistance (derived from absolute flow measured with an ultrasonic flow probe placed around the artery and distal pressure), in the presence or absence of epicardial stenosis (created with an external vascular occluder), before and after disruption of the microcirculation with embolized microspheres.

This index has the advantage that it can be easily derived in the catheterization laboratory. The method of validation which involved disruption of the microcirculation suggests that IMR may be useful in assessing the effect of interventions to prevent microembolization in situations in which this poses a clinical problem. Such scenarios include acute MI where IMR might be useful to assess the effects of pharmacological intervention or the use of distal protection devices to prevent or attenuate the functional consequences of microembolization. Its utility in microvascular dysfunction due to other factors is less certain. Finally, as the authors point out in the limitations section of the paper, the presence of a significant collateral circulation would likely result in measured IMR being substantially higher than the true microcirculatory resistance because the decrease in distal perfusion pressure, related to the epicardial stenosis, would be attenuated. The effects of collaterals and the validity of IMR in patients microvascular dysfunction of varying aetiologies will need to be further explored before IMR can be adopted in clinical practice.

Both FFR and CFR have limitations in the assessment of the functional severity of an epicardial lesion. This group has previously shown that there was discordance, based on their respective cut-off values, between the results of the techniques in 27% of patients |15|. The next paper further explores this issue using a new index that combines information from flow and pressure measurements obtained sequentially.

Hyperaemic stenosis resistance index for evaluation of functional coronary lesion severity.

M Meuwissen, M Siebes, S A J Chamuleau, *et al. Circulation* 2002; **106**: 441–6.

B A C K G R O U N D . Both CFVR and myocardial FFR are used to evaluate the haemodynamic severity of coronary lesions. However, discordant results of CFVR and FFR have been observed in 25–30% of coronary lesions. An index of stenosis resistance based on intracoronary pressure and flow velocity may improve the assessment of functional coronary lesion severity. SPECT was performed in 151 patients with angina to determine reversible perfusion defects within 1 week before cardiac catheterization. Coronary pressure and flow velocity were measured distal to 181 single coronary lesions with a mean diameter stenosis of 56% (range: 32–85%). Maximum hyperaemia was induced by 15–20 µg IC adenosine to determine CFVR, FFR and the hyperaemic stenosis resistance indexes (h-SRv), defined as the ratio of hyperaemic stenosis pressure gradient (mean aorta pressure – mean distal pressure) and hyperaemic average peak-flow velocity. Receiver operating characteristic curves of CFVR, FFR and h-SRv were calculated to evaluate the predictive value for presence of reversible perfusion defects on SPECT with the use of the area under curve (AUC). The AUC was significantly higher for h-SRv (0.90 ± 0.03) than for CFVR (0.80 ± 0.04; *P* = 0.024) and FFR (0.82 ± 0.03; *P* = 0.018) respectively. Agreement with SPECT was particularly higher

than for CFVR (49%, *P* = 0.022) or FFR (51%, *P* = 0.037) in the group of lesions showing discordant results between CFVR and FFR.

INTERPRETATION. This study used reversibility of SPECT perfusion defects as the gold standard to determine the predictive value of FFR, CFVR and the h-SRv a novel parameter derived from simultaneous measurement of pressure and flow, for the presence of a functionally significant epicardial lesion. The highest predictive value was found for h-SRv and the index proved to be particularly useful for lesions with discordant results on FFR and CFVR.

Comment

Both FFR and CFVR have limitations in the assessment of the functional severity of an epicardial lesion. Ideally, flow and pressure should be measured simultaneously permitting calculation of either the coronary stenosis resistance or the instantaneous hyperaemic diastolic flow velocity–pressure relation |**16,17**|. The former measurement has not been applied in humans due to technical limitations, whereas the latter is cumbersome, requiring simultaneous placement of two wires, and the analysis is complicated. The purpose of this study was to test an index the h-SRv, which incorporates information derived from both pressure and flow, using SPECT as a reference. The index proved particularly useful for lesions where there was discordance between CFVR and FFR (Fig. 6.4). With the advent of a new wire allowing simultaneous measurement of flow and pressure, this index may aid clinical decision-making. However, additional prospective studies will be needed to validate the cut-off

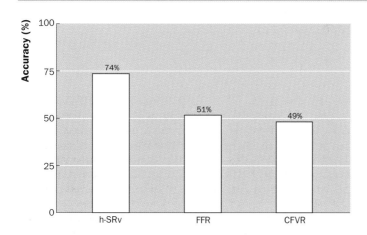

Fig. 6.4 Differences in the predictive accuracy of h-SRv, FFR, and CFVR compared with SPECT outcomes in patients with discordant FFR and CFVR results: either FFR <0.75 with CFVR ≥2.0 or FFR ≥0.75 with CFVR <2.0. h-SRv was significantly better than either FFR (*P* = 0.037) or CFVR (*P* = 0.022). Source: Meuwissen *et al.* (2002).

value for h-SRv and to determine reproducibility and potential haemodynamic dependence of the index.

Assessment of coronary flow reserve by coronary pressure measurement: comparison with flow- or velocity-derived coronary flow reserve.

T Akasaka, A Yamamuro, N Kamiyama, *et al. J Am Coll Cardiol* 2003; **41**: 1554–60.

BACKGROUND. This study sought to assess the reliability of pressure-derived CFR compared with flow- or velocity-derived CFR. Using a pressure guide wire, coronary pressure distal to a stenosis was measured at rest and during hyperaemia in 7 dogs (29 stenoses) with various degrees of stenosis and in 30 patients with angina (34 stenoses). Pressure-derived CFR was calculated by the square root of the pressure gradient across the stenosis (ΔP) during hyperaemia divided by ΔP at rest, using a proprietary software system. At the same time, coronary flow was monitored proximal to the stenosis with a flow meter in the experimental dogs, and coronary flow velocity distal to the stenosis was assessed using a Doppler guide wire in patients with angina. Flow-derived CFR was compared with pressure-derived CFR. Except for one stenosis that had no pressure gradient at rest, a significant correlation was obtained between pressure- and flow-derived CFR in the animal study ($y = 1.05x - 0.03$, $r = 0.92$, $P = 0.0001$). A significant correlation was also seen between pressure- and velocity-derived CFR in the human study, except in three stenoses with no resting pressure gradient ($y = 0.70x + 0.37$, $r = 0.85$, $P = 0.0001$).

INTERPRETATION. Similar to flow (or velocity) measurement, CFR can be assessed by pressure measurement, except in stenoses with minor resting ΔP.

Comment

This paper describes an alternative approach to measure CFR from pressure measurements alone. The mathematical basis for this approach was described in a previous paper |**14**|. Briefly, two fluid dynamic mechanisms (Poiseuille's and Bernouille's laws) can be used to characterize the pressure drop across a stenosis. In most situations, the ratio $\sqrt{P}$ during hyperaemia to $\sqrt{P}$ at rest can be used to derive the CFR. There are several limitations of the algorithm. First, being based on pressure gradient measurements, it is critically dependent on the accuracy of the measurements. An error of 0.5 mmHg in baseline pressure gradient leads to an error of 10 and 20% in CFR for a pressure gradient at rest of 3 and 1.5 mmHg respectively. Second, being based on pressure gradient measurements, it cannot be used to calculate CFR in a normal reference vessel. Third, if the lesion is >25mmHg long and has a tubular configuration, the algorithm is not valid. This suggests that assessment of long lesions or of diffusely diseased vessels is not possible. In this study, there was a good correlation between pressure-derived CFR and Doppler-derived CFR in lesions that were moderate or severe. However, there was a mean 20% difference between the measurements with higher values for Doppler-derived CFR. For lesions with low basal pressure gradients pressure-derived CFR was not feasible and while the authors suggest that this is not a problem in clinical situations as lesions <50% are not candidates for intervention, this is untrue. The potential value of concomitant FFR and CRF is, in fact, greatest in patients with less severe lesions but co-existing microvascular disease. The potential of this method is intrinsically limited by its inability to measure CFR in a normal vessel, by the potential confounding effects of diffuse disease, and by its exquisite dependence on the accuracy of the pressure measurements.

Pulse transmission coefficient: a novel non-hyperemic parameter for assessing the physiological significance of coronary artery stenoses.

D Brosh, S T Higano, M J Slepian, *et al. J Am Coll Cardiol* 2002; **39**: 1012–19.

BACKGROUND. Coronary lesions may impair the transmission of pressure waves across a stenosis, potentially acting as a low-pass filter. The PTC is a novel non-hyperaemic parameter that calculates the transmission of high-frequency components of the pressure signal through a stenosis. Thus, it may reflect the severity of the coronary artery stenosis. This study tested the hypothesis that PTC can serve as a non-hyperaemic physiologic marker for the severity of coronary artery stenosis in humans by examining the correlation between PTC and FFR in patients with coronary artery disease. Pressure signals were obtained with a pressure wire in 56 lesions (49 patients) in the non-hyperaemic state and were analysed using a new algorithm that identifies the high-frequency components in the pressure signal. The PTC was calculated as the ratio between the distal and proximal high-frequency components of the pressure waveform across the lesion. The FFR measurements were assessed with intracoronary adenosine. There was a significant correlation between PTC and FFR ($r = 0.81$, $P <0.001$). By using a receiver operating characteristic analysis, we identified a PTC <0.60 (sensitivity 100%, specificity 98%) to be the optimal cut-off value for predicting an FFR <0.75.

INTERPRETATION. PTC is a novel non-hyperaemic parameter for the physiological assessment of coronary artery stenoses. It correlates significantly with FFR and may predict an FFR <0.75 with high accuracy. PTC may be useful as an adjunct measurement to FFR, especially in patients with microcirculatory disease and impaired maximal hyperaemia.

Comment

This is a fascinating study that applies a concept developed in the peripheral vasculature to the analysis of stenosis severity in the coronary circulation. Previous studies suggested that analysis of the pressure waveform might be used to evaluate the severity of atherosclerosis. The dicrotic notch is a transient upstroke in the pressure waveform reflecting the deceleration in arterial pressure after closure of the aortic valve. Based on the appearance of the dicrotic notch, it was shown that an abnormal pressure waveform with the absence of a discrete dicrotic notch was associated with significant atherosclerotic vascular disease |**18,19**|. More recently, the alteration or disappearance of the dicrotic notch on the carotid pressure waveform was highly correlated with the presence of isolated aortic stenosis |**20,21**|. Similar results were reported in the iliac artery where the disappearance of the dicrotic notch on a pressure waveform recorded distal to a stenosis was highly predictive of a significant iliac artery stenosis, whereas a normal wave form was correlated with normal haemodynamics |**22**|. Spectral analysis of the dicrotic notch segment shows that there are numerous high-frequency components representing reflections from the peripheral circulation. A stenosis acts as a filter limiting transmission of these high-frequency components across the stenosis and the severity of the stenosis can be calculated by determining the degree of attenuation of these high-frequency components. The results show that a PTC <0.60 predicts an FFR <0.75 with a sensitivity of 100% and a specificity of 98%. One advantage of this technique is that it is not dependent on hyperaemia. A disadvantage is that lesions seem to act as a filter with an all-or-none response. For a physiologically significant lesion, there is sharp attenuation, whereas for less severe lesions there is no attenuation. Thus, there is poor correlation with FFR for lesions with a measured FFR >0.75. This obviously limits the use of PTC in the assessment of the results of intervention.

Conclusion

Coronary pressure and flow measurements are now an established and extremely useful tool to aid the interventional cardiologist in decision-making in the catheterization laboratory. Some of the articles reviewed in this chapter have further clarified the relative contribution of both approaches in the setting of intervention. However, a note of caution is warranted regarding the application of these measurements in settings where their use is inappropriate.

It is important to remember that both types of measurement are intended to assess the functional significance of lesions and thus their potential to cause inducible ischaemia. Their ideal field of application is thus in stable patients with single-vessel or multivessel disease in whom the potential physiological significance of one or more lesions is unclear. In other settings such as unstable angina or recent MI, the potential of a lesion to cause inducible ischaemia is an important, but not the only, consideration. The potential of such lesions to cause MACE such as death or MI is the most pressing clinical concern.

Until now, there are no validated methods to determine which of these lesions still have the potential to cause recurrent acute coronary syndromes in patients who are asymptomatic at the time of catheterization. However, the event rate in patients with unstable angina, even with modern therapy, remains at 5–10% in the subsequent year and in asymptomatic patients after thrombolytic therapy for acute MI, up to

30% of lesions reocclude within three months, an event that is generally associated with recurrent infarction.

Deferral of intervention at such lesions, based on pressure measurements has been justified by the fact that it is not associated with an increased clinical event rate. However, the vast majority of events, if intervention is performed, are elective reinterventions for restenosis. With the advent of drug-eluting stents, the need for reintervention has been dramatically reduced. Thus, the role of physiological assessment in the setting of acute coronary syndromes will need to be reassessed.

Finally, the use of drug-eluting stents may also modify the approach to lesions with borderline results on either FFR or CFR measurement or where there is conflict between the two methods. Since the introduction of FFR to aid decision-making, we have seen an increasing number of symptomatic patients, with an FFR that was abnormal but not below the accepted threshold for intervention, referred back for reassessment. FFR is not infallible as some patients may not have achieved maximum vasodilatation. Furthermore, the epicardial and microcirculation are not independent and it cannot be excluded that restoring full epicardial patency may also ameliorate microcirculatory function in some of these patients by improving flow-mediated vasodilator responses. A randomized trial of intervention with drug-eluting stents compared with medical therapy in this group of patients, with assessment of pressure and flow responses before and after intervention, and at follow-up should be performed in such patients, who represent a small but problematic proportion of referrals.

References

1. Kern MJ, Bach RG, Mechem C, *et al.* Variations in normal coronary vasodilator reserve stratified by artery, gender, heart transplantation, and coronary artery disease. *J Am Coll Cardiol* 1996; **28**: 1154–60.

2. Wolford TL, Donohue TL, Bach RG, *et al.* Heterogeneity of coronary flow reserve in the examination of multiple individual allograft coronary arteries. *Circulation* 1999; **99**: 626–32.

3. Wieneke H, Haude M, Ge J, *et al.* Corrected coronary flow reserve: a new concept of assessing coronary perfusion. *J Am Coll Cardiol* 2000; **35**: 1713–20.

4. McGinn AL, White CW, Wilson RF. Interstudy variability of coronary flow reserve: influence of heart rate, arterial pressure, and ventricular preload. *Circulation* 1990; **81**: 1319–30.

5. Marcus ML, Mueller ML, Gascho JA, Kerber RE. Effects of cardiac hypertrophy secondary to hypertension on the coronary circulation. *Am J Cardiol* 1979; **44**: 1023–31.

6. Chauhan A, Millins PA, Petch MC, Schonfield PM. Is coronary flow velocity response really normal in syndrome X? *Circulation* 1994; **89**: 1998–2004.

7. Pijls NHJ. Is it time to measure fractional flow reserve in all patients? *J Am Coll Cardiol* 2003; **41**: 1122–4.

8. Heller GV, Herman SD, Travin MI, *et al*. Independent prognostic value of intravenous dipyridamole with technitium-99m sestamibi tomographic imaging in predicting cardiac events and cardiac-related hospital admissions. *J Am Coll Cardiol* 1995; **26**: 1202–8.

9. Schaler BD, Kegzl JG, Heo J, *et al*. Prognostic implications of normal exercise SPECT thallium images in patients with strongly positive electrocardiograms. *Am J Cardiol* 1993; **72**: 1201–3.

10. Fattah AA, Kamal AM, Pancholy S, *et al*. Prognostic implications of normal exercise tomographic thallium images in patients with angiographic evidence of significant coronary disease. *Am J Cardiol* 1994; **74**: 769–71.

11. Miller DD. Coronary flow studies for risk stratification in multivessel disease; a physiological bridge too far? *J Am Coll Cardiol* 2002; **39**: 859–63.

12. Pijls NHJ, de Bruyne B, Bech GJW, *et al*. Coronary pressure measurement to assess the hemodynamic significance of serial stenoses within one coronary artery. *Circulation* 2000; **102**: 2371–7.

13. Kaski JC. 'Normal' coronary arteriograms, 'abnormal' haemodynamics. *Lancet* 2002; **359**: 1631–2.

14. Shalman E, Barak C, Dgany E, *et al*. Pressure-based simultaneous CRF and FFR measurements: understanding the physiology of a stenosed vessel. *Comp Biol Med* 2001; **31**: 353–63.

15. Meuwissen M, Chamuleau SAJ, Siebes M, *et al*. Role of variability in microvascular resistance on fractional flow reserve and coronary blood flow velocity reserve in intermediate coronary lesions. *Circulation* 2001; **103**: 184–7.

16. Gould KL, Lipscomb K, Calvert C. Compensatory changes of the distal coronary vascular bed during progressive coronary constriction. *Circulation* 1975; **51**: 1085–94.

17. Di Mario C, Krams R, Gil R, *et al*. Slope of the instantaneous hyperaemic diastolic coronary flow-velocity pressure relation. A new index for assessment of the physiologic significance of coronary stenosis in humans. *Circulation* 1994; **90**: 1215–24.

18. Dawber TR, Thomas HE, McNamara PM. Characteristics of the dicrotic notch of the arterial pulse wave in coronary heart disease. *Angiology* 1973; **24**: 244–55.

19. Freis ED, Kyle MC. Computer analysis of carotid and brachial pulse waves. Effects of age in normal subjects. *Am J Cardiol* 1968; **22**: 691–5.

20. O'Boyle MK, Vibhakar NI, Chung J, *et al*. Duplex sonography of the carotid arteries in patients with isolated aortic stenosis: imaging findings and relation to severity of stenosis. *Am J Roentgenol* 1996; **166**: 197–202.

21. Cousins AL, Eddleman EE, Reeves TJ. Prediction of aortic valvular area and gradient by non-invasive techniques. *Am Heart J* 1978; **95**: 308–15.

22. Barringer M, Poole GV, Shircliffe AC, *et al*. The diagnosis of aortoiliac disease: a non-invasive femoral cuff technique. *Ann Surg* 1983; **197**: 204–9.

7

Stent design

Introduction

The utilization of stents during percutaneous coronary intervention (PCI) has dramatically increased in the last 10 years with stenting becoming applicable in a wide variety of lesion morphologies and clinical settings. They provide a scaffold that supports the arterial wall, thereby sealing dissections and eliminating elastic recoil, which, together with enhanced antiplatelet therapy, reduces the rate of abrupt vessel closure compared with balloon angioplasty alone. Stents provide angiographically, a very pleasing result in the short-term; however in the long-term, success is hindered by the development of restenosis that has proven to be extremely difficult to treat effectively.

A lot of research has been undertaken to better understand the pathophysiology behind the formation of neointima. Balloon inflation alone causes relatively uncontrolled stretching and fracturing of the vessel wall, whereas the struts of an expanding stent cause focal deep vascular trauma. The severity of arterial injury has been shown to correlate directly with inflammation and late neointimal growth [1], and stent oversizing relative to the arterial wall is associated with an increase in neointima [2]. The adventitia appears to play a crucial role in the formation of neointima with migration of adventitial myofibroblasts documented in animal models of overstretched vessels [3,4]. The evolution of stent technology has, therefore, been aimed at trying to control and minimize this damage.

In parallel with the increased use of stents and knowledge regarding neointimal formation, has been the evolution of stent technology and design with improved flexibility and deliverability. Worldwide, there are now more than 40 stent designs available for use, with more currently under investigation. Ideal stent characteristics include being thrombo-resistant, being highly trackable with a low unconstrained profile, and providing a scaffold whilst still maintaining side branch access and conforming to the vessel contour. The majority of stents are composed of 316 L stainless steel that is an alloy of predominantly iron (60–65%) with chromium (17–18%) to protect against corrosion, and nickel (12–14%). Other designs have also incorporated nitinol, gold, tantalum and other metals. Whatever the metal used, it must be biocompatible and resistant to corrosion by the (salty) blood, elastic and yet provide high radial strength; radiopacity provides improved visibility during fluoroscopy.

Not all stents are metal; some composed purely of polymer have been found to be strong enough to maintain radial force and withstand the stress imposed by cardiac contractions. They confer the potential advantage of being biodegradable and have the possibility of transporting anti-proliferative drugs to act locally at the site of implantation. However, many of the polymers that have been studied to date have had only limited success as they have been found to invoke a marked inflammatory reaction.

Relation of stent design and stent surface material to subsequent in-stent intimal hyperplasia in coronary arteries determined by intravascular ultrasound.

R Hoffmann, G Mintz, P Haager, *et al. Am J Cardiol* 2002; **89**: 1360–4.

BACKGROUND. This study sought to determine the impact of stent design and gold coating of stents on the subsequent development of neointimal hyperplasia (NIH) in human atherosclerotic coronary arteries. Angiographic and intravascular ultrasound (IVUS) studies were performed at 6-month follow-up, on 311 native coronary lesions of 311 patients treated with 99 Multi-Link stents, 74 InFlow steel stents, 73 InFlow gold-coated stents, 41 Palmaz-Schatz stents, 12 NIR steel stents and 12 gold-coated NIR Royal stents. Lumen and stent cross-sectional area (CSA) were measured at 1-mm axial increments. The mean NIH CSA (stent CSA – lumen CSA) and mean NIH thickness were calculated and averaged over the total stent length. Mean NIH thickness was different for the six stents and ranged from 0.20 ± 0.13 mm for Multi-Link stents to 0.43 ± 0.14 mm for InFlow gold-coated stents (P <0.001). Multivariate analysis proved non-Multi-Link stent design (odds ratio [OR] 3.45, 95% confidence intervals [CI] 1.13–11.11, P <0.034) and gold coating (OR 3.78, 95% CI 1.88–7.54, P <0.001) to be the only independent predictors of NIH thickness >0.3 mm.

INTERPRETATION. Both stent design and surface material make an important contribution to the long-term outcome following PCI by impacting on the risk of developing NIH.

Comment

This study used 6-month angiographic and IVUS examination to assess a variety of stent designs. Although not a randomized study, in accordance with previous evaluations, it confirmed the apparent deleterious effect of a gold coating on restenosis rates. Moreover, despite relatively small numbers of patients (total $n = 311$) a statistically significant difference in the thickness of NIH development was detectable. Characteristics of the stents used (in alphabetical order) are as follows:

InFlow: slotted tube design, strut thickness 80 μm;

InFlow gold: as above but with a 5 μm coating of gold;

Multi-Link: a 56 μm stainless steel wire with a corrugated-ring design;

NIR: continuous multicellular design, strut-thickness 75 μm;

NIR-Royale: as above, with a gold coating;

Palmaz-Schatz: slotted tube design, strut thickness 70 μm.

Intimal hyperplasia thickness was lowest with the Multi-Link stent that, notably, has a different design to the others, and the smallest sized struts. Results of all the stents are presented in Fig. 7.1.

This study follows on from two reports assessing the influence of stent design on restenosis. The first was a randomized study assessing five stainless steel stents (Inflow, Multi-Link, NIR, Palmaz-Schatz and PURA-A) |5|. Although the 30-day outcome was not different, both the 6-month angiographic and 1-year clinical results were dependent of the stent type implanted. Even after adjusting for baseline character-istics that differed between the groups, the stent type remained an independent pre-dictor of event-free survival ($P = 0.013$). The results remained anonymous as to which stent was best, but did confirm the importance of stent design.

A further study from the same author, although not randomized, comprised a very large cohort of consecutive patients (>4500) with a follow-up angiography rate of 80% |6|. The stents assessed were the InFlow, InFlow gold, Jostent, Multi-Link, Palmaz-Schatz and PURA-A. There was a clear difference in the 6-month restenosis rates between the stent types ranging from 20.0 to 50.3%. Once again, the best results were with the Multi-Link stent, and the worst with the gold-coated InFlow stent.

In summary, therefore, it appears that stent design plays an important role in determining the long-term outcome. In the above studies, all stents were stainless steel and based on a slotted-tube design except for the Multi-Link stent, which, notably, had the best results. Its design, which uses wire just 56 μm in diameter (compared with the thicker struts of the other stents), may induce less trauma to the vascular wall and thereby minimize the degree of inflammation and subsequent restenosis relating to the development of NIH. One important conclusion, therefore, is that when evaluating trials in interventional cardiology, the results of a study that uses one particular type of stent cannot necessarily be extrapolated to the perform-ance of other stents in the same situation.

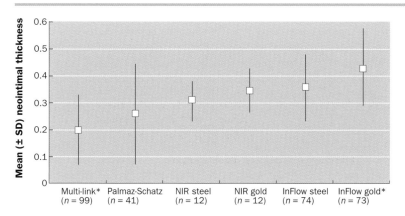

Fig. 7.1 Mean ($\pm$ SD) neointimal thickness for the different stent types. *Multi-Link stent versus InFlow gold stent, $P <$0.001. Source: Hoffman *et al.* (2002).

Effects of gold coating of coronary stents on neointimal proliferation following stent implantation.

J vom Dahl, P Haager, E Grube, *et al. Am J Cardiol* 2002; **89**: 801–5.

BACKGROUND. Experimental studies suggest a reduction in neointimal tissue proliferation when vascular stainless steel stents are coated with gold. This prospective multicentre trial evaluated the impact of gold coating on neointimal tissue proliferation in patients undergoing elective stent implantation. The primary end-point was in-stent tissue proliferation measured by IVUS at 6 months comparing stents of identical design with or without gold coating (InFlow). Two hundred and four patients were randomized to receive uncoated (group A, $n = 101$) or coated (group B, $n = 103$) stents. Baseline parameters did not differ between the groups. Stent length and balloon size were comparable, whereas inflation pressure was slightly higher in group A (14 ± 3 atm vs 13 ± 3 atm, $P = 0.013$). Procedural success was similar (A, 97%; B, 96%). The acute angiographic result was better for group B (remaining stenosis $4 \pm 12\%$ vs $10 \pm 11\%$, $P = 0.002$). Six-month ultrasound examination revealed more neointimal proliferation in group B, the neointimal volume within the stent was 47 ± 25 mm^3 versus 41 ± 23 mm^3 ($P = 0.04$), with a ratio of neointimal volume-to-stent volume of 0.45 ± 0.12 versus 0.40 ± 0.12 ($P = 0.003$). The angiographic minimal luminal diameter was smaller in group B (1.47 ± 0.57 mm vs 1.69 ± 0.70 mm, $P = 0.04$), with a higher late luminal loss of 1.17 ± 0.51 mm versus 0.82 ± 0.56 mm ($P = 0.001$).

INTERPRETATION. The results of experimental studies suggest that a gold-coated coronary stent induces less inflammation and thereby restenosis due to neointima formation. However, contrary to this, results in clinical practice are significantly worse than with an identical non-coated stainless steel stent.

Comment

Gold is used to manufacture many types of implants commonly used in medical practice such as dental prostheses; and gold-coated stainless steel prostatic stents and endovascular stents have shown good results with a reduction in associated inflammation. In the animal model, gold-plated stents deployed in the aorta have been shown to induce minimal reaction within the wall compared with identical stents plated with silver or copper, or coated with silicone or Teflon |7|. Moreover, gold has been shown *in vitro* to reduce thrombus formation and platelet aggregation compared with stainless steel |8|. It is highly visible on fluoroscopy thus aiding accurate stent placement and the hypothesis of the current study, therefore, was that a gold coating would confer significant advantages in the reduction of adverse cardiac events. Both stents used were an identical slotted-tube stainless steel design, with patients randomized prior to the procedure as to whether or not they received one with a 5-μm thick gold coating. All those included had stable angina symptoms, with a coronary lesion >50% stenosis which could be covered by a single stent ≤15 mm long. All lesions were pre-dilated. The results are interesting in that they are contrary to what was predicted at the start of the study in that the gold-coated stent group fared worse, with significantly more NIH and a higher angiographic diameter stenosis at follow-up.

In addition to these results, Kastrati *et al.* have previously published similar adverse data regarding gold-coated stents |9|. They randomized more than 700 patients treated irrespective of clinical presentation or lesion morphology to either a stainless steel stent or an identical gold-coated one. A significantly lower event-free survival was evident in the gold-coated stent group, and was apparent from 4 months after the procedure – long before the scheduled date for follow-up angiography at 6 months. Indeed, the study reported one of the highest ever restenosis rates.

The explanation as to why, in the setting of coronary intervention, coating a stainless steel stent with gold does not convey an advantage (indeed, is disadvantageous) is unclear. Theoretically, it could relate to a problem with the galvanizing process or an inability of the coating to stand up to the pressure used during stent deployment and subsequent mechanical strain. This may then lead to surface defects and inhomogeneity of the coating, and induction of an inflammatory reaction. Whatever the reason, the evidence teaches us that the presence of good theoretical advantages together with encouraging pre-clinical work do not necessarily always translate into superior outcomes in clinical practice.

Stent design-related coronary artery remodelling and patterns of neointima formation following self-expanding and balloon-expandable stent implantation.

A Konig, T Schiele, J Rieber, *et al. Cathet Cardiovasc Intervent* 2002; **56**: 478–86.

B A C K G R O U N D . The self-expanding Wallstent and balloon-expandable Palmaz-Schatz stents display different mechanical and dynamical stent properties. This study analysed the impact of these stent designs on coronary wall geometry using quantitative coronary angiography (QCA) and IVUS measurements in 50 patients (25 Wallstent, 25 Palmaz-Schatz). Relative changes for each parameter in both stent designs were calculated (Mann–Whitney U-test; 95% CI). The luminal net gain in Wallstent was not significantly higher than in Palmaz-Schatz (1.63 ± 1.11 mm vs 1.44 ± 0.63 mm; $P = 0.2554$). The respective loss indexes were also similar (0.38 ± 0.42 vs 0.36 ± 0.23; $P = 0.8578$). The Wallstent segments showed significant post-interventional stent expansion with positive vessel remodelling. The neointima formation at 6.5 ± 1.2 months was significantly higher in Wallstent segments (4.23 ± 2.07 mm^2 vs 2.22 ± 2.22 mm^2, $P < 0.0001$).

I N T E R P R E T A T I O N . The coronary wall morphology and stent geometry at follow-up were related to the stent design. In Wallstent segments, the increased neointima formation was balanced by post-interventional stent expansion, resulting in a comparable relative lumen loss in both stent types.

Comment

The degree of vascular injury during stent implantation is directly related to the subsequent development of NIH. The self-expanding Wallstent exerts a chronic radial force on the vessel wall, whereas the Palmaz-Schatz stent remains geometrically stable. In this study, the size of Wallstent used was 20–40% greater than the mean angiographic vessel reference diameter (stent-to-artery ratio 1.4 ± 0.3), and in both stent groups high-pressure dilatation was carried out to achieve an optimal angiographic result with residual diameter stenosis <10% (balloon-to-artery ratio 1.2 ± 0.2, mean pressure 16 bar). At follow-up, the Wallstent showed significantly more stent expansion with positive vessel remodelling, however, there was a positive correlation between this and neointima formation. The Wallstent was noted to shorten with, overall, twofold more neointima compared with the Palmaz-Schatz stent (Fig. 7.2). IVUS examination revealed that the neointima in the Wallstent was most prominent in the medial part of the stent with exaggerated stent expansion at this site, perhaps related to increased barotrauma leading to more extensive vessel injury. The Palmaz-Schatz stented segments did not show any evidence of significant remodelling, and neointima formation within the Palmaz-Schatz stent was more homogeneously distributed. The overall lumen result was not significantly different between the two groups. Further studies are needed to assess whether in the long-term,

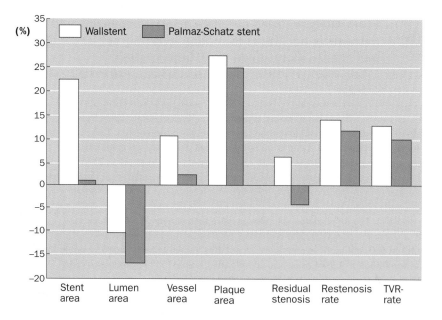

Fig. 7.2 Relative stent segment area change during follow-up of the Wallstent and Palmaz-Schatz stent. Source: Konig et al. (2002).

the continuing radial force exerted by the Wallstent might lead to a disadvantageous overall result. However, the positive remodelling associated with the Wallstent, if combined with other modalities to reduce neointima formation (such as drug elution) might, in the future, prove to be advantageous.

Nickel and molybdenum contact allergies in patients with coronary in-stent restenosis.

R Koster, D Vieluf, M Kiehn, *et al. Lancet* 2000; **356**: 1895–8.

BACKGROUND. Coronary in-stent restenosis might be triggered by contact allergy to nickel, chromate or molybdenum ions released from stainless steel stents. This study therefore investigated the association between allergic reactions to stent components and the occurrence of in-stent restenosis. A group of consecutive patients with coronary stainless steel stents undergoing angiography for suspected restenosis were included. QCA for analysis of percentage diameter stenosis was performed on 131 patients (mean age 62 years [SD 9]) with 171 stents, a mean of 6.1 months after stent implantation. All patients underwent epicutaneous patch tests (Finn chamber method) for nickel, chromate, molybdenum, manganese and small 316 L stainless steel plates. Patch tests were independently assessed by dermatologists blinded to the angiographic data after 48 h, 72 h and when necessary 96 h of contact with the potential allergen. In-stent restenosis (≥50% diameter stenosis) was present in 89 patients. All ten patients with positive patch test results had restenosis ($P = 0.03$). Four male patients had positive reactions to molybdenum, and seven patients (four male, three female) had reactions to nickel. No patient had a positive reaction to the stainless steel plates.

INTERPRETATION. Inflammation related to allergy to nickel and molybdenum increases the likelihood of restenosis after stent implantation.

Comment

In-stent restenosis reflects an excessive fibroproliferative and inflammatory response to injury to the arterial wall. Histological examination shows the presence of macrophages, histiocytes, eosinophils and T lymphocytes with focal inflammation evident around stent struts. This focal reaction suggests that a reaction to foreign material may play an important role. The vast majority of stents used in coronary intervention are made from 316 L stainless steel that contains nickel (12%), chromium (17%) and molybdenum (2%); ions of these metals are eluted from the stent. In this study, patients underwent patch testing to determine evidence of an allergic reaction and its relationship to clinically important in-stent restenosis. Eighty-nine per cent of patients with restenosis had a negative patch test result suggesting that other mechanisms were involved in the pathogenesis. However, all those with a positive patch test result ($n = 10$) had clinically significant restenosis requiring further intervention. Moreover, only one of these patients had a clinically apparent history of contact allergy suggesting that history alone is not sufficient to assess the potential for reaction. The authors suggest that those with a history of restenosis should be tested for allergy to metals before further stent implantation is carried out. In those with a history of metal hypersensitivity, there may be a role for the use of stents composed of materials other than metal such as carbon or biodegradable stents.

Stent and artery geometry determine intimal thickening independent of arterial injury.
J Garasic, E Edelman, J Squire, *et al. Circulation* 2000; **101**: 812–18.

BACKGROUND. **Clinical trials show that larger immediate post-deployment stent diameters provide greater ultimate luminal size, whereas animal data show that arterial injury and stent design determine late neointimal thickening. At deployment, a stent stretches a vessel, imposing a cross-sectional polygonal luminal shape that depends on the stent design, with each strut serving as a vertex. This study evaluated whether this design-dependent post-deployment luminal geometry affected late neointimal thickening independently of the extent of strut-induced injury. Stainless steel stents of three different configurations were implanted in rabbit iliac arteries for 3 or 28 days. Stents designed with twelve struts per cross-section had 50–60% less mural thrombus and twofold less neointimal area than identical stents with only eight struts per cross-section. Sequential histological sectioning of individual stents showed that immediate post-deployment luminal geometry and subsequent neointimal area varied along the course of each stent subunit. Mathematical modelling of the shape imposed by the stent on the artery predicted late neointimal area, based on the re-creation of a circular vessel lumen within the confines of the initial stent-imposed polygonal luminal shape.**

INTERPRETATION. Stent design, with differing immediate post-deployment geometry, has a significant impact on subsequent NIH. Stents designed with twelve struts, which give rise to a more circular geometric shape than those with just eight struts, are associated with significantly less neointima formation.

Comment

Stent deployment induces vascular injury that is thought to dictate the extent of subsequent intimal thickening. This study evaluated the influence of the number of struts and thus the stent geometry, in determining the extent of neointimal formation. The authors used a rabbit model, whereby the iliac arteries were denuded using an embolectomy catheter and then stented with either an eight- or twelve-strut design. Furthermore, the effect of strut thickness was evaluated by using twelve-strut designed stents composed of either 125- or 200-μm thick struts. All eight-strut designs were 200 μm thick. A mathematical model was developed which assumed that when deployed, a stent takes up the geometric shape of a polygon with the struts marking each vertex. The more struts, the closer the polygonal shape becomes to the circular shape of the vessel (Fig. 7.3). Blood flow dynamics suggest areas of turbulence exist in the vicinity of stent struts, thus a more circular shape with optimized flow characteristics might be expected to be associated with less platelet and inflammatory cell adhesion and a better outcome.

After 3 days, stents were harvested and the area of mural thrombus was assessed and found to be significantly less in the twelve-strut design than the eight-strut design. Furthermore, similar advantageous results of the twelve-strut design regarding extent of neointima formation were found at 28 days (Fig. 7.4). Interestingly, unlike evidence from other studies, no significant differences between the 125- or 200-μm thick struts were found suggesting that the most important factor is the

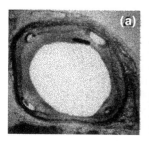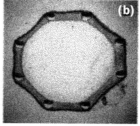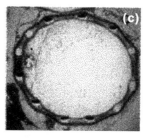

Fig. 7.3 Photomicrographs of cross-sections of rabbit iliac artery 28 days following balloon injury and stent implantation. (a) An eight-strut stent at a confluence of struts where four struts create a square form. (b) An eight-strut stent where the equally spaced struts impose an octagonal shape. (c) A twelve-strut stent creates a more circular shape. Source: Garasic *et al.* (2000).

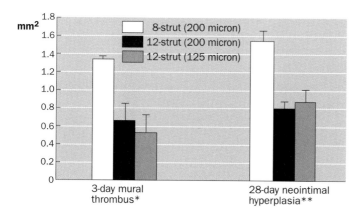

Fig. 7.4 Area of mural thrombus at 3 days and neointimal formation at 28 days. *Eight-strut versus twelve-strut, 200 μm, $P <0.01$, and versus 125 μm, $P <0.004$. **Eight-strut versus twelve-strut, 200 μm, $P <0.002$, and versus 125 μm, $P <0.005$. Source: Garasic *et al.* (2000).

geometric shape. In clinical practice, however, stents are deployed into arteries with atherosclerotic and sometimes calcified plaque and it is unlikely that they deploy with equidistant, radially distributed struts. Perhaps in this scenario, strut diameter becomes more important.

Could stent design affect platelet activation? Results of the Platelet Activation in Stenting (PAST) study.

P Gurbel, K Callahan, A Malinin, *et al. J Invas Cardiol* 2002; **14**: 584–9.

BACKGROUND. This prospective, randomized pilot study of 54 elective patients studied whether platelet activation induced by coronary artery stenting was related to stent design. Platelet activation was analysed before and at 2 h, 24 h, 5 days and 30 days post implantation of either a closed-cell (NIR) or open-cell (TETRA) stent. Platelet activation was less following NIR implantation as indicated by reduced aggregation to 5 µmol adenosine diphosphate at 30 days (32.3 ± 6.1% vs 94.5 ± 18.9%; $P = 0.02$) and reduced expression of multiple surface markers (log mean fluorescence intensity): at 2 h, CD 107a (22 ± 13 vs 18 ± 5; $P = 0.045$); at 24 h, CD 31 (136 ± 48 vs 110 ± 48; $P = 0.04$), CD 151 (104 ± 45 vs 91 ± 31; $P = 0.048$), platelet leukocyte aggregates (95 ± 40 vs 77 ± 24; $P = 0.018$) and CD 107a (24 ± 12 vs 17 ± 4; $P = 0.03$); and at 30 days, CD 151 (99 ± 33 vs 81 ± 32; $P = 0.03$), platelet leukocyte aggregates (84 ± 35 vs 72 ± 31; $P = 0.045$) and PAC-1 (88 ± 91 vs 72 ± 30; $P = 0.025$). *Ex vivo* studies in explanted swine hearts revealed that the NIR stent produced less intimal prolapse and thus a smoother stent-vessel wall interface than the TETRA stent.

INTERPRETATION. Closed-cell designed stents appear to induce less platelet activation than open-cell stents perhaps related to superior scaffolding resulting in a smoother luminal contour. This infers that their usage may, therefore, be associated with a lower rate of thrombotic complications, and may be beneficial in reducing restenosis.

Comment

Platelet activation is a major factor affecting both short- and long-term outcome after stenting. The formation of large platelet aggregates bound to the stent surface may lead to subacute closure |**10,11**|, and the release of platelet-derived mitogenic factors affects restenosis |**2,12**|. Different stent designs may result in different shear forces on platelets and thereby affect activation. In this study, all patients were on aspirin and received a loading dose of clopidogrel 300 mg in the catheterization laboratory followed by 75 mg for 30 days. The two groups of patients were similar with respect to number and length of stents implanted. There were no episodes of subacute thrombosis, Q-wave myocardial infarction (MI) or death during the 30-day follow-up period. Baseline assessment of platelet activation was similar, however, indices showed significantly more platelet activation following implantation of the TETRA open-cell design stent. This was apparent at 2 h (Fig. 7.5) and was sustained at 30 days (Fig. 7.6).

The NIR stent is a closed-design whereby the cell is bound on all sides with the junction of each strut pair joined to another strut pair junction. The open-cell design of the TETRA stent means that some junction nodes are unattached within the stent structure. To determine the effect of each design on vessel geometry, stents were implanted into explanted swine hearts within a straight vessel segment. The arteries were then filled with a solution of 2% agarose gel that was allowed to solidify thus forming a cast. The artery stented with a TETRA stent exhibited multiple irregular areas created by invagination of the vessel wall between the struts, whereas the NIR stent created a smoother stent-vessel wall interface.

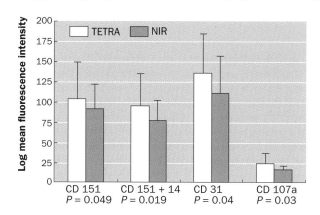

Fig. 7.5 Markers of platelet activation at 24 h. Source: Gurbel *et al.* (2002).

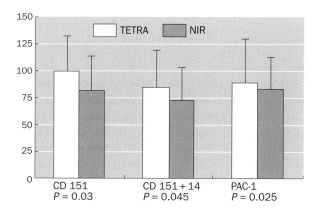

Fig. 7.6 Markers of platelet activation at 30 days. Source: Gurbel *et al.* (2002).

This study appears to correlate with the study of Garasic *et al.* (see above) who demonstrated that an increased number of struts per cross-section gave rise to a more circular lumen, and exhibited the least degree of mural thrombus. A smoother stent-vessel wall interface, seen here with the NIR stent is likely to induce less shear stress and thereby reduce platelet activation.

Intracoronary Stenting and Angiographic Results: Strut Thickness Effect on Restenosis Outcome (ISAR-STEREO-2) trial.

J Pache, A Kastrati, J Mehilli, *et al. J Am Coll Cardiol* 2003; **41**: 1283–8.

B A C K G R O U N D . This study sought to evaluate whether strut thickness is a determinant of restenosis in the presence of different stent designs. In total 611 patients with symptomatic coronary artery disease were randomly assigned to receive either the thin-strut ACS RX MultiLink stent (Guidant): strut thickness 50 μm, interconnected ring design, *n* = 309, or the thick-strut BX Velocity stent (Cordis): strut thickness 140 μm, closed cell design, *n* = 302. The primary end-point was angiographic restenosis (≥50% diameter stenosis) at 6-month follow-up. Secondary end-points were the incidence of target vessel revascularization (TVR) and the combined rate of death and MI at 1 year. The incidence of angiographic restenosis was 17.9% in the thin-strut group compared with 31.4% in the thick-strut group, relative risk (RR) 0.57 (95% CI, 0.39–0.84), *P* <0.001. A TVR due to restenosis was required in 12.3% of the thin-strut group versus 21.9% of the thick-strut group, RR 0.56 (95% CI, 0.38–0.84), *P* = 0.002. No significant difference was observed in the combined incidence of death and MI at 1 year.

I N T E R P R E T A T I O N . When two stents of different design are compared, the one with thinner struts elicits less clinical and angiographic restenosis than the stent with thicker struts.

Comment

Stents with thicker struts have higher radial strength and may therefore incur long-term benefit by resisting elastic vessel recoil. However, they also induce a greater degree of vascular injury, which correlates closely with the subsequent development of NIH. The first ISAR-STEREO study |13| was a randomized assessment of stents of comparable design (interconnected ring design) but different strut thickness (50 or 140 μm) in native vessels >2.8 mm. At 1 year, there was a significant reduction (42% risk reduction) in angiographic and clinical restenosis with the thinner strut device.

Following on from this, this study evaluated whether this difference occurred irrespective of stent design. Achievement of procedural success with the assigned device was higher with the thick-strut BX Velocity than with the thin-strut ACS RX Multi-link (99 vs 87%, *P* <0.001). This might relate to the stent design although lesions

Table 7.1 Six-month angiographic follow-up data, and 1-year clinical data comparing use of thin-strut (50 μm) interconnected ring-design stent and thick-strut (140 μm) closed-cell design stent.

	Thin strut $n = 229$	Thick strut $n = 236$	P
Minimal luminal diameter (mm)	1.96 ± 0.76	1.70 ± 0.83	<0.001
Diameter stenosis (%)	33.4 ± 21.5	42.4 ± 24.1	<0.001
Late lumen loss (mm)	0.93 ± 0.61	1.19 ± 0.69	<0.001
Loss index	0.51 ± 0.37	0.65 ± 0.44	<0.001
Incidence of restenosis (%)	17.9	31.4	<0.001
Death at 1 year (%)	3.9	4.6	0.66
Death or MI at 1 year (%)	4.9	6.3	0.46
TVR at 1 year (%)	12.3	21.9	0.002

Source: Pache *et al.* (2003).

treated with the thinner strut device were more complex with a rate of B2/C lesions of 82 versus 70% for the thick-strut BX-Velocity (P <0.001). There were no differences in early lumen gain or post-procedural diameter stenosis between the two groups.

Angiography at 6 months was carried out in those with a successful initial procedure and clearly demonstrated a reduction in restenosis with the thinner strut device (Table 7.1). Clinical follow-up demonstrated a reduced need for TVR. Taken together, the results of the two ISAR-STEREO trials suggest that strut thickness is an important factor in the development of restenosis that is independent of stent design.

In-stent restenosis in small coronary arteries: impact of strut thickness.

C Briguori, C Sarais, P Pagnotta, *et al. J Am Coll Cardiol* 2002; **40**: 403–9.

BACKGROUND. Small vessel size (<3.0 mm) is an independent risk factor for the occurrence of in-stent restenosis. This study retrospectively evaluated all patients who had successful stenting in small native vessels between March 1996 and April 2001. The strut was defined as thin when <0.10 mm and thick when ≥0.10 mm. A total of 821 (57%) of 1447 patients had angiographic follow-up available and were included in the analysis. The thin group included 400 patients with 505 lesions. The thick group included 421 patients with 436 lesions. The restenosis rate was 28.5% in the thin group and 36.6% in the thick group (P = 0.009; OR 1.44, 95% CI 1.09–1.90). The study group was classified into three subgroups according to the reference vessel diameter: ≤2.50, 2.51–2.75 and 2.76–2.99 mm. Strut thickness influenced the restenosis rate only in the subgroup with a reference vessel diameter between 2.76 and 2.99 mm, with rates of 23.5% in the thin group and 37% in the thick group (P = 0.006). Using logistic regression analysis, predictors of restenosis were stent length (OR 1.03, 95% CI

1.01–1.04; *P* = 0.001), strut thickness (OR 1.68, 95% CI 1.23–2.29; *P* = 0.001) and diabetes mellitus (OR 2.10, 95% CI 1.21–3.68; *P* = 0.007).

INTERPRETATION. Strut thickness is an independent predictor of restenosis in coronary arteries with a reference diameter of 2.75–2.99 mm though is of less importance in very small arteries.

Comment

This study was a retrospective analysis of a series of patients who underwent success-ful angioplasty and stent implantation in small coronary vessels of <3.0 mm in dia-meter and had follow-up angiography at 6 months (or earlier if symptomatic). A large variety of stents was used, both the slotted-tube and multicellular design, and divided into those with struts <0.10 or ≥0.10 mm in diameter. In this study, logistic regression analysis showed three predictors of restenosis: diabetes mellitus, stent length ≥16 mm and strut thickness ≥0.10 mm in diameter. Moreover, the restenosis rate observed in the thin-strut group was lower even though patients in this group were significantly more likely to be diabetic and have a longer final stent length.

These results corroborate those of the ISAR-STEREO trials (see above). However, coronary arteries of ≤2.75 mm in diameter have a small lumen and stenting is there-fore associated with a relatively higher metal/vessel ratio. In this study, subgroup analysis showed that the advantage conferred by using thin-strut stents was not evident in those with small vessels (Fig. 7.7).

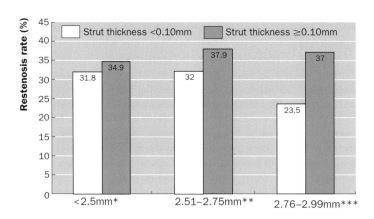

Fig. 7.7 Restenosis rates of lesions relative to strut thickness and reference vessel diameter. *P = 0.57, **P = 0.30, ***P = 0.006. Source: Briguori *et al.* (2002).

Initial and 6-month results of biodegradable poly-L-lactic acid coronary stents in humans.

H Tamai, K Igaki, E Kyo, *et al. Circulation* 2000; **102**: 399–404.

BACKGROUND. Compared with metallic stents, poly-L-lactic acid (PLLA) stents are biodegradable and can deliver drugs locally. Fifteen patients electively underwent PLLA Igaki–Tamai stent implantation for coronary artery stenoses. The Igaki–Tamai stent is made of a PLLA monopolymer, has a thickness of 0.17 mm, and has a zigzag helical coil pattern. A balloon-expandable covered sheath system was used, and the stent expanded by itself to its original size with an adequate temperature. Twenty-five stents were successfully implanted in 19 lesions in 15 patients, and angiographic success was achieved in all procedures. No stent thrombosis and no major cardiac event occurred within 30 days. Coronary angiography and IVUS were serially performed 1 day, 3 months and 6 months after the procedure. Angiographically, both the restenosis rate and TLR rate per lesion were 10.5% (2 lesions of 19); the rates per patient were 6.7% (1 of 15) at 3 months, with no further restenosis between 3 and 6 months. IVUS findings revealed no significant stent recoil at 1 day, with maintained stent expansion at follow-up. No major cardiac event, except for repeat angioplasty, developed within 6 months.

INTERPRETATION. Preliminary evidence suggests that PLLA stents are a feasible alternative to metallic stents in treating coronary disease.

Comment

Stents provide a scaffold following coronary angioplasty thereby eliminating elastic recoil and improving long-term results compared with balloon angioplasty alone. However, in some people, hypersensitivity to component metals may potentiate the risk of restenosis and moreover, the presence of a long segment of stented artery could be a problem should therapy such as bypass surgery be contemplated. The use of a biodegradable stent could, therefore, be an attractive alternative. However, initial studies using several different polymers in an animal model showed significant degrees of inflammation and neointimal formation, which had not been predicted from previous *in vitro* tests |**14**|. Subsequent investigation suggested that high molecular mass PLLA utilized in this study was biocompatible in porcine coronary models. In this study, balloon inflation was performed with heated dye (50°C at the target site) to ensure adequate stent expansion and potentially minimize vessel injury caused by a heated balloon. The stent is a self-expanding coil design with gold markers at either end to facilitate positioning. After deployment the stent continues to expand until equilibrium is obtained between the dilating radial force of the stent and the elastic resistance of the arterial wall. There were no episodes of stent thrombosis, no MI, death or need for coronary artery bypass grafting (CABG). At 6 months, arteries had a mild layer of NIH; a single patient developed restenosis in two lesions and underwent TLR (Tables 7.2 and 7.3).

Table 7.2 Results of the angiographic QCA analysis of the PLLA Igaki–Tamai stent

	Before stenting	After stenting	24 h	3 months	6 months
Number of lesions	19	19	19	19	18
Reference vessel diameter (mm)	2.85 ± 0.34	2.95 ± 0.35	3.00 ± 0.40	2.75 ± 0.49	2.69 ± 0.49
Minimum lumen diameter (mm)	1.02 ± 0.36	2.59 ± 0.35	2.58 ± 0.32	1.88 ± 0.59	1.84 ± 0.66
% DS	64 ± 11	12 ± 8	13 ± 11	33 ± 14	33 ± 18
Loss index				0.44 ± 0.30	0.48 ± 0.32

Source: Tamai *et al.* (2000).

Table 7.3 Quantitative IVUS results of the PLLA Igaki–Tamai stent

	After stenting	24 h	3 months	6 months
Number of lesions	19	19	18	18
Stent CSA (mm^2)	7.42 ± 1.51	7.37 ± 1.44	8.18 ± 2.42*	8.13 ± 2.52*
Neointimal area (mm^2)			2.51 ± 0.94	2.50 ± 0.65
Lumen CSA (mm^2)	7.42 ± 1.51	7.37 ± 1.44	5.67 ± 2.42†	5.63 ± 2.70§

*$P < 0.1$ versus after stenting; †$P < 0.005$ versus after stenting; §$P < 0.001$ versus after stenting.
Source: Tamai *et al.* (2000).

Stents must maintain their scaffolding strength for >6 months to overcome late vessel remodelling, thus any biodegradable stent must not break down until after this period. However, long-term evaluation is needed to determine the interaction between the process of dissolution of the struts and restenosis mechanisms. Recently, the long-term results of a related biodegradable stent composed of a self-reinforced copolymer of *l*- and *d*-lactide, used in a rabbit model, have been published. The stent was found to have disintegrated at 24 months and been replaced by fibrous tissue; encouragingly, lumen patency was maintained |**15**|.

Modern stent technology is concentrating on the delivery of anti-proliferative drugs that act locally to inhibit the development of NIH and restenosis. Restenosis is directly related to the trauma induced when a stent is deployed and is most prominent at/around the struts. Most drug-eluting stents rely on covering the stents' metallic struts with a polymer coating that is loaded with drug. Biodegradable stents are composed of polymer, and if this can be combined with effective anti-proliferative medication then this may confer the advantage that drug delivery would be greatest at the very site where it is most needed – the site of injury caused by the struts.

Conclusion

The main problem hindering successful outcome after coronary stent implantation is restenosis. The degree of injury induced by stent deployment relates to a more pronounced inflammatory reaction and subsequently more NIH. In animal restenosis models, design determines endothelial denudation during stent expansion and the depth of stent strut incision. Vessel injury has been found to relate to strut thickness, the number of struts and tubular-slotted versus corrugated-ring design |**16,17**|.

Stents with a high number of struts deploy, at least in the animal model, with a more circular geometry thus more closely representing that of the vessel itself; this is associated with reduced neointima formation at follow-up. However, obtaining a circular geometry is likely to be more difficult when stents are deployed in clinical practice in diseased vessels with eccentric plaque, particularly in the presence of calcification. Evidence also suggests that to minimize neointima formation the best stents are those with thin struts; however, any reduction in strut diameter must not be at the expense of losing radial force, which would lead to negative remodelling and a reduction in luminal area. Small vessels unfortunately continue to pose a problem; the benefit obtained by utilizing stents with thin struts does not override the small residual lumen present.

Coatings, by necessity, will increase strut thickness and alter the expansion dynamics. Problems may arise particularly if the stent and coating are of different material strengths. Stent design or the presence of a coating may also influence the interaction with the circulating blood, with evidence of different degrees of platelet activation and the potential for inducing thrombosis.

The possible role of hypersensitivity to stent components in causing restenosis requires further evaluation, but may provide a niche for biodegradable stents, particularly if these are combined with the capability of drug elution. The development of stents that elute anti-proliferative agents such as paclitaxol and sirolimus has revolutionized coronary intervention with dramatically reduced rates of restenosis when used in relatively simple *de novo* lesions. However, results of these stents in more complex disease, though encouraging, show us that the problem of restenosis has not been completely abolished. It is likely that a combination of optimizing stent design together with drug-elution properties will remain an important area of research.

References

1. Virmani R, Farb A. Pathology of in-stent restenosis. *Curr Opin Lipidol* 1999; **10**: 499–506.

2. Farb A, Sangiorgi G, Carter AJ, Walley VM, Edwards WD, Schwartz RS, Virmani R. Pathology of acute and chronic coronary stenting in humans. *Circulation* 1999; **99**: 44–52.

3. Scott NA, Cipolla GD, Ross CE, Dunn B, Martin FH, Simonet L, Wilcox JN. Identification of a potential role for the adventitia in vascular lesion formation after balloon overstretch injury of porcine coronary arteries. *Circulation* 1996; **93**: 2178–87.

4. Shi Y, O'Brien JE, Fard A, Mannion JD, Wang D, Zalewski A. Adventitial myofibroblasts contribute to neointimal formation in injured porcine coronary arteries. *Circulation* 1996; **94**: 1655–64.

5. Kastrati A, Dirschinger J, Boekstegers P, Elezi S, Schuhlen H, Pache J, Steinbeck G, Schmitt C, Ulm K, Neumann FJ, Schomig A. Influence of stent design on 1-year outcome after coronary stent placement: a randomized comparison of five stent types in 1,147 unselected patients. *Catheter Cardiovasc Interven* 2000; **50**: 290–7.

6. Kastrati A, Mehilli J, Dirschinger J, Pache J, Ulm K, Schuhlen H, Seyfarth M, Schmitt C, Blasini R, Neumann FJ, Schomig A. Restenosis after coronary placement of various stent types. *Am J Cardiol* 2001; **87**: 34–9.

7. Tanigawa N, Sawada S, Kobayashi M. Reaction of the aortic wall to six metallic stent materials. *Acad Radiol* 1995; **2**: 379–84.

8. Beythien C, Gutensohn K, Kuehnl P, Hamm CW, Alt E, Terres W. Influence of 'diamond-like' and gold coating on platelet activation: a flow cytometry analysis in a pulsed floating model (abstract). *J Am Coll Cardiol* 1998; 413A.

9. Kastrati A, Schomig A, Dirschinger J, Mehilli J, von Welser N, Pache J, Schuhlen H, Schilling T, Schmitt C, Neumann FJ. Increased risk of restenosis after placement of gold-coated stents: results of a randomized trial comparing gold-coated with uncoated steel stents in patients with coronary artery disease. *Circulation* 2000; **101**: 2478–83.

10. Steinhubl SR, Ellis SG, Wolski K, Lincoff AM, Topol EJ. Ticlopidine pre-treatment before coronary stenting is associated with sustained decrease in adverse cardiac events: data from the Evaluation of Platelet IIb/IIIa Inhibitor for Stenting (EPISTENT) Trial. *Circulation* 2001; **103**: 1403–9.

11. Schomig A, Neumann FJ, Kastrati A, Schuhlen H, Blasini R, Hadamitzky M, Walter H, Zitzmann-Roth EM, Richardt G, Alt E, Schmitt C, Ulm K. A randomized comparison of antiplatelet and anticoagulant therapy after the placement of coronary-artery stents. *N Engl J Med* 1996; **334**: 1084–9.

12. Le Breton H, Plow EF, Topol EJ. Role of platelets in restenosis after percutaneous coronary revascularization. *J Am Coll Cardiol* 1996; **28**: 1643–51.

13. Kastrati A, Mehilli J, Dirschinger J, Dotzer F, Schuhlen H, Neumann FJ, Fleckenstein M, Pfafferott C, Seyfarth M, Schomig A. Intracoronary stenting and angiographic results: strut thickness effect on restenosis outcome (ISAR-STEREO) trial. *Circulation* 2001; **103**: 2816–21.

14. van der Giessen WJ, Lincoff AM, Schwartz RS, van Beusekom HM, Serruys PW, Holmes DR, Jr., Ellis SG, Topol EJ. Marked inflammatory sequelae to implantation of biodegradable and nonbiodegradable polymers in porcine coronary arteries. *Circulation* 1996; **94**: 1690–7.

15. Hietala EM, Salminen US, Stahls A, Valimaa T, Maasilta P, Tormala P, Nieminen MS, Harjula AL. Biodegradation of the copolymeric polylactide stent. Long-term follow-up in a rabbit aorta model. *J Vasc Res* 2001; **38**: 361–9.

16. Rogers C, Tseng DY, Squire JC, Edelman ER. Balloon-artery interactions during stent placement: a finite element analysis approach to pressure, compliance, and stent design as contributors to vascular injury. *Circ Res* 1999; **84**: 378–83.

17. Rogers C, Edelman ER. Endovascular stent design dictates experimental restenosis and thrombosis. *Circulation* 1995; **91**: 2995–3001.

8

Percutaneous coronary intervention and statins

Introduction

Recurrent cardiac events occur in approximately 40% of patients undergoing percutaneous coronary interventions (PCI), by 5 years. Treatments with statins do not reduce the 6-month restenosis rate following intervention |1–3|, but may influence later changes at the treated site |4|. Almost a decade ago, the Scandinavian Simvastatin Survival Study (4S) trial convincingly demonstrated the benefit of simvastatin treatment in patients with coronary disease and an elevated cholesterol level |5|. Similar findings with pravastatin |6,7| suggested that the benefit was likely to be a class effect.

Two major studies published during the last year extend this data further, first, by including patients up to 80 years of age, and secondly, by including those with a total cholesterol level in the 'normal' range, >3.5 mmol/l. The findings of the large Heart Protection Study (HPS) in particular, although not specifically a study of patients undergoing PCI, have major implications for the long-term treatment of all such patients. The smaller Lescol Intervention Prevention Study (LIPS) trial provides important corroborating data, evaluating another statin in interventional patients.

MRC/BHF Heart Protection Study of cholesterol lowering with simvastatin in 20 536 high-risk individuals: a randomized placebo-controlled trial.
Heart Protection Study Collaborative Group. *Lancet* 2002, **360**: 7–22.

B ᴀ ᴄ ᴋ ɢ ʀ ᴏ ᴜ ɴ ᴅ . Statins are effective for the secondary prevention of vascular events in patients with elevated cholesterol levels. The Heart Protection Study evaluated those 'at substantial 5 year risk of death from coronary heart disease'. Patients were eligible for enrolment if their total cholesterol level was >3.5 mmol/l and if they were under 80 years of age. Two-thirds of patients had a history of coronary disease; of the remainder, 25% had cerebrovascular disease, 38% had peripheral vascular disease and 56% had diabetes. A 2 × 2 factorial design evaluated simvastatin 40 mg daily and antioxidant vitamins, compared with placebo. The study population of 20 536 was followed for a mean of 5 years. The mean cholesterol level at enrolment was

5.9 mmol/l. At the end of the study, 82% of those randomized to simvastatin and 32% of those on placebo were taking a statin. There was a mean absolute difference between the statin and placebo groups in total cholesterol level of 1.2 mmol/l. Total mortality was 12.9% in the simvastatin group, compared with 14.7% in the placebo group, mainly due to an 18% relative reduction in the coronary death rate (Fig. 8.1). The incidence of non-fatal first myocardial infarction (MI) was reduced by 38%, from 5.6% in the placebo group to 3.5% in the simvastatin group. The benefit appeared consistent across all subgroups analysed (Fig. 8.2). Simvastatin treatment reduced the incidence of first stroke by 25% (from 5.7% with placebo to 4.3% with simvastatin). The need for coronary, carotid or other peripheral revascularization was reduced by a similar amount in the simvastatin treatment group. Adverse effects related to statin treatment were infrequent; the incidence of myopathy was estimated at 0.01%. Antioxidant vitamins had no effect on cardiac events.

INTERPRETATION. Simvastatin 40 mg daily reduces all-cause mortality and major vascular events in patients with or at high risk for vascular disease. The benefit was demonstrated in those with a total cholesterol >3.5 mmol/l, and up to the age of 80 years.

Comment

This is the largest randomized trial of statin treatment in high-risk patients with or without established coronary or other vascular disease. It convincingly demonstrates the efficacy and safety of statin treatment in such patients. Although the study did not

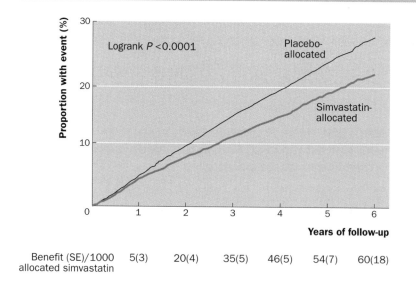

Fig. 8.1 Life table plot of major vascular events, showing the benefit of simvastatin treatment. Source: Heart Protection Study Collaborative Group (2002).

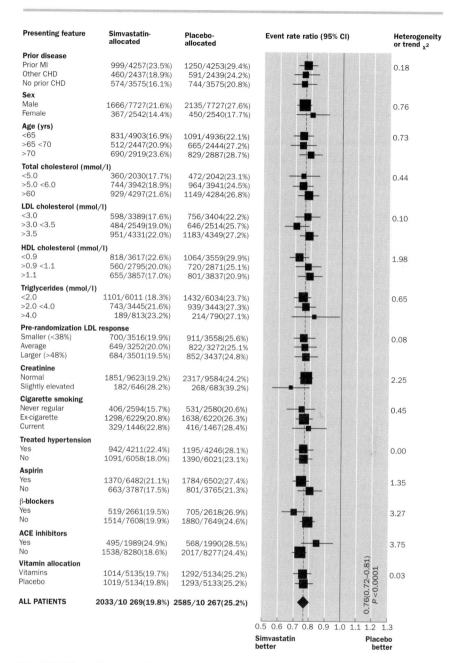

Presenting feature	Simvastatin-allocated	Placebo-allocated	Event rate ratio (95% CI)	Heterogeneity or trend χ^2
Prior disease				
Prior MI	999/4257(23.5%)	1250/4253(29.4%)		0.18
Other CHD	460/2437(18.9%)	591/2439(24.2%)		
No prior CHD	574/3575(16.1%)	744/3575(20.8%)		
Sex				
Male	1666/7727(21.6%)	2135/7727(27.6%)		0.76
Female	367/2542(14.4%)	450/2540(17.7%)		
Age (yrs)				
<65	831/4903(16.9%)	1091/4936(22.1%)		0.73
>65 <70	512/2447(20.9%)	665/2444(27.2%)		
>70	690/2919(23.6%)	829/2887(28.7%)		
Total cholesterol (mmol/l)				
<5.0	360/2030(17.7%)	472/2042(23.1%)		0.44
>5.0 <6.0	744/3942(18.9%)	964/3941(24.5%)		
>60	929/4297(21.6%)	1149/4284(26.8%)		
LDL cholesterol (mmol/l)				
<3.0	598/3389(17.6%)	756/3404(22.2%)		0.10
>3.0 <3.5	484/2549(19.0%)	646/2514(25.7%)		
>3.5	951/4331(22.0%)	1183/4349(27.2%)		
HDL cholesterol (mmol/l)				
<0.9	818/3617(22.6%)	1064/3559(29.9%)		1.98
>0.9 <1.1	560/2795(20.0%)	720/2871(25.1%)		
>1.1	655/3857(17.0%)	801/3837(20.9%)		
Triglycerides (mmol/l)				
<2.0	1101/6011 (18.3%)	1432/6034(23.7%)		0.65
>2.0 <4.0	743/3445(21.6%)	939/3443(27.3%)		
>4.0	189/813(23.2%)	214/790(27.1%)		
Pre-randomization LDL response				
Smaller (<38%)	700/3516(19.9%)	911/3558(25.6%)		0.08
Average	649/3252(20.0%)	822/3272(25.1%)		
Larger (>48%)	684/3501(19.5%)	852/3437(24.8%)		
Creatinine				
Normal	1851/9623(19.2%)	2317/9584(24.2%)		2.25
Slightly elevated	182/646(28.2%)	268/683(39.2%)		
Cigarette smoking				
Never regular	406/2594(15.7%)	531/2580(20.6%)		0.45
Ex-cigarette	1298/6229(20.8%)	1638/6220(26.3%)		
Current	329/1446(22.8%)	416/1467(28.4%)		
Treated hypertension				
Yes	942/4211(22.4%)	1195/4246(28.1%)		0.00
No	1091/6058(18.0%)	1390/6021(23.1%)		
Aspirin				
Yes	1370/6482(21.1%)	1784/6502(27.4%)		1.35
No	663/3787(17.5%)	801/3765(21.3%)		
β-blockers				
Yes	519/2661(19.5%)	705/2618(26.9%)		3.27
No	1514/7608(19.9%)	1880/7649(24.6%)		
ACE inhibitors				
Yes	495/1989(24.9%)	568/1990(28.5%)		3.75
No	1538/8280(18.6%)	2017/8277(24.4%)		
Vitamin allocation				
Vitamins	1014/5135(19.7%)	1292/5134(25.2%)		0.03
Placebo	1019/5134(19.8%)	1293/5133(25.2%)		
ALL PATIENTS	**2033/10 269(19.8%)**	**2585/10 267(25.2%)**		

0.76(0.72–0.81)
P <0.0001

0.5 0.6 0.7 0.8 0.9 1.0 1.1 1.2 1.3

Simvastatin better   Placebo better

Fig. 8.2 Effect of simvastatin allocation on first major vascular event in different categories of participant. Source: Heart Protection Study Collaborative Group (2002).

specifically evaluate patients undergoing PCI, the findings can appropriately be applied to such patients, all of whom have coronary disease.

The study used a fixed dosage of 40 mg daily of simvastatin. The relative efficacy of higher or lower dosages is unknown. The effect of dosage titration to a cholesterol target, particularly in those with higher cholesterol levels, is also unknown.

Fluvastatin for prevention of cardiac events following successful first percutaneous coronary intervention.

P W J C Serruys, P de Feyter, C Macaya, *et al. JAMA* 2002; **287**: 3215–22.

BACKGROUND. The LIPS trial was a randomized comparison of fluvastatin 80 mg per day with placebo in 1677 patients with stable or unstable angina, or silent myocardial ischaemia, following a successful first PCI procedure. Patients had baseline cholesterol levels between 3.5 and 7.0 mmol/l with a fasting triglyceride level <4.5 mmol/l. They were enrolled a median of 2.0 days post-intervention, and followed for a median of 3.9 years. The median reduction in low density lipoprotein (LDL) cholesterol with treatment was 27%. Cardiac death, non-fatal MI or re-intervention occurred in 21.4% of the fluvastatin group and 26.7% of the placebo group (relative risk reduction 0.78, $P = 0.01$). The benefit was independent of baseline cholesterol levels, and the risk reduction was greater in those with diabetes and with multivessel disease.

INTERPRETATION. Fluvastatin treatment significantly reduces adverse cardiac events in patients following a successful PCI procedure. The effect was seen in patients with 'normal' to moderately elevated cholesterol levels.

Comment

This is the largest randomized, controlled trial of statin therapy specifically in patients undergoing PCI. The findings are consistent with the Heart Protection Study trial, which had the same lower threshold for total cholesterol level at patient enrolment. The 5.3% absolute reduction and 22% relative reduction in fatal and non-fatal major adverse cardiac events is similar to that observed in other secondary prevention trials of statin therapy. The benefit was unlikely to be due to reduced 6-month restenosis as re-intervention was not decreased and the major adverse cardiac event-free survival curves did not diverge until around 18 months post intervention.

Statin treatment following coronary artery stenting and one-year survival.

A Schomig, J Mehilli, H Holle, *et al. J Am Coll Cardiol* 2002; **40**: 854–61.

BACKGROUND. This registry study evaluated 12-month outcomes by statin treatment in patients undergoing stent deployment. The study population was 4520 patients under the age of 80 years surviving to discharge from hospital over a 4-year period from 1995 to 1999. The majority (79%) of patients received statins, with that proportion increasing over the study duration. Simvastatin was used in one half and atorvastatin in one quarter. There were significant differences between the two study groups. Those on statins were younger, had more hypertension, had a higher mean cholesterol level, had more previous MIs, had more complex lesions, had more severely narrowed lesions pre-intervention, and had a greater length of stent implanted. Furthermore, there were large differences between groups in the use of other medications at the time of stent deployment and at hospital discharge. Those on statins were more likely to receive abciximab (33.4 vs 21.8%), and were more likely to be discharged on beta-blockers (91.9 vs 44.1%) and angiotensin converting enzyme (ACE) inhibitors (78.8 vs 40.9%). Logistic regression was used to create a propensity score for each patient in an attempt to control for differences between groups. The cumulative 1-year mortality was 2.6% for patients on statins at hospital discharge and 5.6% for those who were not, giving an odds ratio (OR) of 0.46 (Fig. 8.3). Mortality did not differ between those on statins prior to admission and those started after admission. There was an interaction with beta-blocker therapy, with the lowest mortality in those on both a beta-blocker and a statin. Statin therapy did not appear to reduce recurrent MI or repeat target vessel revascularization (TVR).

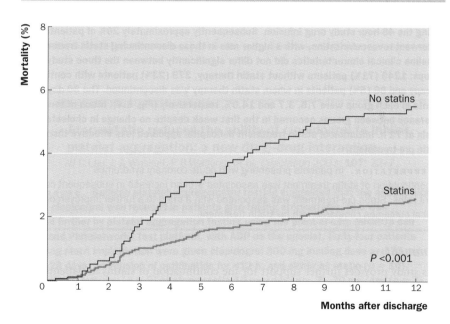

Fig. 8.3 Cumulative 1-year mortality curves for patients with and without statins. Source: Schomig *et al.* (2002).

INTERPRETATION. Atorvastatin may inhibit the antiplatelet effects of clopidogrel. Other statins not metabolized by CYP 3A4 may have a clinical advantage in patients taking clopidogrel.

Comment

This study reports an interaction between atorvastatin and clopidogrel, as assessed by one test of platelet function. The two drugs are commonly used in patients undergoing stent deployment, so the finding is of potential clinical importance.

A subsequent editorial |8| criticized various aspects of the study design including the small sample size, lack of control for other medications affecting CYP 450 3A4, and use of a single method to assess platelet function. Another evaluation of platelet inhibition in 100 patients undergoing PCI found that approximately 20% of patients did not achieve profound platelet inhibition with clopidogrel, but that this appeared unrelated to whether the patient was on a statin or which particular statin was used |9|. Apart from the study methodology limitations, it remains uncertain whether the interaction is clinically important.

Use of secondary preventive drugs in patients with acute coronary syndromes treated medically or with coronary angioplasty: results from the nationwide French PREVENIR survey.

N Danchin, O Grenier, J Ferrieres, C Cantet, J-P Cambon. *Heart* 2002; **88**: 159–62.

BACKGROUND. This registry study evaluated the use of secondary prevention drugs in patients with acute coronary syndromes managed conservatively or treated by PCI admitted to participating French hospitals and clinics in January 1998. Approximately 15% of French hospitals managing such patients were included. Of 1394 patients, almost one half underwent PCI during the initial hospital admission. At admission, 16% were taking statins and 10% fibrates. At hospital discharge 35% were on statins, 6% on fibrates, 90% on aspirin, 68% on beta-blockers, 41% on ACE inhibitors and 28% on calcium antagonists. Compared with those treated medically, patients undergoing PCI were more likely to receive statins (OR 1.7), aspirin (OR 2.9) and beta-blockers (OR 1.5). Six months later there was a 10% absolute increase in the percentage of patients on statins.

INTERPRETATION. This registry from 5 years ago demonstrated that only one third of patients presenting with acute coronary syndromes in France were treated with statins. Patients undergoing PCI were more likely to receive statins, aspirin and beta-blockers than those treated conservatively.

Comment

This study demonstrates that there remains a gap between trial data demonstrating drug efficacy in the secondary prevention of coronary artery disease, and the use of these drugs in clinical practice. It reinforces the potential for improved clinical outcomes if the HPS and LIPS trial findings are applied across high-risk populations. The reason why patients undergoing PCI were more likely to receive 'evidence-based' treatment compared with patients treated medically is unclear. An interventional procedure is one point of patient care in a longstanding and chronic disease, and does offer an opportunity for comprehensive risk factor assessment and modification.

Conclusion

The HPS and LIPS trial data firmly establish the role of statin treatment in almost all patients undergoing PCI. Both trials extend the lower cholesterol threshold for treatment to 3.5 mmol/l, and the upper age threshold to 80 years. The benefit appears sustained in all subgroups. There are a number of unresolved issues. Should treatment be with a fixed dose of statin or to a target cholesterol level, as many treatment guidelines recommend? Should patients over 80 years of age be treated? Is there a role for fibrates, particularly in patients with a low HDL cholesterol and high triglyceride levels, either instead of or combined with statins?

The finding that the magnitude of benefit of statin treatment appeared unrelated to the pre-treatment cholesterol level should provide a further impetus for studies on the non-cholesterol lowering effects of statins. They reduce non-specific markers of inflammation such as high-sensitivity C reactive protein, which have been associated with adverse cardiac outcomes in patients with unstable coronary syndromes, including those undergoing stent deployment [10].

The potential drug interaction between statins and other drugs commonly used during stent deployment is interesting but of uncertain clinical significance. A related issue is whether antiplatelet drug regimens used clinically may be optimized by platelet function testing, particularly at point of care. Higher dosages of clopidogrel might be more effective, at least in those patients who are resistant to standard clopidogrel regimens. There is some evidence that a 600 mg loading dose and 150 mg/day has a greater effect on platelet function than standard regimens of half that dosage [11].

These important trial findings must be translated into clinical practice. The PRE-VENIR survey suggests that there is some way to go, despite increased prescription of statins over the last decade. The European Action on Secondary Prevention by Intervention to Reduce Events (EUROASPIRE) survey of nine European countries in 1995–1996 found statins prescribed in 18.5% of patients with established coronary disease. By the time of EUROASPIRE II in 1999–2000 the use of statins had increased to 58% [12]. With the level of evidence now available, in 2003 this figure should be over 90%.

References

1. Bertrand ME, McFadden EP, Fruchart JC, *et al.* Effect of pravastatin on angiographic restenosis after coronary balloon angioplasty. *J Am Coll Cardiol* 1997; **30**: 863–9.

2. Weintraub WS, Boccuzzi SJ, Klein JL, *et al.* Lack of effect of lovastatin on restenosis after coronary angioplasty. *N Engl J Med* 1994; **331**: 1331–7.

3. Serruys PW, Foley DP, Jackson G, *et al.* A randomized placebo-controlled trial of fluvastatin for prevention of restenosis after successful coronary balloon angioplasty: final results of the Fluvastatin Angiographic Restenosis (FLARE) trial. *Eur Heart J* 1999; **20**: 58–69.

4. Mulder HJ, Bal ET, Jukema JW, Zwinderman AH, Schalij MJ, van Boven AJ, Bruschke AVG. Pravastatin reduces restenosis two years after percutaneous transluminal coronary angioplasty (REGRESS trial). *Am J Cardiol* 2000; **86**: 742–6.

5. The Scandinavian Simvastatin Survival Study (4S) Investigators. Randomized trial of cholesterol lowering in 4444 patients with coronary heart disease: the Scandinavian Simvastatin Survival Study (4S). *Lancet* 1994; **344**: 1383–9.

6. Sacks FM, Pfeffer MA, Moye LA, *et al.* for the Cholesterol and Recurrent Events Trial Investigators. The effect of pravastatin on coronary events after myocardial infarction in patients with average cholesterol levels. *N Engl J Med* 1996; **335**: 1001–9.

7. The Long-Term Intervention with Pravastatin in Ischaemic Disease (LIPID) Study Group. Prevention of cardiovascular events and death with pravastatin in patients with coronary heart disease and a broad range of initial cholesterol levels. *N Engl J Med* 1998; **339**: 1349–57.

8. Serebruany VL, Steinhubl SR, Hennekens CH. Are antiplatelet effects of clopidogrel inhibited by atorvastatin? A research question formulated but not yet adequately tested. *Circulation* 2003; **107**: 1568–9.

9. Serebruany VL, Malinin AI, Kallahan KP, *et al.* Statins do not affect platelet inhibition with clopidogrel during coronary stenting. *Atherosclerosis* 2001; **239**: 259–61.

10. Walter DH, Fichtlscherer S, Britten MB, *et al.* Statin therapy, inflammation and recurrent coronary events in patients following coronary stent implantation. *J Am Coll Cardiol* 2001; **38**: 2006–12.

11. Muller I, Seyfarth M, Rudiger S, Wolf B, Pogatsa-Murray G, Schomig A, Gawaz M. Effect of a high loading dose of clopidogrel on platelet function in patients undergoing coronary stent placement. *Heart* 2001; **85**: 92–3.

12. EUROASPIRE I and II Group. Clinical reality of coronary prevention guidelines: a comparison of EUROASPIRE I and II in nine countries. *Lancet* 2001; **357**: 995–1001.

9

Percutaneous coronary intervention and diabetes mellitus

Introduction

Patients with diabetes have an increased risk of coronary artery disease (CAD), and are at an increased risk of mortality and morbidity with coronary revascularization procedures. This is due to various modifications associated with diabetes, such as endothelial dysfunction (an abnormal response of the cells of the vascular wall), and a greater risk of thrombotic events. In 1995, the report of the results from the Bypass Angioplasty Revascularization Investigation (BARI) raised doubts about the use of angioplasty in diabetic patients [1,2]. The data showed that the 5-year survival rate of diabetics with multivessel coronary lesions was better after coronary artery bypass grafting (CABG) than after angioplasty. This was supported by results from the Emory Angioplasty versus Surgery Trial (EAST) and the Coronary Angioplasty versus Bypass Revascularization Investigation (CABRI) trial [3,4].

Since these reports extensive research has been undertaken to understand the reason(s) for this poor outcome of diabetic patients after percutaneous coronary revascularization. More recently, new tools and approaches to percutaneous coronary intervention (PCI) have been developed, including stents, glycoprotein (GP) IIb/IIIa inhibitors and brachytherapy. These new techniques have been evaluated in diabetic patients and the purpose of this review is to report the major findings related to the outcome of diabetics after PCI during the year 2002.

Recent analyses derived from the BARI trial

Coronary bypass graft patency in patients with diabetes in the Bypass Angioplasty Revascularization Investigation (BARI).

L Schwartz, K E Kip, R L Frye, E L Alderman, H V Schaff, K M Detre; Bypass Angioplasty Revascularization Investigation. *Circulation* 2002; **106**: 2652–8.

BACKGROUND. In the BARI trial, 5- and 7-year follow-up demonstrated that survival of diabetic patients with multivessel CAD was better after bypass surgery than after coronary balloon angioplasty. The survival advantage of bypass surgery suggested sustained graft patency in diabetic patents despite their propensity to accelerate atherosclerosis. However, no data were available on this issue.

INTERPRETATION. Among 1526 patients in the BARI trial who underwent bypass surgery as initial revascularization, 34% with treated diabetes and 38% without treated diabetes had follow-up angiography. Follow-up angiography was performed a mean of 3.9 years after surgery and was performed in two circumstances: by protocol in about 30% of patients or as clinically indicated (70%). Internal mammary artery grafts were more likely to be stenosis-free than vein grafts. However, the percentage of internal mammary artery grafts free of stenoses was similar between diabetic and non-diabetic patients (89 vs 85%). The patency rate of vein grafts was also similar between patients with or without diabetes (71 vs 75%).

Comment

These data suggest that diabetes does not appear to adversely affect patency of mammary or vein grafts over a 4-year period. This is completely different to what is observed on the patency of native artery after coronary balloon angioplasty. These results might partly explain the clinical benefit of bypass surgery versus coronary angioplasty in diabetic patients with multivessel coronary artery disease.

Differential influence of diabetes mellitus on increased jeopardized myocardium after initial angioplasty or bypass surgery.

K E Kip, E L Alderman, M G Bourassa, *et al. Circulation* 2002: **105**: 1914–20.

BACKGROUND. In the BARI trial, 5- and 7-year follow-up demonstrated that survival of diabetic patients with multivessel CAD was better after bypass surgery than after coronary balloon angioplasty. The reason(s) for this protection observed after bypass surgery in diabetic patients, but not in non-diabetic patients is unclear.

INTERPRETATION. Change in jeopardized myocardium was analysed in patients enrolled in the BARI trial with: (1) reduction in jeopardized myocardium at the time of revascularization and (2) angiographic follow-up. The total percentage of jeopardized myocardium was determined by the overall percentage of the coronary perfusion territory compromised by stenosis ≥50%. Among 128 patients with 1-year protocol angiography in the percutaneous transluminal coronary angioplasty (PTCA) arm, the mean percentage of jeopardized myocardium was similar between patients with or without diabetes both at study entry (58 vs 60%) and immediately after initial revascularization (13 vs 15%). However, at 1-year follow-up, patients with diabetes had a higher percentage increase in jeopardized myocardium than patients without diabetes (42 vs 24%, $P = 0.05$). In the bypass surgery arm, the percentage of jeopardized myocardium was higher in diabetic than in non-diabetic patients at study entry (66 vs 60%, $P = 0.05$), but was similar immediately after initial revascularization (7 vs 7%). In contrast to the PTCA arm, at 1-year follow-up the percentage of jeopardized myocardium was similar between coronary artery bypass graft (CABG) patients with or without diabetes (11 vs 15%).

Comment

These data suggest that diabetes is associated with an increase in jeopardized myocardium at midterm follow-up after PTCA but not after bypass surgery. Several explanations might be proposed for this effect specifically seen in the PTCA arm. This might be related to the increased restenosis associated with diabetes while it has no or little effect on graft patency (see Schwartz *et al.*). This might also partly be related to atherosclerosis progression in non-instrumented segments that would not increase the area of myocardium at risk when a graft is implanted in that segment.

Influence of the bypass angioplasty revascularization investigation National Heart, Lung, and Blood Institute diabetic clinical alter on practice patterns.

D K McGuire, K J Anstrom, E D Peterson. *Circulation* 2003; **107**: 1864–70.

BACKGROUND. In 1995, the BARI study found that patients with diabetes had a survival advantage when treated with bypass surgery versus balloon angioplasty, prompting a National Heart, Lung, and Blood Institute 'clinical alert'. The purpose of this study was to analyse the impact of this 'clinical alert' on clinical practice in the USA.

INTERPRETATION. Using the National Cardiovascular Network Coronary Revascularization Database (13 US hospitals), the authors evaluate rates of percutaneous versus surgical revascularization among diabetics meeting BARI eligibility criteria before and after the Clinical Alert release (1994–1997). Over the 4-year period of the study, the 'clinical alert' had no significant impact on the proportion of diabetic patients undergoing percutaneous revascularization (28.6% before vs 26.8% after the clinical alert). Among those surveyed, although 91% were aware of the clinical alert and 76% felt that it was valid, more than 50% felt that the clinical alert had limited or no impact on their practice.

Comment

This study demonstrates that the results of the BARI trial had little or no impact on clinical practice in the US. The most frequent explanation proposed by physicians to explain this apparent contradictory result is that technological advances in revascularization make the BARI results obsolete (67%). Interestingly, although 50% of cardiac surgeons viewed the BARI results as 'still relevant', only 20% of interventional cardiologists felt that the study applied to current practice as a result of therapeutic advances. These views by physicians were based on little evidence. Indeed by 1997, little was known on the benefit of coronary stenting and glycoprotein (Gp) IIb/IIIa in diabetic patients. This very interesting study demonstrates how it is difficult to change medical practice, especially when the findings are not as the physician would like them to be.

Benefit from technical and pharmacological adjunct during PCI in diabetics

 Effects of coronary stenting on vessel patency and long-term clinical outcome after percutaneous coronary revascularization in diabetic patients.
E Van Belle, M Perie, D Braune, *et al. J Am Coll Cardiol* 2002; **40**: 410–17.

BACKGROUND. Although coronary stenting is associated with a lower restenosis rate than balloon angioplasty in diabetic patients, the effect of coronary stenting on long-term outcome is unclear in this population.

INTERPRETATION. Comparison of clinical outcome of diabetic patients after coronary stenting or balloon angioplasty was investigated by individual matching of 314 diabetic patients treated with either coronary stenting or balloon angioplasty. Matching criteria were gender, anti-diabetic regimen, stenosis location, reference diameter and minimal luminal diameter. At 6 months coronary stenting was associated with a lower restenosis rate (27 vs 62%) and a lower occlusion rate of the target site (4 vs 13%) compared with balloon angioplasty. Four-year follow-up demonstrated that the combined rate of cardiac death and non-fatal myocardial infarction (MI) was lower in the stent group than in the balloon group (14.8 vs 26%), as was the need for repeat revascularization (35.4 vs 52.1%).

Comment

These data demonstrate that in diabetic patients, the use of coronary stents rather than balloon angioplasty is associated with an improved clinical outcome. These results extend the results of the EPISTENT trial, showing that among diabetics receiving abciximab, those randomized to coronary stent implantation had a trend toward a reduced rate of death and large MI at 1 year compared with those treated with balloon angioplasty (4.9 vs 10.4%). It is of note, however, that most of the patients were treated on a single vessel and that angioplasty was performed in relatively large vessels (mean vessel diameter = 3.06 mm). It is unclear whether these improved results associated with stent implantation would extend to more severely diseased diabetics.

Impact of different platelet glycoprotein IIb/IIIa receptor inhibitors among diabetic patients undergoing percutaneous coronary intervention. Do Tirofiban And ReoPro Give similar Efficacy outcomes Trial (TARGET) 1-year follow-up.

M Roffi, D J Moliterno, B Meier, *et al. Circulation* 2002; **105**: 2730–6.

BACKGROUND. The platelet Gp IIb/IIIa inhibitor abciximab has been associated with an improved long-term survival when used as an adjunct to percutaneous coronary revascularization in diabetic patients. It is unclear whether a similar benefit may be achieved with other Gp IIb/IIIa inhibitors. Analysis of the subgroup of diabetic patients enrolled in the TARGET trial (do Tirofiban And ReoPro Give similar Efficacy outcomes Trial), a head-to-head comparison between tirofiban and abciximab used at the time of percutaneous coronary stent implantation could provide some insight into this issue.

INTERPRETATION. In the TARGET trial, randomization was stratified according to diabetic status to allow a similar distribution of diabetic patients among the two treatment arms. Overall, 1117 patients (23% of the total population) had diabetes. At 1 year, mortality tended to be higher in diabetics than in non-diabetic patients (2.5 vs 1.6%). In the diabetic subgroup, major baseline clinical and procedural characteristics were well balanced between the two treatment groups. The rate of events (death, MI, target vessel revascularization) at 6 months and 1 year was not different between diabetics treated with tirofiban or abciximab. In particular the 1-year mortality rate was 2.9% in diabetics treated with abciximab and 2.1% in diabetics treated with tirofiban.

Comment

These data suggest that tirofiban provides a similar benefit to abciximab when used at the time of coronary stent implantation in diabetic patients. Although there was no placebo control group in this study and it is difficult to compare one study with another, it should be mentioned that the 1-year mortality rate in diabetic patients receiving abciximab in the TARGET trial (2.9%) was similar to that seen in diabetic patients receiving abciximab in meta-analysis of the EPIC, EPILOG and EPISTENT trials (2.5%).

Primary angioplasty in diabetic patients with acute MI

Comparison of outcomes of diabetic and non-diabetic patients undergoing primary angioplasty for acute myocardial infarction.

K J Harjai, G W Stone, J Boura, *et al. Am J Cardiol* 2003; **91**: 1041–5.

BACKGROUND. Few studies have focused on the outcome of diabetic patients undergoing primary angioplasty for acute MI. The Gusto IIb trial included only 95 diabetic patients randomized to primary angioplasty.

INTERPRETATION. This study reports the outcome of the 626 diabetic patients included in the seven PAMI trials (PAI-1, PAMI-2, PAMI Stent Pilot, Stent PAMI, Local PAMI, Air PAMI and PAMI-No SOS) who were intended to be treated by primary angioplasty. Diabetic patients had more severe baseline clinical and angiographic characteristics, longer pain onset, longer to-hospital arrival and longer door-to-balloon time. Diabetics were more likely to die in hospital (4.6 vs 2.5%) and by 6 months (8.1% vs 4.2%). After adjusting for other co-factors of mortality, diabetes remained associated with 6-month mortality (Hazard ratio = 1.53) but not with in-hospital mortality (Hazard ratio = 1.1).

Comment

In patients referred for primary angioplasty for an acute MI, diabetic patients have more severe baseline characteristics and the application of treatment is delayed compared with non-diabetic patients. These differences explain the increased in-hospital mortality in diabetic patients compared with non-diabetics, and suggest that reduction of delay in treatment application could improve in-hospital mortality in this high-risk group of patients.

Clinical outcome of patients with diabetes mellitus and acute myocardial infarction treated with primary angioplasty or fibrinolysis.

L F Hsu, K H Mak, K W Law, *et al. Heart* 2002; **88**: 260–5.

BACKGROUND. A *post hoc* analysis of the Gusto IIb trial including 177 diabetic patients with an acute MI suggests that primary angioplasty is associated with a modest improvement in short- and long-term outcome compared with fibrinolysis. It is unclear if the same figure is seen in a non-selected population.

INTERPRETATION. Two hundred and two consecutive diabetic patients with acute MI were treated with fibrinolysis (*n* = 99) or primary angioplasty (*n* = 103) according to patient and physician preference. In patients treated with fibrinolysis, 80% received streptokinase. In patients treated with primary angioplasty 94 received adjunct coronary stenting and 63% received Gp IIb/IIIa inhibitors. Thirty-day follow-up was not different between groups. By 1 year the composite rate of death and re-infarction was lower in the angioplasty group (17.5 vs 31.3%).

Comment

This interesting study reports the outcome of a consecutive series of diabetic patients treated with 'modern' primary angioplasty (stent + Gp IIb/IIIa inhibitors) and suggests a benefit of this strategy over fibrinolysis. It has to be noted, however, that in this study, fibrinolytic treatment was performed with streptokinase in the majority of cases, which is not the best fibrinolytic agent.

PCI in diabetic patients with additional high-risk factors

PCI in diabetics with renal insufficiency

Outcome of patients with chronic renal insufficiency in the bypass angioplasty revascularization investigation.

L A Szczech, P J Best, E Crowley, *et al. Circulation* 2002; **105**: 2253–8.

BACKGROUND. Although severe chronic kidney diseases and diabetes are independent predictors of mortality among patients with CAD, the impact of mild chronic kidney disease in conjunction with diabetes in patients who undergo myocardial revascularization is unknown. Data from the BARI trial allowed provision of such information.

INTERPRETATION. Chronic kidney disease defined as serum creatinine >1.5 mg/dl was observed in 76 (2.1%) of the 3608 patients with multivessel CAD enrolled in the BARI trial and registry. The presence of diabetes defined by treatment with oral hypoglycaemics or insulin at baseline was found in 641 patients (18%). Seven-year all-cause mortality was markedly different for patients on the basis of both the presence and absence of diabetes and chronic kidney disease. Among patients without diabetes, mortality at 7 years was 39% among patients with chronic kidney disease and 12% among patients without chronic kidney disease. Mortality was higher among patients with diabetes, at 28% for patients without chronic kidney disease and 67% for patients with chronic kidney disease. In the fully adjusted model that included the interaction between the presence of chronic kidney disease and diabetes treated with insulin, chronic kidney disease was associated with an even greater risk of mortality among patients with insulin-treated diabetes (relative risk = 3.3) than among those without insulin-treated diabetes (relative risk = 1.88).

Comment

These data clearly demonstrate that diabetic patients with 'moderate' renal insufficiency are at very high risk of death after myocardial revascularization with fewer than a third of patients surviving by 7 years. Because of the lack of power, it is not possible to conclude on the advantage/disadvantage of bypass surgery versus angioplasty in this group of patients. This study suggests that, besides myocardial revascularization, the combination of diabetes and renal insufficiency identifies a group of patients that probably need a very aggressive treatment for atherosclerosis and very close clinical follow-up in an attempt to prevent these complications. This also suggests that further research is required in that field and that new modalities of treatment and follow-up need to be developed for these patients.

Comparative survival of dialysis patients in the United States after coronary angioplasty, coronary artery stenting, and coronary artery bypass surgery and impact of diabetes.

C A Herzog, J Z Ma, A J Collins. *Circulation* 2002; **106**: 2207–11.

BACKGROUND. The optimal method of coronary revascularization in diabetics with chronic kidney disease is unknown. This study investigating the survival of dialysis patients after coronary angioplasty, coronary artery stenting and coronary artery bypass surgery provides some insights to this issue.

INTERPRETATION. Using the US Renal Data system, the outcome of 15 784 chronic dialysis patients undergoing revascularization procedures from January 1995 to December 1998 was investigated. End-stage renal disease was secondary to diabetes in about 45% of cases. Three revascularization procedures were compared: PTCA ($n = 4836$), coronary stenting ($n = 4280$) and bypass surgery ($n = 6668$). In the overall population there was a higher in-hospital mortality rate in the bypass surgery group (8.6%) compared with the two other groups (6.4 and 4.1%). However, by 2 years, survival was better in patients treated by bypass surgery (56%) than in patients treated by PTCA (48%) or stent (48%). After adjustment for confounding factors, the survival advantage of bypass surgery was observed in non-diabetic and diabetic patients. When PTCA and stent patients were compared it appeared that stent implantation reduced total mortality by 10% (relative reduction) and cardiac mortality by 13% (relative reduction) in non-diabetic patients. In the diabetic group, however, coronary stent implantation was not associated with a reduction in mortality compared with balloon angioplasty.

Comment

These data clearly demonstrate that, even in the stent era there is still a survival advantage of bypass surgery versus percutaneous coronary revascularization in patients with end-stage renal disease with or without diabetes. It is unclear, however, how these data apply to patients with less severe renal disease.

PCI in diabetics with a previous bypass surgery

Comparative outcome of percutaneous coronary interventions in diabetics vs non-diabetics with prior coronary artery bypass grafting.

V Mathew, S H Wilson, G W Barsness, R L Frye, R Lennon, D R Holmes.
Eur Heart J 2002; **23**: 1456–64.

BACKGROUND. Diabetic patients have a higher mortality rate after percutaneous coronary revascularization performed on native coronary artery. There is limited information on the outcome of percutaneous coronary revascularization performed in patients with a previous bypass graft.

INTERPRETATION. From January 1996 to 31 August 2000, 1153 patients with a previous bypass surgery underwent a percutaneous coronary revascularization procedure at the Mayo Clinic. Patients with acute MI or cardiogenic shock were excluded. Diabetics represent 28% ($n = 326$) of the population. The procedure was performed in a bypass graft in 42% of cases; stents were used in 82% of cases and Gp IIb/IIIa inhibitors in 40% of cases. Overall, diabetes was associated with an increased mortality (hazard ratio = 1.58). However, when patients were treated for a single-territory coronary artery disease (30% of diabetics), or when complete revascularization was achieved, mortality of diabetic and non-diabetic patients was comparable.

Comment

The high rate of coronary stenting and use of Gp IIb/IIIa inhibitors is highly relevant to the current practice of the majority of centres. This study highlights the importance of achieving complete revascularization in diabetic patients with a previous bypass graft.

Outcome of repeat revascularization in diabetic patients with prior coronary surgery.

J H Cole, E L Jones, J M Craver, *et al. J Am Coll Cardiol* 2002; **40**: 1968–75.

BACKGROUND. The method of revascularization of choice in diabetic patients with multivessel CAD is bypass surgery. However, some diabetic patients with a previous bypass surgery may need repeat revascularization. There is a lack of data on the outcome of such patients after repeat bypass surgery or percutaneous intervention.

INTERPRETATION. The study population was drawn from all patients presenting to Emory University Hospitals from 1985 to 1999. It included 1721 with the diagnosis of diabetes who had previously undergone bypass surgery; 1123 underwent PCI and 598 underwent re-CABG according to physician and patient preference. Hypertension and prior MI were more prevalent in the bypass group. PCI patients had more two- and three-vessel disease. Only 25% of PCI patients underwent coronary stenting and 43% of bypass procedures involved saphenous vein graft. In-hospital outcome was significantly better in PCI patients with lower rates of death (1.6 vs 11%), Q-wave MI (1.25 vs 3.18%) and stroke (0.09 vs 4.68%). However, mortality differences were no longer significant by 5 years (38 vs 39%) or 10 years (68 vs 74%). In diabetic patients with cardiac heart failure, long-term outcome tended to be better when re-CABG was performed rather than PCI. The opposite trend was seen in diabetic patients without cardiac heart failure.

Comment

This study suggests that when repeat revascularization is considered in diabetic patients with a previous bypass surgery and no cardiac heart failure, there is no clear survival advantage to performing a new bypass rather than a percutaneous coronary revascularization procedure. In patients with cardiac heart failure a new bypass may be preferred but at the price of a higher in-hospital complication rate. There are some limitations to the generalization of these data; indeed the rate of stent use was low, whereas the rate of saphenous vein graft use was high in this population.

Percutaneous coronary intervention versus coronary bypass graft surgery for diabetic patients with unstable angina and risk factors for adverse outcomes with bypass. Outcome of diabetic patients in the AWESOME randomized trail and registry.

S P Sedlis, D A Morrison, J D Lorin, *et al. J Am Coll Cardiol* 2002; **40**: 1555–66.

BACKGROUND. In current guidelines, the method of revascularization of choice in diabetic patients with multivessel coronary artery disease is bypass surgery. However, some patients may be high-risk candidates for bypass surgery for various reasons. Analysis of the diabetic subgroup of the Angina With Extremely Serious Operative Mortality Evaluation (AWESOME) trial and registry may provide some insights to this issue.

INTERPRETATION. The AWESOME trial was conducted from 1995 to 2000 and compared survival after percutaneous coronary revascularization or bypass surgery for patients with refractory angina and who were relatively poor candidates for bypass surgery because of at least one of the following risk factors: prior CABG, MI within 7 days, left ventricular ejection fraction <35%, age >70 years or requiring intra-aortic balloon pumping. Data of the diabetic subgroup of patients included in the randomized trial and the associated registry were analysed ($n = 144$ in the randomized trial and $n = 614$ in the registry). In the randomized trial, baseline characteristics were well balanced between treatment groups. In the bypass surgery group, about 80% received at least one mammary artery graft. The proportion of patients treated with stents in the PCI group is unknown. In the registry, diabetic patients referred for bypass surgery tended to be sicker than those referred for angioplasty. In both the trial and the registry, 3-year survival was similar between diabetics treated by bypass surgery or angioplasty (72 vs 81% in the trial and 73 vs 71% in the registry).

Comment

This study suggests that when considering diabetics with a relative high risk for bypass surgery, percutaneous coronary revascularization is a relatively safe alternative to bypass surgery with similar mid-term (3-year) outcome.

Conclusion

Every year provides new findings and new hopes in the treatment of diabetic patients with coronary artery disease, in particular, in the treatment of diabetic patients using percutaneous techniques. The results published this year provide some light and suggest that, although diabetes remains a major risk factor after PCI, stents and Gp IIb/IIIa may provide some benefit in this population, while PCI seems a very reasonable alternative to bypass surgery in diabetics with additional risk factors as demonstrated in the AWESOME trial. Similarly, primary PCI for an acute MI seems an efficient alternative to fibrinolysis in this population.

We are confident that 2003 will provide additional exciting information, including the use of drug-eluting stents in diabetic patients.

References

1. The BARI Investigators. Comparison of coronary bypass surgery with angioplasty. *N Engl J Med* 1996; **335**: 217–25.

2. The BARI Investigators. Seven-year outcome in the BARI by treatment and diabetic status. *J Am Coll Cardiol* 2000; **35**: 1122–9.

3. King S B, Lembo N J, Weintraub W S. A randomized trial comparing coronary angioplasty with coronary bypass surgery. *N Engl J Med* 1994; **331**: 1044–50.

4. Cabri-Trial Participants. First-year results of CABRI (Coronary Agnioplasty versus Bypass Revascularization Investigation). *Lancet* 1995; **346**: 1179.

Part IV

New developments

10

Brachytherapy

Introduction

Brachytherapy is the technique of intravascular delivery of γ- or β-radiation to the vessel wall to inhibit restenosis following percutaneous coronary intervention (PCI). This is achieved by delivery of a radioactive source into a catheter situated within the injured vessel segment following the revascularization procedure. The equipment available for this procedure has been refined in recent years such that most lesions are accessible and brachytherapy has now become a standard tool for the coronary interventionalist.

It has certainly been an interesting year for brachytherapy. The clinical evidence base for this percutaneous treatment has grown over the past 12 months, with many impressive studies serving to consolidate brachytherapy as the 'gold standard', and indeed the only proven therapy for in-stent restenosis. Yet, with the introduction of stents which elute drugs inhibiting neointimal hyperplasia, many commentators have cast doubts over the future of brachytherapy, predicting its early demise with drug-eluting stents becoming the first-line treatment for in-stent restenosis |**1–3**|. The literature supporting brachytherapy continues to grow and the length of follow-up post-irradiation treatment has increased with no obvious long-term ill effects emerging.

In this chapter, we have selected ten studies published in the past year which have advanced our knowledge of brachytherapy and the natural history of in-stent restenosis after treatment with γ- or β-radiation.

Routine intracoronary beta-irradiation; acute and one year outcome in patients at high risk for recurrence of stenosis.
E Regar, K Kozuma, G Sianos, *et al. Eur Heart J* 2002; **23**(13): 1038–44.

BACKGROUND. Intracoronary radiation is a promising therapy potentially reducing restenosis following catheter-based interventions. Currently, only limited data on this treatment are available. The feasibility and outcome in daily routine practice, however, are unknown. In 100 consecutive patients, intracoronary β-radiation was performed with a ⁹⁰Strontium system (Novoste Beta-Cath™) following angioplasty. Predominantly complex (73% type B2 and C) and long lesions (length 24.3 ± 15.3 mm) were included (37% *de novo*, 19% restenotic and 44% in-stent restenotic lesions).

This was an important analysis which helped to extend the brachytherapy evidence base firmly into one patient population in which it is needed most.

Intracoronary beta-radiation to reduce restenosis after balloon angioplasty and stenting; the Beta Radiation in Europe (BRIE) study.

P W Serruys, G Sianos, W van der Giessen, *et al. Eur Heart J* 2002; **23**(17): 1351–9.

B A C K G R O U N D . The Beta Radiation in Europe (BRIE) trial is a registry evaluating the safety and performance of ^{90}Sr delivered locally (Beta-Cath™ system of Novoste) to *de novo* and restenotic lesions in patients with up to two discrete lesions in different vessels. In total, 149 patients (175 lesions) were enrolled; 62 were treated using balloons and 113 using stents. The restenosis rate, the minimal luminal diameter and the late loss were determined in three regions of interest: (a) in a sub-segment of 5 mm containing the original minimal luminal diameter pre-intervention termed target segment; (b) the irradiated segment, 28 mm in length; and (c) the entire analysed segment, 42 mm in length, termed the vessel segment.

I N T E R P R E T A T I O N . Binary restenosis rate was 9.9% for the target segment, 28.9% for the irradiated segment and 33.6% for the vessel segment. These angiographic results include 5.3% total occlusions. Excluding total occlusions binary restenosis rate was 4.9, 25 and 29.9%, respectively. At 1 year the incidence of major adverse cardiac events placed in a hierarchical ranking were: death 2%, MI 10.1%, CABG 2%, and TVR 20.1%. The event-free survival rate was 65.8%. Non-appropriate coverage of the injured segment by the radioactive source, termed geographical miss, affected 67.9% of the vessels, and increased edge restenosis significantly (16.3 vs 4.3%, *P* = 0.004). It accounted for 40% of the treatment failures. The results of this registry reflect the learning process of the practitioner. The full therapeutic potential of this new technology is reflected by the restenosis rate at the site of the target segment. It can only be unravelled once the incidence of late vessel occlusion and geographical miss has been eliminated by the prolonged use of thienopyridine, the appropriate training of the operator applying this new treatment for restenosis prevention, and the use of longer sources.

Comment

This registry of β-radiation brachytherapy using a ^{90}Sr source and the Novoste Beta-Cath™ delivery system is limited in its support of the efficacy of brachytherapy. It includes patients with *de novo* lesions and restenosis following 'plain old balloon angioplasty' (POBA), two groups in whom brachytherapy would not be universally used in most centres today. There is no control group with which to compare and the use of historical controls is not a robust enough method on which to base or change clinical practice. However, the study does address many of the important milestones in the evolution of the technique, partly because patients were enrolled during a period (July 1998 to June 1999) when important concepts of intracoronary radiation treatment were emerging. These include:

Geographical miss, the term given to a balloon- or stent-injured vessel which is not subsequently irradiated. As experience with brachytherapy grew, it became apparent that low-dose irradiation, at the edges of the source, could actually stimulate cellular proliferation in the injured vessel wall |**11**| and that this was the reason for the 'candy wrapper' effect of proximal and distal edge restenosis, seen particularly after the use of radioactive stents |**12**|. An appreciation of geographical miss led to more care being taken with coverage of the injured vessel segment with the radioactive source and a recommendation that the balloon-to-source ratio should be 1:2, particularly in the absence of any evidence to suggest harm was done by irradiating segments of normal vessel proximal or distal to the injured segment. Geographical miss in this study occurred in 67.9% of vessels analysed and was responsible for 40% of the restenosis observed in the treated segment. This high incidence was thought to be due in part to the high proportion (73.8%) of vessels treated post irradiation and the recommendation was made that the delivery of the radiation therapy should be planned as the last intervention.

Quantitative coronary angiographic analysis, which has to be much more complex to analyse these effects and to this end, this paper divides the treated vessel into a number of subsections in order to give an appreciation of where any treatment failure was occurring.

Late stent thrombosis, which was 5.3% at the beginning of the study, but dropped to 2.1% in 1999 with the prolongation of antiplatelet treatment up to 6 months. In keeping with the concept of delayed stent endothelialization after brachytherapy, the incidence of occlusion was much higher (7.3%) after the placement of a stent than compared with balloon angioplasty alone (1.7%). This supports the current clinical practice of avoiding the placement of new stents if possible.

This registry was acquired during the formative phase for brachytherapy and although the results do not greatly influence today's practice, the data carry a number of important messages.

Twelve versus six months of clopidogrel to reduce major cardiac events in patients undergoing gamma-radiation therapy for in-stent restenosis: Washington Radiation for In-Stent Restenosis Trial (WRIST) 12 versus WRIST PLUS.

R Waksman, A E Ajani, E Pinnow, et al. *Circulation* 2002; **106**(7): 776–8.

BACKGROUND. Intracoronary γ-radiation reduces recurrent ISR. Late thrombosis was attenuated with 6 months of aspirin and clopidogrel. We aimed to find out whether 12 months of aspirin plus clopidogrel is superior to a strategy of 6 months following radiation therapy for patients with ISR. One hundred and twenty consecutive patients with diffuse ISR in native coronaries and vein grafts with lesions <80 mm in length underwent percutaneous transluminal coronary angioplasty (PTCA), laser ablation or

Comment

This was a study in a pig coronary model examining the use of an extended radiation source, effectively irradiating normal artery proximal and distal to a stented segment, to conquer the 'edge effect'. As discussed above, edge restenosis appears to be due to the stimulatory effect of low-dose irradiation (dose fall-off) on the intima of injured vessels. The phenomenon was first witnessed with radioactive stents, which often produced a 'candy wrapper' restenotic process |**16**|. The current study used brachy-therapy administered immediately after stent placement in normal swine coronary arteries and therefore must be interpreted with all the caveats of using animal models to understand a biologically different human disease process. However, the edge effect was created in this model and was effectively prevented by lengthening the radiation margins. Indeed, lack of radiation coverage was associated with a 2.3-fold increase in neointimal formation when compared with full treatment beyond the stent margins. The other important observation is that extension of the radiation source beyond the stent margins did not provoke any adverse effect. There had been concerns that radiation may stimulate aberrant neointimal formation in normal vessel segments, particularly if delivered in sub-optimal doses, but this did not appear to be the case in the absence of vascular injury.

The study protocol included the placement of a second stent after delivery of radiation therapy, overlapping with the first and this was shown to stimulate excess neointimal proliferation at the point of overlap. This is in keeping with a worse clinical course in patients who have another stent placed at the time of brachytherapy,

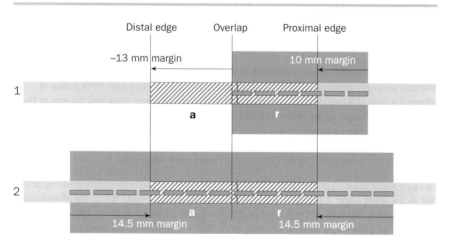

Fig. 10.2 Illustration of procedure. Implantation of reference stent (r) is overlapped by implantation of additional stent (a). 1, ^{192}Ir irradiation with 6-seed train (tip on distal boundary of reference stent). 2, Irradiation with 14-seed train (middle of source on distal boundary of reference stent). Overlap segment is not covered by ^{192}Ir source in 1 (margin, 0 mm) and is fully covered in 2 (margin, 27.5 mm). Source: Cheneau *et al.* (2002).

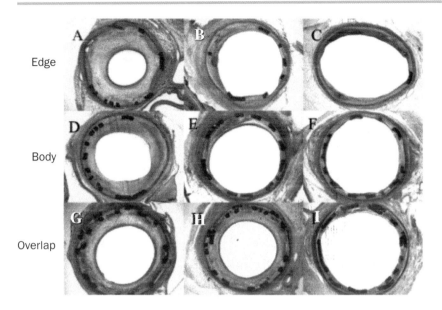

Fig. 10.3 Representative stented segments 28 days after radiation. Lack of radiation coverage provokes an edge effect (A, edge segment with –13-mm radiation margin at 15 Gy). The edge effect is prevented by adequate radiation coverage of 14.5 mm at 15 Gy (B) and 22 Gy (C). In the body of the stent, neointimal proliferation is induced by stent implantation (D, radiation margin, –13 mm at 15 Gy) but is inhibited by radiation coverage (E, radiation margin, 14.5 mm at 15 Gy; F, radiation margin, 14.5 mm at 22 Gy). Intimal proliferation is stimulated at overlapping segments at 15 Gy independently of radiation coverage (G, radiation margin, 0 mm; H, radiation margin, 27.5 mm) but is inhibited by higher radiation dose (I, radiation margin, 27.5 mm, 22 Gy). Source: Cheneau *et al.* (2002).

and this diminished clinical outcome is not completely accounted for by late stent thrombosis. There appears to be a higher TVR rate in patients who undergo additional stent deployment at the time of irradiation providing a further disincentive to use stents at this stage.

Cost-effectiveness of gamma radiation for treatment of in-stent restenosis: results from the Gamma-1 trial.

D J Cohen, R S Cosgrove, R H Berezin, *et al. Circulation* 2002; **106(6)**: 691–7.

BACKGROUND. Recently, several randomized trials have demonstrated that intracoronary brachytherapy can reduce the rates of both angiographic and clinical

restenosis in patients undergoing PCI for in-stent restenosis. Whether this practice is cost-effective is unknown. Between December 1997 and July 1998, 252 patients with in-stent restenosis were randomized to receive brachytherapy or placebo after successful PCI as part of the Gamma-1 trial. We collected detailed resource utilization and cost data for each patient's initial hospitalization and for 1 year after randomization.

INTERPRETATION. Compared with conventional treatment, intracoronary brachytherapy increased procedure duration, physician services and equipment costs. As a result, initial costs were increased by nearly $4100 per patient ($15 724 vs $11 675, $P < 0.001$). Over the 1-year follow-up period, brachytherapy reduced the need for repeat revascularization by 21% and reduced the need for bypass surgery by 44%. Although follow-up medical care costs were $2200/patient lower with brachytherapy, total costs remained higher at 1 year ($28 543 vs $26 737, $P = 0.46$). In a sensitivity analysis that incorporated recent technical modifications and the use of prolonged antiplatelet therapy to prevent late thrombotic occlusion, follow-up cost savings increased to $3600/patient, and 1-year costs were slightly lower with brachytherapy ($26 352 vs $26 729, $P = 0.87$). Subgroup analysis demonstrated significant cost savings in patients with diabetes and patients who did not undergo repeat stenting. As performed in the Gamma-1 trial, coronary brachytherapy for in-stent restenosis improved clinical outcomes but increased 1-year costs compared with standard therapy. If late thrombosis can be eliminated, however, this technology has the potential to reduce overall medical care costs.

Comment

This is a particularly timely study, given the ramifications of the costing of drug-eluting stents in most countries and the debates that this issue has generated. New therapies/devices in interventional cardiology tend to be expensive and brachytherapy is no exception. In order to be accepted as standard practice and to be reimbursed by healthcare systems, these new therapies must not only be efficacious, but must also be cost-effective so that short-term expense can be justified to the health economists by longer term savings. This study prospectively utilized the patient cohort of the Gamma-1 trial |17| to analyse the total costs of patient treatment up to 1 year after randomization in the placebo and γ-brachytherapy arms and it represents the first detailed cost-effectiveness analysis of brachytherapy.

In the basic cost analysis, although the increased initial cost of the technique ($4100 per patient) was partially offset by the saving due to decreased target vessel revascularization ($2100 per patient), the overall cost remained higher ($1800 per patient) in the brachytherapy group than the placebo group. However, as a result of evolution of the technique during the course of the Gamma-1 trial, a number of features confound the cost analysis such as routine use of intravascular ultrasound (IVUS) to determine radiation dose and the high incidence of late stent thrombosis with only 8 weeks of combined antiplatelet therapy. Indeed, it was apparent that late stent thrombosis was a critical determinant of the cost-effectiveness of brachytherapy. A secondary, rather speculative 'sensitivity analysis' was used to determine costs making the assumptions that late stent thrombosis would be reduced by prolonged antiplatelet therapy to the rate observed in the placebo group and that routine IVUS

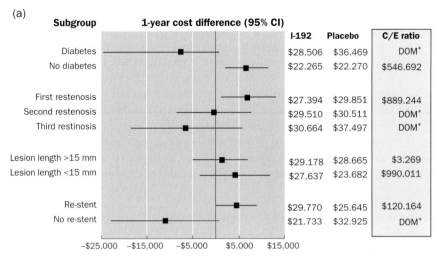

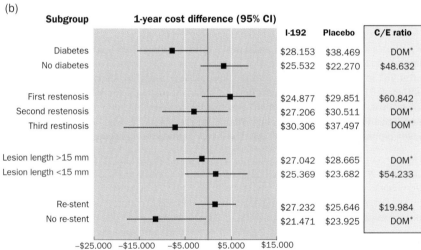

Fig. 10.4 Subgroup analysis of 1-year treatment costs and cost-effectiveness (C/E) with brachytherapy (I-192) or placebo based on primary Gamma-1 trial results (a) or updated treatment and outcome assumptions (b). Each plot indicates the difference in 1-year treatment costs between brachytherapy and conventional treatment along with 95% CI for difference. Shaded column indicates cost-effectiveness ratio for brachytherapy compared with conventional treatment (in dollars per repeat revascularization avoided). *DOM indicates those subgroups for which brachytherapy was economically dominant (i.e. lower aggregate cost and better clinical outcomes). Source: Cohen *et al.* (2002).

would not be required for dosimetry. With these assumptions, the cost saving during the follow-up period post brachytherapy increased to $3600 per patient with the result that there was no longer a significant difference in aggregate 1-year medical care costs between the groups.

An interesting subgroup analysis was performed which showed that brachytherapy was more cost-effective in certain groups of patients. These included groups in whom brachytherapy leads to a greater reduction in clinical events, such as diabetics and lesion lengths of >15 mm. However, cost-effectiveness was also greater in those patients in whom no further stent was deployed at the time of irradiation. This provides another disincentive for repeat coronary stenting in this setting.

It is worth noting that this study used γ-radiation, which requires a greater capital cost for alteration of catheter laboratory facilities to protect personnel and longer procedural times. The cost of β-radiation brachytherapy would have been less in this respect.

Two-year angiographic follow-up of intracoronary Sr^{90} therapy for restenosis prevention after balloon angioplasty.

D Meerkin, M Joyal, J C Tardif, *et al. Circulation* 2002; **106**(5): 539–43.

BACKGROUND. Post-coronary angioplasty VBT has emerged as a successful intervention for restenosis prevention in some clinical scenarios. Longer-term follow-up after VBT in *de novo* non-stented lesions has not been reported. Thirty patients treated with post-PTCA VBT with Sr^{90} underwent clinical and angiographic follow-up at 6 and 24 months. Specific vessel segment quantitative coronary angiographic analyses were performed to identify radiation edge effects. Nineteen patients who had not undergone index procedure stenting or TVR over the 2-year period were analysed separately.

INTERPRETATION. Of the 30 patients, 3 underwent TVR by 6-month follow-up. An additional 4 patients required TVR between 6 and 24 months. In the total cohort of 26 patients undergoing angiographic follow-up at 6 and 24 months, an increase in minimal lumen diameter of the initial target segment was noted at 6 months compared with post-procedure analysis (2.31 ± 0.48 vs 2.04 ± 0.43 mm, *P* <0.05). At 24 months, this was no longer significant (2.19 ± 0.61 mm). In the proximal segments of the entire cohort and the non-intervened subgroup, the principal late loss occurred over the first 6 months with no additional late loss at 2-year follow-up. The distal segments remained stable over the entire follow-up period. Although some late failures of post-PTCA VBT are seen between 6 and 24 months, most treated vessels remain stable with no late loss or additional luminal increase beyond the 6-month period. This suggests that late aneurysm formation and significant late edge restenosis are unlikely in VBT after PTCA of *de novo* lesions for up to 2 years.

Comment

This study provides long-term follow-up of *de novo* brachytherapy after balloon angioplasty. Biologically, radiation therapy would be expected to be more potent in the treatment of ISR (which is due in large part to neointimal hyperplasia) than restenosis after balloon angioplasty alone (a process due to a combination of neo-intimal hyperplasia, vascular recoil and negative remodelling of the vessel wall). Despite this, initial studies of *de novo* brachytherapy were encouraging |**4,18,19**|, showing a reduction in the incidence of restenosis. However, the only randomized controlled trial of *de novo* brachytherapy was confounded by the inclusion of both *de novo* lesions and vessels with restenosis following a previous intervention |**19**|. More-over, the decline in the use of POBA is continuing with >80% stent rates in most centres worldwide, making the results of these studies less relevant to current prac-tice. The introduction of drug-eluting stents into clinical practice, with substantially lower restenosis rates has probably sounded the death knell for *de novo* brachythera-py as a useful clinical tool.

Nevertheless, this study adds to the pool of evidence confirming the absence of significant long-term complications after brachytherapy. It also provides informa-tion about the natural history of restenosis after brachytherapy: both the 6-month luminal gain at the intervened segment and the luminal loss at the edges remain unaltered from 6 months to 2 years post intervention, allaying concerns about a late 'catch-up' phenomenon in restenosis (brachytherapy *delaying* rather than abolishing restenosis).

As with other studies reviewed in this chapter, the practice of brachytherapy was changing during patient recruitment and an appreciation of the importance of geo-graphic miss was not present during the treatment of these patients. Detailed docu-mentation of balloon and radiation source positioning was not performed and this complicated subsequent quantitative angiographic analysis and the assessment of edge restenosis.

Five-year clinical follow-up after intracoronary radiation: results of a randomized clinical trial.

M A Grise, V Massullo, S Jani, *et al. Circulation* 2002; **105**(23): 2737–40.

BACKGROUND. Several clinical trials indicate that intracoronary radiation is safe and effective for the treatment of restenotic coronary arteries. We previously reported 6-month and 3-year clinical and angiographic follow-up demonstrating significant decreases in TLR and angiographic restenosis after γ-radiation of restenotic lesions. The objective of this study was to document the clinical outcome 5 years after treatment of restenotic coronary arteries with catheter-based iridium-192 (^{192}Ir). A double-blind, randomized trail compared ^{192}Ir with placebo sources in patients with restenosis after coronary angioplasty. Over a 9-month period, 55 patients were enrolled; 26 were randomized to ^{192}Ir and 29 to placebo.

INTERPRETATION. At 5-year follow-up, TLR was significantly lower in the ^{192}Ir group (23.1 vs 48.3%, *P* = 0.05). There were two TLRs between years 3 and 5 in patients in the ^{192}Ir group and none in patients in the placebo group. The 5-year event-free survival rate (freedom from death, MI or TLR) was greater in ^{192}Ir-treated patients (61.5 vs 34.5%,

$P = 0.02$). Despite apparent mitigation of efficacy over time, there remains a significant reduction in TLR at 5 years and an improvement in event-free survival in patients treated with intracoronary [192]Ir. The early clinical benefits after intracoronary γ-radiation with ^{192}Ir seem durable at 5-year clinical follow-up.

Comment

This study reports long-term (5-year) follow-up of the original SCRIPPS (Scripps Coronary Radiation to Inhibit Intimal Proliferation Post Stenting) trial patient cohort |**20**|. Although patient numbers are small, it represents the longest follow-up of a randomized, placebo-controlled trial of γ-radiation for the treatment of coronary restenosis. The authors also achieve 100% clinical follow-up. There were no mandated coronary angiograms after year 3 and subsequent events reported in this study were clinically driven. Whilst there appeared to be some attrition in efficacy of brachytherapy over time (there was no longer a significant difference in the combined end-point of death, MI or TVR at 5 years between the groups, which there had been at 3 years |**21**|), there was a significantly better event-free survival over the 5-year period in treatment compared with placebo patients (see Fig. 10.5). Significant differences in target lesion revascularization also persisted over the entire follow-up

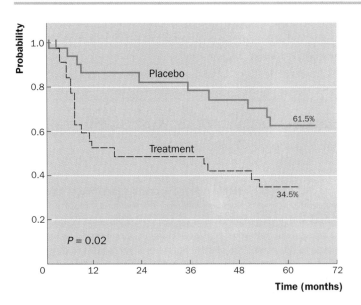

Fig. 10.5 Kaplan–Meier curves for event-free survival in ^{192}Ir and placebo groups. Event-free survival was defined as survival without MI or repeated revascularization of target lesion. The two curves begin to separate at 3 months, and the differences persist throughout the follow-up period. Source: Grise *et al.* (2002).

period. Reassuringly, no long-term ill effects of brachytherapy became apparent in this patient cohort.

It is worth noting that these groups comprised patients with both ISR (62% of patients in each group) and restenosis after balloon angioplasty alone. This may not be entirely representative of the patients treated in current clinical practice in most centres, the majority of whom will have ISR. However, these data suggest that brachytherapy continues to be an effective and safe treatment for at least 5 years.

Intravascular gamma radiation for in-stent restenosis in saphenous-vein bypass grafts.

R Waksman, A E Ajani, R L White, *et al. N Engl J Med* 2002; **346**(16): 1194–9.

B A C K G R O U N D . Intracoronary radiation therapy is effective in reducing the recurrence of ISR in native coronary arteries. We examined the effects of intravascular γ-radiation in patients with ISR of saphenous vein bypass grafts. A total of 120 patients with ISR in saphenous vein grafts (SVG), the majority of whom had diffuse lesions, underwent balloon angioplasty, atherectomy, additional stenting or a combination of these procedures. If the intervention was successful, the patients were randomly assigned in a double-blind fashion to intravascular treatment with a ribbon containing either ^{192}Ir or non-radioactive seeds. The prescribed dose, delivered at a distance of 2 mm from the source, was 14–15 Gy in vessels that were 2.5–4.0 mm in diameter and 18 Gy in vessels with a diameter that exceeded 4.0 mm. The primary end-points were death from cardiac causes, Q wave MI, revascularization of the target vessel, and a composite of these events at 12 months.

I N T E R P R E T A T I O N . Revascularization and radiation therapy were successfully accomplished in all patients. At 6 months, the restenosis rate was lower in the 60 patients assigned to the ^{192}Ir group than in the 60 assigned to the placebo group (21 vs 44%, $P = 0.005$). At 12 months, the rate of revascularization of the target lesion was 70% lower in the ^{192}Ir group than in the placebo group (17 vs 57%, $P < 0.001$), and the rate of major cardiac events was 49% lower (32 vs 63%, $P < 0.001$). The results of our study support the use of γ-radiation therapy for the treatment of ISR in patients with bypass grafts.

Comment

This elegant study definitively extends the evidence base for the use of brachytherapy for ISR from native coronary arteries to SVGs. In contrast to many of the other studies, it has very few confounding features and studies a homogenous patient population with (mainly diffuse) ISR in a SVG. Such patients pose a significant challenge to the interventional cardiologist and as the authors point out, acceptable alternative treatments for these patients are limited. This is a randomized, placebo-controlled trial and all patients in the treated group received γ-radiation in a standardized way. Angiographic follow-up is provided at 6 months with clinical data to 12 months and the results are impressive: the minimum lumen diameter is significantly greater in the brachytherapy group, the late loss significantly lower and the risk of a cardiac event significantly lower in this group at 12 months (see Fig. 10.6). The decrease in major adverse cardiac event (MACE) rate in the treated group is driven by a dramatic reduction in TLR (70% reduction) and TVR (55% reduction). Safety was confirmed both peri-procedurally and up to 12 months. Owing to increased awareness of geographic miss there was no evidence of edge restenosis, emphasizing the effectiveness of adequate coverage of injured vessel with the radiation source in avoiding this complication.

An appreciation of the need for prolonged antiplatelet therapy to avoid late stent thrombosis was gained during the patient recruitment for this trial (the latter 35 patients received 6 months of antiplatelet therapy) suggesting that the benefit of brachytherapy could have been underestimated, with better results if all irradiated patients had received the more prolonged course. However, the absolute rates of late thrombosis were lower in the brachytherapy group than in the placebo group, despite the use of additional stenting in 50% of the patients in both groups.

Although longer term follow-up is obviously required in this group of patients, these findings strongly support the use of brachytherapy for ISR in vein grafts.

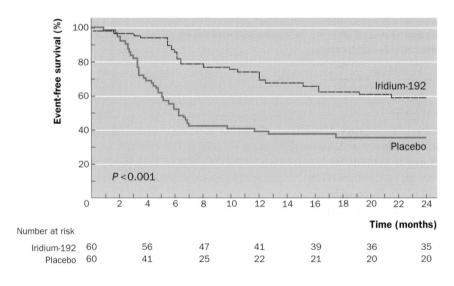

Fig. 10.6 Event-free survival at 24 months. Event-free survival was defined as survival without Q wave myocardial infarction or revascularization of the target vessel. Data were available for 79 of 120 patients at 24 months. Source: Waksman *et al.* (2002).

Long-term outcome of patients treated with repeat percutaneous coronary intervention after failure of gamma-brachytherapy for the treatment of in-stent restenosis.

R Prpic, P S Teirstein, J P Reilly, *et al. Circulation* 2002; **106**(18): 2340–5.

BACKGROUND. **Although ¹⁹²Ir intracoronary brachytherapy has been demonstrated to dramatically reduce the recurrence of ISR, up to 24% of these patients will still require repeat TVR. The short- and long-term outcomes of repeat PCI in this population have not been characterized. Analysis was performed of all patients enrolled in the GAMMA-I and GAMMA-II brachytherapy trials who underwent repeat percutaneous TLR because of restenosis. Subjects were divided into two cohorts: those who had received ¹⁹²Ir brachytherapy and those randomized to placebo.**

INTERPRETATION. Forty-five (17.6%) of a total of 256 patients whose index treatment was intracoronary radiation therapy and 36 (29.8%) of 121 patients whose index treatment was placebo required repeat percutaneous TLR. The mean time to this first TLR was 295 ± 206 days in the irradiated group and 202 ± 167 days in the placebo group ($P = 0.03$). Acute procedural success occurred in 100% of irradiated patients and 94% of placebo controls ($P = 0.19$). After the first TLR, a subsequent TLR was required in 15 (33.3%) of 45 brachytherapy patients versus 17 (47.2%) of 36 placebo failure patients ($P = 0.26$). There was no significant difference in time to second TLR between the two groups. Other long-term major adverse event rates in both groups were comparable with those of other contemporary angioplasty/stenting series. In those patients who 'fail' ¹⁹²Ir intracoronary brachytherapy for ISR, treatment with ¹⁹²Ir delays the time to first TLR. Also, repeat percutaneous intervention in these patients is safe and efficacious in the short-term, with acceptable long-term results.

Comment

Despite the efficacy of brachytherapy, a certain proportion of treated patients will suffer recurrent restenosis and require TLR and this will be the case even in the era of prolonged antiplatelet therapy and the avoidance of geographic miss. Although coronary artery bypass surgery will be indicated in some, repeat percutaneous therapy will maintain considerable appeal in terms of procedural morbidity and mortality, particularly in the setting of single-vessel disease. This study helps to elucidate the natural history of patients who 'fail' brachytherapy and require repeat TLR, comparing them with those who 'fail placebo'.

The study utilizes the patient cohorts from GAMMA-I |**17**| and GAMMA-II |**22**| to determine outcomes of those patients who required TLR having had brachytherapy and those requiring TLR who had placebo. This TLR following the trial was termed the index TLR. There was no significant difference in the *repeat* TLR rate following index TLR in these two groups. Indeed, there was a trend to a lower TLR (33.3%) in the brachytherapy group than that in the placebo group (47.2%), i.e. of the 45 irradi-

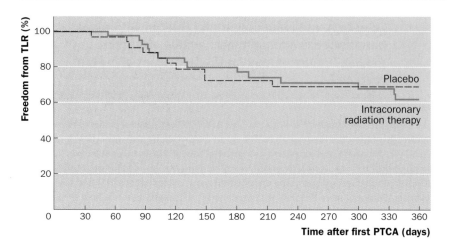

Fig. 10.7 Kaplan–Meier curves demonstrating survival free from second TLR for patients who had PTCA as their first TLR. In irradiated group, 33.3% underwent second TLR compared with 47.2% of placebo group. Plots demonstrate no significant difference between IRT and placebo cohorts ($P = 0.72$). Source: Prpic *et al.* (2002).

ated patients who required repeat TLR by percutaneous means, 33.3% required a further TLR. The fact that this compared favourably with the placebo group and the fact that 66.7% required no further TLR indicates that repeat percutaneous treatment of such cases is a reasonable strategy.

The mean time to first TLR was 295 days in the irradiated group, compared with 202 days in the placebo group, suggesting that brachytherapy may have *delayed* recurrent in-stent restenosis. It is also interesting to note that none of the traditionally accepted risk factors for clinical restenosis were predictive of the need for additional TLR.

Conclusion

Brachytherapy is an effective technique for the treatment of a difficult clinical problem which has evolved alongside a carefully acquired evidence base. Lessons about late stent thrombosis and geographic miss have been learnt quickly and practice has changed accordingly. Indeed, so fast-moving is this field that analysis of studies such as those outlined above is confounded because practice has changed during patient recruitment or shortly afterwards. As a result, treatment within study groups has been heterogeneous and the beneficial effects of radiation treatment have perhaps been underestimated.

In the excitement surrounding the introduction of drug-eluting stents many have sounded the death knell for brachytherapy, assuming that these devices will prove more effective than radiation for the treatment of ISR. This may turn out to be the case, but just as brachytherapy has been rigorously evaluated at every stage of its introduction into clinical practice, drug-eluting stents should be also. Currently, there is no solid evidence base on which to justify the use of these newer devices in the treatment of ISR. In contrast, early reports of the use of sirolimus-eluting stents have been mixed and rather sobering. Although the Brazilian group reported only 1 patient from 25 developing in-stent restenosis at 1-year follow-up with no stent thromboses, deaths or repeat revascularizations |**23**|, the initial European experience has been less encouraging. Degertekin *et al.* |**24**| described 16 patients with ISR also treated with sirolimus-eluting stents: by 9 months two patients had died, one had suffered a Q wave MI and 3 had developed in-stent/in-lesion restenosis. Results with stents eluting other agents have been even more disappointing. The use of a stent eluting a paclitaxel derivative in 15 patients resulted in 61.5% angiographic restenosis at 12 months |**25**|. There are currently no randomized trials comparing drug-eluting stents with the current gold standard, i.e. brachytherapy.

Whilst drug-eluting stents may yet become the gold standard for the treatment of ISR, we would suggest that it is premature to write off brachytherapy at this stage and it is certainly too soon to advocate the routine use of drug-eluting stents in this situation with the current lack of evidence. The past year's evidence has served to consolidate brachytherapy as a safe and efficacious treatment for ISR. However, a year is a long time in interventional cardiology and it remains to be seen whether next year's literature will alter this balance.

References

1. Williams DO. Intracoronary brachytherapy. Past, present and future. *Circulation* 2002; **105**: 2699–700.

2. Seabra-Gomes R. Intracoronary brachytherapy for restenosis: an efficient technique in the struggle for survival? *Eur Heart J* 2002; **23**: 1319–21.

3. Di Mario C, Toutouzas K. No room for radiant dreams in the real world. *Eur Heart J* 2002; **23**: 999–1001.

4. Verin V, Popowski Y, De Bruyne B *et al.* Endoluminal beta-radiation therapy for the prevention of coronary restenosis after balloon angioplasty. *N Engl J Med* 2001; **344**: 243–9.

5. Costa MA, Sabate M, Van der Giessen WJ *et al.* Late coronary occlusion after intracoronary brachytherapy. *Circulation* 1999; **100**: 789–92.

6. Waksman R, Bhargava B, Mintz GM *et al.* Late total occlusion after intracoronary brachytherapy for patients for in-stent restenosis. *J Am Coll Cardiol* 2000; **36**: 65–8.

7. Waksman R, White RL, Chan RC *et al.* Intracoronary gamma-radiation therapy after angioplasty inhibits recurrence in patients with in-stent restenosis. *Circulation* 2000; **10:** 2165–71.

8. Raizner AE, Oesterle SN, Waksman R *et al.* Inhibition of restenosis with beta-emitting radiotherapy: report of the Proliferation Reduction with Vascular Energy Trial (PREVENT). *Circulation* 2000; **102:** 951–8.

9. Teirstein PS, Massullo V, Jani S *et al.* Three-year clinical and angiographic follow-up after intracoronary radiation: results of a randomized clinical trial. *Circulation* 2000; **101:** 360–5.

10. Waksman R, Bhargava B, White L *et al.* Intracoronary beta-radiation therapy inhibits recurrence of in-stent restenosis. *Circulation* 2000; **10:** 1895–8.

11. Carter AJ, Laird JR, Bailey LR *et al.* Effects of endovascular radiation from a beta-particle-emitting stent in a porcine coronary restenosis model. A dose response study. *Circulation* 1996; **94:** 2364–8.

12. Albiero R, Adamian M, Kobayashi N *et al.* Short- and intermediate-term results of ^{32}P radioactive β-emitting stent implantation in patients with coronary artery disease: the Milan dose–response study. *Circulation* 2000; **101:** 18–26.

13. Waksman R, Ajani AE, White RL *et al.* Prolonged antiplatelet therapy to prevent late thombosis after intracoronary gamma-radiation in patients with in-stent restenosis. *Circulation* 2001; **103:** 2332–5.

14. Mehta SR, Yusuf S, Peters RJ *et al.* Effects of pre-treatment with clopidogrel and aspirin followed by long term therapy in patients undergoing percutaneous coronary intervention: the PCI-CURE study. *Lancet* 2001; **358:** 527–33.

15. Steinhubl SR, Berger PB, Mann JT 3rd *et al.* Early and sustained dual oral antiplatelet therapy following percutaneous coronary intervention: a randomized controlled trial. *JAMA* 2002; **288:** 2411–20.

16. Albiero R, Nishida T, Adamian M *et al.* Edge restenosis after implantation of high activity ^{32}P radioactive β-emitting stents. *Circulation* 2000; **101:** 2454–7.

17. Leon MB, Teirstein PS, Moses JW *et al.* Localized intracoronary gamma-radiation therapy to inhibit the recurrence of restenosis after stenting. *N Engl J Med* 2001; **344:** 250–6.

18. Meerkin D, Tardif JC, Crocker IR et al. Effects of intracoronary beta-radiation therapy after coronary angioplasty. An intravascular ultrasound study. *Circulation* 1999; **99:** 1660–5.

19. Raizner AE, Oesterle SN, Waksman R *et al.* Inhibition of restenosis with beta-emitting radiotherapy. Report of the proliferation reduction with vascular energy trial (PREVENT). *Circulation* 2000; **102:** 951–8.

20. Teirstein PS, Massullo V, Jani S *et al.* Catheter-based radiotherapy to inhibit restenosis after coronary stenting. *N Engl J Med* 1997; **336:** 1697–703.

21. Teirstein PS, Massullo V, Jani S *et al.* Three-year clinical and angiographic follow-up after intracoronary radiation: results of a randomized clinical trial. *Circulation* 2000; **101:** 360–5.

22. Wong SC, Teirstein PS, Moses JW *et al.* Nine-month clinical outcomes after intravascular radiation therapy for in-stent restenosis: a report from the GAMMA-II registry. *Am J Cardiol* 2000; **86(suppl. 1):** 8A.

23. Sousa JE, Costa MA, Abizaid A *et al.* Sirolimus-eluting stent for the treatment of in-stent restenosis. A quantitative coronary angiography and three-dimensional intravascular ultrasound study. *Circulation* 2003; **107:** 24–7.

24. Degertekin M, Regar E, Tanabe K *et al*. Sirolimus-eluting stent for treatment of complex in-stent restenosis. *J Am Coll Cardiol* 2003; **41**: 184–9.

25. Liistro F, Stankovic G, Di Mario C *et al*. First clinical experience with a paclitaxel derivative-eluting polymer stent system implantation for in-stent restenosis: immediate and long-term clinical and angiographic outcome. *Circulation* 2002; **105**: 1883–6.

11

No-reflow and distal protection in percutaneous coronary intervention

Introduction

With high-pressure stent deployment, modern anti-platelet therapy, and now the advent of drug-eluting stents, effective and sustained patency of the target vessel can be reliably achieved during percutaneous coronary intervention (PCI). However, vessel patency does not necessarily imply normal myocardial perfusion. The no-reflow phenomenon is defined as the presence of inadequate tissue perfusion in the absence of mechanical vessel obstruction, and complicates 2–5% of all PCI procedures [1]. However, in two specific patient groups its frequency is far higher, and the clinical consequences are considerable.

During PCI for acute coronary syndromes (ACS), no-reflow has an incidence of around 5% in unstable angina, and up to 30% in acute myocardial infarction (AMI) [1,2]. After PCI for AMI, no-reflow is the main predictor of adverse short- and long-term outcome. Myocardial recovery is impaired, in-hospital MI and death are increased up to 10-fold, and the long-term incidence of heart failure, malignant arrhythmias and cardiac death is significantly higher [2,3].

No-reflow is also common during saphenous vein graft (SVG) intervention, and is associated with peri-procedural non Q wave MI in up to a quarter of cases [1,4]. The occurrence of a significant rise in cardiac enzymes after vein graft intervention heralds a worse long-term outcome, including an increase in cardiac death [4].

Understanding the pathophysiology of the no-reflow phenomenon is crucial to developing effective therapeutic interventions. Electron microscopy findings from animal ischaemia/reperfusion models of no-reflow have implicated microvascular dysfunction due to a number of mechanisms. Endothelial dysfunction, vasospasm, tissue oedema, myocyte contracture and intravascular plugging by fibrin, platelets and leukocytes have all been identified [5]. However, strategies that have been successful in preventing or treating experimental models of no-reflow have not worked in human trials. It is possible that the mechanisms of no-reflow in experimental and clinical settings are different. In particular, mechanical disruption of thrombus and atheroma, with subsequent distal embolization, is likely to be an important factor in no-reflow during PCI that is not recognized in pure ischaemia/reperfusion models.

In addition to mechanical obstruction of small vessels and capillaries by embolic material, platelet emboli release vasoactive substances, whereas atheromatous debris rich in thrombogenic tissue factor may also contribute to no-reflow [6,7]. The observation that no-reflow is most prevalent in the context of AMI, when thrombus burden is highest, and SVG PCI, when lesions are most friable, is consistent with a role for distal embolization. The advent of distal protection devices (DPDs) has enabled the contribution of distal embolization to be better defined. Embolic material was retrieved in 100% of procedures in SVGs, and 73% in native coronary arteries during initial clinical experience with 33 patients using the FilterWire DPD [8]. In 26% of cases platelets or fibrin only were retrieved; 74% also had plaque material.

Initial efforts to establish an effective treatment for no-reflow focused on the contribution of vasospasm, and the potential benefit of vasodilator therapy. Many agents have been evaluated in the setting of no-reflow, predominately in relatively small observational studies. Verapamil, adenosine, sodium nitroprusside, nicorandil and papaverine have all been shown to have the potential to improve coronary flow and/ or myocardial perfusion [9]. However, there are as yet no firm data from large randomized trials that vasodilator therapy improves outcome following no-reflow.

Because of the role of platelet emboli, glycoprotein (Gp) IIb/IIIa platelet receptor inhibitors may be beneficial in the prevention of no-reflow. These drugs are known to reduce the rate of death/MI following PCI [10], and have been found to improve no-reflow in the setting of AMI [11]. However, the major contribution of atheromatous debris to embolic material retrieved from distal protection devices, particularly from vein grafts, emphasizes the limited potential of Gp IIb/IIIa inhibitors. Indeed, a recent meta-analysis indicated that Gp IIb/IIIa inhibitors have no impact on clinical outcome during SVG PCI [12].

With increasing recognition of the role of distal embolization, attention has shifted to the potential of mechanical interventions to prevent no-reflow. Thrombectomy devices can remove *in situ* thrombus prior to angioplasty and stent deployment, whereas DPDs aim to prevent embolic material reaching the microvascular bed. Preliminary studies with DPDs in particular have been encouraging [8,13].

Over the past year several papers have been published which have increased our understanding of the no-reflow phenomenon, and which have explored the therapeutic options available. In particular, seminal studies evaluating the role of DPDs have presented their findings, with consequent major changes in clinical practice. We present the key findings of these papers, and attempt to put them into context to summarize the current status of no-reflow and DPDs in clinical interventional practice.

No-reflow is an independent predictor of death and myocardial infarction after percutaneous coronary intervention.

F S Resnic, M Wainstein, M K Y Lee, *et al. Am Heart J* 2003; **145**: 42–6.

BACKGROUND. The objectives of this study were to determine the effect of no-reflow on clinical outcomes after PCI, to identify risk factors for its development, and to assess the effect of pharmacological interventions for no-reflow on clinical outcome. The study was a prospective observational review of 4264 patients undergoing PCI in a single centre. One hundred and thirty-five patients (3.2%) developed no-reflow. No-reflow was more common in patients with unstable angina (multivariate odds ratio [OR] 1.5), AMI (OR 3.5) and SVG intervention (OR 5.3). Rates of peri-procedural death and/or MI were much higher in patients in whom no-reflow developed (Fig. 11.1). Even after multivariate logistic regression, no-reflow remained a strong predictor of death and MI (OR 3.6). The risk of death/MI was much lower in patients in whom no-reflow complicated SVG intervention than after native vessel PCI (7.7 vs 19.4%, *P* = 0.018). Although use of nitroprusside (but not verapamil) resulted in a greater improvement in flow than patients treated conservatively, neither nitroprusside nor verapamil influenced clinical outcome (OR for death/MI 1.04 for patients treated with nitroprusside, 0.94 for verapamil).

INTERPRETATION. This study confirms previous findings that the risk of no-reflow during PCI is greatest in SVG intervention and in AMI, and is also increased in unstable angina. The occurrence of no-reflow is associated with a much higher rate of death/MI, particularly

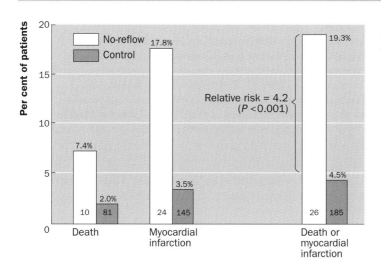

Fig. 11.1 The risk of death or MI in patients with no-reflow compared with patients without no-reflow. Source: Resenic *et al.* (2003).

after native vessel PCI. Although pharmacological interventions may improve flow, this study suggests that they have no effect on clinical outcomes.

Comment

This study provides further evidence for the adverse consequences of no-reflow during PCI, with high rates of death/MI, particularly after native vessel intervention for ACS (primarily AMI). The poor outcome of no-reflow during native vessel PCI is accompanied by the absence of effective treatment. A number of studies have shown beneficial effects on flow with vasodilators, but none has provided firm evidence of improved outcome. This study found no effect on clinical outcome with vasodilator therapy, despite improved flow with nitroprusside. Outcome after no-reflow in SVG PCI is less poor, and, as discussed below, proven effective mechanical interventions to prevent no-reflow and improve outcome are now available.

Angiographic morphologic features of infarct-related arteries and timely reperfusion in acute myocardial infarction.

HK Yip, MC Chen, HW Chang, *et al. Chest* 2002; **122**: 1322–32.

B A C K G R O U N D . No-reflow complicating PCI for AMI is associated with a poor outcome. The aim of this study was to evaluate whether pre-revascularization angiographic characteristics of the infarct-related artery could be used to predict the occurrence of no-reflow. The study was a retrospective observational review of 825 patients undergoing PCI for AMI in a single centre. One hundred and twenty patients (15.1%) developed no-reflow (Thrombolysis in Myocardial Infarction [TIMI] flow grade <3). Eight pre-specified angiographic morphological features were evaluated to determine the association with occurrence of no-reflow. Six of these features were strongly predictive of the development of no-reflow (Table 11.1): reference lumen diameter (RLD) ≥4 mm, cut-off pattern of occlusion, presence of floating thrombus proximal to occlusion, presence of accumulated thrombus, presence of persistent dye staining distal to obstruction, incomplete obstruction with angiographic thrombus >3× RLD in length (Type II lesion).

I N T E R P R E T A T I O N . Large vessels and heavy thrombus burden are associated with increased risk of no-reflow during PCI for AMI. Specific angiographic morphological features can be used to identify a heavy thrombus burden, and consequently to predict the risk of no-reflow.

Comment

Death and MI are frequent consequences when no-reflow complicates PCI in AMI. Identification of patients at greatest risk would allow targeting of adjunctive pharmacological or mechanical interventions to prevent no-reflow. Intravascular

Table 11.1 Multiple stepwise logistic regression analysis of angiographic morphologic features of infarct-related arteries (IRAs) in predicting slow-flow or no-reflow reperfusion after coronary angioplasty

Variables	Odds ratio	95% Confidence interval	P value
Type II lesion	1.56	1.23–1.98	0.0003
Cutoff pattern	7.09	3.88–12.98	0.0001
Presence of accumulated thrombus	3.45	2.09–5.826	0.003
Presence of floating thrombus proximal to occlusion	4.34	1.24–15.14	0.021
Presence of persistent dye staining distal to obstruction	3.22	1.02–10.15	0.046
RLD ≥4.0 mm	4.14	2.439–7.2	0.0001

RLD, reference lumen diameter.
Source: Yip *et al.* (2002).

ultrasound (IVUS) lesion characteristics, in particular lesion elastic membrane cross-sectional area (i.e. vessel size) and a lipid-pool-like image, have previously been shown to predict risk of no-reflow in AMI |**14**|. However, most centres performing infarct angioplasty will not routinely use IVUS. The characterization of angiographic features that predict risk of no-reflow is, therefore, an important advance.

Intracoronary verapamil for reversal of no-reflow during coronary angioplasty for acute myocardial infarction.

G S Werner, K Lang, H Kuehnert, H R Figulla. *Cathet Cardiovasc Intervent* 2002; **57**: 444–51.

BACKGROUND. Retrospective observational studies have demonstrated improved microvascular perfusion and myocardial salvage using the vasodilator verapamil. This was a prospective observational study of the effects of verapamil on coronary flow in patients with no-reflow complicating PCI for AMI. In a consecutive series of 212 patients undergoing primary or rescue PCI for AMI, 23 (10.8%) developed no-reflow. All 23 patients were treated with intracoronary verapamil, administered distal to the target lesion via a perfusion catheter. Coronary flow was assessed by TIMI flow grade and TIMI frame count before and after verapamil. TIMI flow grade improved after verapamil in 20 patients (87%) and was TIMI-3 in 15 (65%). TIMI frame count improved from 90 ± 65 frames to 28 ± 17 frames (*P* <0.001) (Fig. 11.2).

INTERPRETATION. In a small observational study, intracoronary verapamil administered distal to the target lesion improves coronary flow in patients with established no-reflow during PCI for AMI.

Comment

Because microvascular spasm is believed to be one mechanism responsible for no-reflow, many studies have evaluated the effects of vasodilator therapy. Adenosine, verapamil, nitroprusside, nicorandil and papaverine have all been shown to improve flow in patients with no-reflow complicating PCI [9]. This study provides further evidence that verapamil is effective in increasing coronary flow. However, the majority of published studies have been observational, and, although vasodilators can improve flow, there is little or no evidence that clinical outcome is affected. In addition, whether prophylactic vasodilator therapy, as opposed to treatment for established no-reflow, might be effective also remains unclear from the available literature. In the VAPOR (VAsodilator Prevention On no-Reflow) trial of 22 patients undergoing vein graft PCI, no-reflow was reduced in patients randomized to pre-treatment with intragraft verapamil [15]. In another small, randomized study, routine administration of intra-coronary adenosine during primary PCI for AMI resulted in less frequent occurrence of no-reflow, reduced Q-wave MI and improved left ventricular (LV) function [16]. However, larger randomized studies are required to assess the effects of vasodilator therapy on no-reflow and clinical outcome during PCI, to establish which vasodilator agent is most effective, and to determine whether a strategy of prophylactic or treatment use of vasodilators is more beneficial.

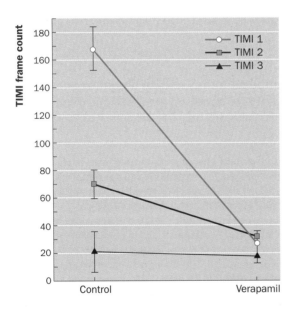

Fig. 11.2 Comparison of the effect of verapamil on TIMI frame count in patients with different severity of no-reflow or unimpaired flow (TIMI 1–3) after percutaneous transluminal coronary angioplasty for AMI. Source: Stone *et al.* (2002).

Randomized trial of a distal embolic protection device during percutaneous coronary intervention of saphenous vein aorto-coronary bypass grafts. (SAFER [Saphenous vein graft Angioplasty Free of Emboli Randomized] trial.)

D S Baim, D Wahr, B George, *et al. Circulation* 2002; **105**: 1285–90.

BACKGROUND. Distal embolization of atherothrombotic debris has been proposed as a major factor in the occurrence of no-reflow and subsequent adverse outcome in SVG intervention. Preliminary studies with DPDs demonstrated almost universal recovery of atherosclerotic plaque debris, as well as fewer adverse events with device use |8,13|. In this study, 801 eligible patients undergoing SVG PCI were randomly assigned to stent placement using a PercuSurge Guardwire DPD, or a conventional angioplasty guidewire. The Guardwire incorporates a distal occlusion balloon inflated for the duration of the procedure, with subsequent aspiration of blood and any embolic material. The primary end-point of the study was 30-day major adverse cardiac event (MACE; death/MI/target lesion revascularization). There was a 42% relative reduction in 30-day MACE in the Guardwire patients compared with controls (9.6 vs 16.5%, *P* = 0.004), owing primarily to reduced incidence of non-Q wave MI (7.4 vs 13.7%) (Table 11.2). The trial was not powered to show a significant reduction in mortality, but there was a trend (1.0 vs 2.3%,

Table 11.2 Clinical outcomes of 801 patients with saphenous vein graft lesions treated by stenting assigned to receive Guardwire embolic protection or conventional guidewire

Clinical end-point	Guardwire (*n* = 406)	Control (*n* = 395)	*P*
Primary end-point (30 day)	39 (9.6)	65 (16.5)	0.004
Myocardial infarction (30 day)	35 (8.6)	58 (14.7)	0.008
Q wave MI	5 (1.2)	5 (1.3)	
Non-Q wave MI (>3 times normal)	30 (7.4)	54 (13.7)	
CK-MB fraction 3–8 times upper limit normal	19 (4.7)	31 (7.8)	
CK-MB fraction >8 times upper limit normal	12 (3.0)	19 (4.8)	
Any CK-MB elevation above upper limit of normal	66 (16.3)	95 (24.1)	0.006
Death (30 day)	4 (1.0)	9 (2.3)	0.17
Emergent bypass surgery (30 day)	0	2 (0.5)	0.24
Subgroup analyses			
In patients with intent to use IIb/IIIa antagonist	25/232 (10.8)	42/232 (18.1)	0.03
In patients with intent *not* to use IIb/IIIa antagonist	14/174 (8.0)	23/163 (14.1)	0.08
Actual use of a IIb/IIIa antagonist (*n* = 244)	26/244 (10.7)	48/247 (19.4)	0.008
No actual use of a IIb/IIIa antagonist (*n* = 162)	13/162 (8.0)	17/148 (11.5)	0.34

Values are *n* (%) or *n*/total subset (%). CK-MB = creatinine kinase-myocardial band.
Some patients had >1 event.
Source: Baim *et al.* (2002).

P = 0.17). No-reflow was also significantly reduced (3 vs 9%, *P* = 0.001). Technical success with the Guardwire was achieved in 90.1%. Use of Gp IIb/IIIa inhibitors was at the discretion of the operators, and did not affect the benefit seen with the Guardwire.

INTERPRETATION. This large randomized trial demonstrates that the Guardwire balloon occlusion/aspiration distal protection device considerably reduces no-reflow and non-Q wave MI during SVG intervention.

Comment

The results of this study provide powerful evidence for the benefit of distal protection devices in vein graft intervention, and have dramatically altered clinical practice. Most centres now consider the use of a DPD mandatory during vein graft PCI. Criticism has been made of the differences in procedural characteristics of the patient groups, in particular the higher rate of direct stenting in the Guardwire group (79.4 vs 67.7%, *P* = 0.0002), which may have influenced outcome |**17**|. However, further analysis provided by the authors showed that the beneficial effect of the Guardwire was also seen in the direct stent subgroup |**17**|. Some reservations persist after this study regarding distal protection. Patients were only eligible if the target lesion was located in the mid-portion of a vein graft. The Guardwire is not appropriate for distal lesions, for which deployment of the device proximal to the graft insertion is not possible. There was technical failure of the Guardwire in 10% of eligible patients, in whom outcomes were the same as in the control group. For these two groups of patients technical modifications of available protection devices, or alternative strategies, will be necessary.

Distal filter protection during saphenous vein graft stenting: technical and clinical correlates of efficacy.

G W Stone, C Rogers, S Ramee, *et al. J Am Coll Cardiol* 2002; **40**: 1882–8.

BACKGROUND. Although the SAFER trial clearly demonstrated the efficacy of balloon occlusion and aspiration systems such as the Guardwire in reducing atherothrombotic embolization and peri-procedural MI, no such data existed to support the use of the alternative filter-based DPDs. This paper reported both the phase I and phase II prospective observational multicentre registries of the FilterWire EX DPD in vein graft PCI. In the phase I study, 48 eligible patients underwent intervention of 60 SVG lesions with FilterWire distal protection. After analysis of the 30-day results, 230 consecutive patients subsequently underwent PCI of 248 SVG lesions. Adverse event rate in phase I was higher than expected, with a 30-day MACE of 21.3%, and non-Q wave MI 17.1%. Detailed procedural and angiographic analysis identified four correctable technical errors associated with adverse events, leading to five specific technique and operator instructions incorporated into phase II. Outcomes in phase II were much improved (Fig. 11.3), with 30 day MACE 11.3%, and non-Q wave MI 9.6%. No-reflow occurred in

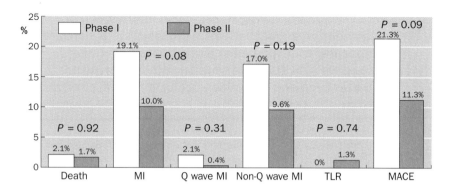

Fig. 11.3 Cumulative 30-day MACE rates in 48 patients in the phase I study compared to 230 patients in the phase II study. TLR = target lesion revascularization. Source: Stone *et al.* (2002).

5.0%. These results were better than seen with historical controls, and similar to outcomes of the Guardwire group in the SAFER study. Technical success was achieved in 96.5% of cases.

INTERPRETATION. In an observational study these findings indicate that the FilterWire filter-based DPD has acceptable safety and efficacy in vein graft intervention. Adherence to specific technical aspects of device use is essential to optimize outcome.

Comment

After presentation and publication of the SAFER study, use of DPDs in vein graft intervention became widespread. Because of their relative ease of use and maintenance of perfusion, distal filters were employed by many interventional cardiologists in preference to the balloon occlusion/aspiration Guardwire system, despite no evidence of equivalent efficacy. This study provides some evidence for the efficacy and safety of the FilterWire EX. The data also illustrate the importance of correct procedure in utilization of the device, in order to achieve satisfactory outcomes. The awaited second-generation FilterWire EZ has an improved design, which should make some of these technical considerations less important, and should potentially, therefore, improve 'real-world' outcomes. The results of this study do not provide an equivalent evidence base to the randomized-controlled trial demonstrating the efficacy of the Guardwire. The subsequent phase III non-inferiority randomized comparison of the FilterWire EX and Guardwire was designed to determine the true relative efficacy of these devices. The results are discussed below.

FIRE (FllterWiRE during transluminal intervention of saphenous vein grafts) study: a prospective randomized multicenter trial comparing distal protection during saphenous vein graft intervention with a filter-based catheter compared to balloon occlusion and aspiration.

G W Stone, C Rogers, J B Hermiller Jr, *et al.* for the FIRE investigators. ACC Scientific Sessions. Late breaking trials. Chicago, 31 March 2003.

BACKGROUND. The phase II trial of the FilterWire EX filter-based DPD demonstrated satisfactory results, with similar outcomes to those achieved by the Guardwire balloon occlusion/aspiration system in the SAFER trial. The FIRE study was a randomized controlled trial comparing the FilterWire and Guardwire DPDs in SVG intervention, and was designed to show non-inferiority of the FilterWire with a primary end-point of 30-day MACE. Six hundred and fifty-one patients were randomized to FilterWire EX or Guardwire. At 30-day follow-up there was no significant difference between the FilterWire and the Guardwire in rate of MACE (9.9 vs 11.6%, *P* = 0.53) or non-Q wave MI (8.1 vs 9.7%). In both groups the device was successfully deployed in >95% of cases (*P* = NS).

INTERPRETATION. The FilterWire EX filter-based distal protection device is safe and effective in SVG PCI, with similar rates of major adverse cardiac events at 30 days to the Guardwire balloon occlusion and aspiration system.

Comment

The SAFER trial provided powerful evidence that the Guardwire distal protection device has a major impact on rate of non-Q wave MI after SVG intervention, and that distal protection should be considered mandatory in SVG PCI. Filter based devices such as the FilterWire are easier to use, and have the inherent advantage of maintained perfusion. The FIRE study provides a sound evidence base for equal efficacy of the FilterWire. Like the Guardwire, however, it cannot be used to protect distal vein graft lesions during PCI.

A prospective, randomized trial of thromboatherectomy during intervention of thrombotic native coronary arteries and saphenous vein grafts: the X-TRACT (X-sizer for TReatment of thrombus and Atherosclerosis in Coronary interventions Trial) trial.

G W Stone, D A Cox, J D Babb, *et al*. ACC Scientific Sessions. Late breaking trials. Chicago, 31 March 2003.

BACKGROUND. During native coronary artery PCI, no-reflow and subsequent adverse outcome is most frequent in thrombotic lesions. Degenerative SVG commonly have friable lipid-rich atheroma with adherent thrombus. Preliminary studies of thromboatherectomy devices have suggested they may reduce no-reflow and improve outcome in these patient groups |19,20|. In the multicentre X-TRACT trial, 800 consecutive patients with diseased SVGs (72%), or native coronary lesions containing thrombus (28%) were prospectively randomized to conventional PCI versus thromboatherectomy using the X-SIZER system. The primary end-point was 30-day MACE. The X-SIZER is a dual-lumen catheter with a helical cutter within the inner lumen, and a vacuum connected to the outer lumen to allow removal of fragmented thrombus. Thrombectomy was performed immediately prior to angioplasty and/or stenting. Gp IIb/IIIa inhibitors were administered in 78% of each group. There was no difference in 30-day MACE (death/MI/target vessel revascularization) between the X-SIZER and control groups (17.0 vs 17.4%, P = NS). The X-SIZER did, however, lower the rate of pre-specified large MI (Q wave MI or CK-MB >8× normal) by 41% (5.5 vs 9.6%, P = 0.03).

INTERPRETATION. Adjunctive thromboatherectomy with the X-SIZER system did not reduce 30-day MACE in a mixed cohort of SVG PCI and PCI in thrombotic native coronary lesions. The X-SIZER system did reduce rate of large MI.

Comment

A number of small observational and randomized studies, primarily in the setting of AMI, have suggested that adjunctive treatment with the X-SIZER and other thrombectomy devices may improve flow, and potentially outcome, following PCI |**19,20**|. The X-TRACT trial is the first major randomized trial of adjunctive thrombectomy, and the results are clearly disappointing. In SVG PCI routine use of distal protection devices has been shown to dramatically reduce non-Q wave MI and MACE, whereas no such benefit was shown with the X-SIZER. It seems clear that DPDs are the adjunctive mechanical intervention of choice during vein graft intervention. If thrombectomy is to have a place, it is likely to be for PCI in native vessels with a heavy thrombus burden, primarily in AMI. Future studies should focus on this patient group, perhaps selecting those patients with high-risk angiographic and/or IVUS criteria for embolization and no-reflow |**14,21**|.

Effect of percutaneous coronary intervention for in-stent restenosis in degenerated saphenous vein grafts without distal embolic protection.

D T Ashby, G Dangas, E A Aymong, *et al. J Am Coll Cardiol* 2003; **14**: 749–52.

BACKGROUND. Unequivocal evidence exists that distal embolization frequently leads to no-reflow and peri-procedural MI during percutaneous intervention for *de novo* lesions in degenerated SVGs, and that DPDs reduce the incidence of these adverse outcomes. The pathology of in-stent restenosis (ISR), including in SVGs, is distinct, consisting predominantly of neointimal smooth muscle cells and extracellular matrix, and may be less likely to result in distal embolization of debris during the PCI procedure. The investigators, therefore, hypothesized that distal protection might not be necessary in the treatment of ISR in degenerated vein grafts. This was a single-centre retrospective observational study of 54 patients undergoing PCI without distal protection for ISR in SVGs. Patients were treated by angioplasty alone, cutting balloon angioplasty, or deployment of a further stent, with brachytherapy in a minority of cases. There were no cases of no-reflow, slow flow, or in-hospital non-Q wave MI (Table 11.3). There was only one MACE: a patient had non-cardiac death due to respiratory failure from pneumonia and chronic obstructive pulmonary disease.

INTERPRETATION. In contrast to PCI for *de novo* lesions, treatment of ISR in vein grafts is not associated with distal embolization, no-reflow and peri-procedural MI. Hence, distal protection is unnecessary.

Comment

Because distal protection is now considered mandatory for PCI to *de novo* vein graft disease, this study sought to address whether it should also be considered in the treatment of ISR in SVGs. Although there is some evidence of conventional athero-sclerotic disease causing ISR in vein grafts |22|, most ISR is caused by pathologically distinct neointima. Intuitively, therefore, distal embolization would not be con-sidered a likely complication of PCI for ISR. The findings of this study support the theory that PCI for ISR of SVGs is not associated with distal embolization, and distal protection is not required.

Table 11.3 Procedural outcomes and in-hospital events

Variables	Values
Procedural outcomes	
Procedural success	98.1% (53/54)
No-reflow/slow flow*	0% (0/54)
Dissection	1.9% (1/54)
Threatened/abrupt closure	0% (0/54)
Final ACT (s)	283 ± 76
CK-MB fraction 1–3 times upper limit of normal	3.7% (2/54)
CK-MB fraction >3 times upper limit of normal	0% (0/54)
In-hospital events	
MACE	2% (1/54)
Death	2% (1/54)
Cardiac death	0% 0/54)
Q wave MI	0% (0/54)
Non-Q wave MI	0% (0/54)
Repeat target lesion PCI	0% (0/54)
Length of stay in-hospital	2.2 ± 2.3 days (range 1–11 days)

* No-reflow = TIMI 0–1 flow; slow flow = TIMI 2 flow.
ACT = activated clotting time.
Source: Ashby *et al.* (2003).

Conclusion

Recognition that no-reflow following PCI is distinct from traditional experimental animal models, with distal embolization the central factor, has been key to recent progress in treatment. Embolic material causes mechanical obstruction, and can trigger microvascular dysfunction via vasospasm, *in situ* thrombosis, capillary plugging and endothelial dysfunction.

During vein graft PCI distal protection with either a filter-based device or a distal occlusion/aspiration system should be used in every case unless technically not feasible. Where the target lesion is too distal to allow deployment of a DPD no effective alternative is yet available. There is no evidence to support a role for thrombectomy.

Although no-reflow complicating native vessel PCI for AMI has a particularly poor outcome, no adjunctive therapy has yet been proven to be effective. Results from the first large trial of thrombectomy were disappointing. Preliminary studies using distal protection devices have reported favourable results [23,24], while some investigators have advocated the use of thrombectomy and distal protection in tandem [25]. Our practice is to employ a DPD in large vessels and when there is angiographic evidence of a heavy thrombus burden. We would reserve thrombectomy for cases of refractory thrombus. Further randomized trials are required to determine the optimal adjunctive mechanical therapy for PCI in AMI.

The precise role of vasodilator therapy is also unclear. On current evidence, prophylactic treatment with verapamil or adenosine, administered distal to the target lesion, is recommended in high-risk native vessel PCI. For treatment of established no-reflow, verapamil, adenosine or nitroprusside can be used. Larger trials are needed.

Recognition of the no-reflow phenomenon has established normal myocardial perfusion as the new therapeutic goal for PCI. The challenge of the next decade will be to develop further adjunctive treatment modalities to achieve this goal.

References

1. Piana RN, Paik GY, Moscucci M, *et al.* Incidence and treatment of 'no-reflow' after percutaneous coronary intervention. *Circulation* 1994; **90**: 2514–18.

2. Morishima I, Sone T, Okumura K, *et al.* Angiographic no-reflow phenomenon as a predictor of adverse long-term outcome in patients treated with percutaneous transluminal coronary angioplasty for first acute myocardial infarction. *J Am Coll Cardiol* 2000; **36**: 1202–9.

3. Abbo KM, Dooris M, Glazier S. Features and outcome of no-reflow after percutaneous coronary intervention. *Am J Cardiol* 1995; 75: 778–82.

4. Hong MK, Mehran R, Dangas G, *et al.* Creatine kinase-MB enzyme elevation following successful saphenous vein graft intervention is associated with late mortality. *Circulation* 1999; **100**: 2400–5.

5. Rezkalla SH, Kloner RA. No-reflow phenomenon. *Circulation* 2002; **105**: 656–62.

6. Kotani J, Nanto S, Mintz GS, *et al.* Plaque gruel of atheromatous coronary lesion may contribute to the no-reflow phenomenon in patients with acute coronary syndrome. *Circulation* 2002; **106**: 1672–7.

7. Bonderman D, Teml A, Jakowitsch J, *et al.* Coronary no-reflow is caused by shedding of active tissue factor from dissected atherosclerotic plaque. *Blood* 2002; **99**: 2794–800.

8. Popma JJ, Cox N, Hauptmann KE, *et al.* Initial clinical experience with distal protection using the FilterWire in patients undergoing coronary artery and saphenous vein graft percutaneous intervention. *Cathet Cardiovasc Intervent* 2002; **57**: 125–34.

9. Kandzari DE, Tcheng JE. Double negatives. *Am Heart J* 2003; **145**: 9–12.

10. Brener SJ, Barr LA, Burchenal JEB, *et al.* Randomized, placebo-controlled trial of platelet glycoprotein IIb/IIIa blockade with primary angioplasty for acute myocardial infarction. *Circulation* 1998; **98**: 734–41.

11. Giri S, Mitchel JF, Hirst JA, *et al.* Synergy between intracoronary stenting and abciximab in improving angiographic and clinical outcomes of primary angioplasty in acute myocardial infarction. *Am J Cardiol* 2000; **86**: 269–74.

12. Roffi M, Mukherjee D, Chew DP, *et al.* Lack of benefit from intravenous platelet glycoprotein IIb/IIIa receptor inhibition as adjunctive treatment for percutaneous interventions of aortocoronary bypass grafts: a pooled analysis of five randomized clinical trials. *Circulation* 2002; **106**: 3063–7.

13. Webb JG, Carere RG, Virmani R, *et al.* Retrieval and analysis of particulate debris following saphenous vein graft intervention. *J Am Coll Cardiol* 1999; **34**: 461–7.

14. Tanaka A, Kawarabayashi T, Nishibori Y, *et al.* No-reflow phenomenon and lesion morphology in patients with acute myocardial infarction. *Circulation* 2002; **105**: 2148–52.

15. Michaels AD, Appleby M, Otten MH, *et al.* Pre-treatment with intragraft verapamil prior to percutaneous intervention of saphenous vein graft lesions: results of the randomized, controlled vasodilator prevention on no-reflow (VAPOR) trial. *J Invasive Cardiol* 2002; **14**: 303–4.

16. Marzilli M, Orsini E, Marraccini P, *et al.* Beneficial effects of intracoronary adenosine as an adjunct to primary angioplasty in acute myocardial infarction. *Circulation* 2000; **101**: 2154–9.

17. Leborgne L, Cheneau E, Waksman R, *et al.* Randomized trial of a distal embolic protection device during percutaneous coronary intervention of saphenous vein aorto-coronary bypass grafts. Correspondence. *Circulation* 2002; **106**: 68.

18. Baim DS, Wahr D, George B, *et al.* Randomized trial of a distal embolic protection device during percutaneous coronary intervention of saphenous vein aorto-coronary bypass grafts. Response. *Circulation* 2002; **106**: 68.

19. Rinfret S, Katsiyiannis PT, Ho KK, *et al.* Effectiveness of rheolytic thrombectomy with the AngioJet catheter. *Am J Cardiol* 2002; **90**: 470–6.

20. Beran G, Lang I, Schreiber W, *et al.* Intracoronary thrombectomy with the X-sizer catheter system improves epicardial flow and accelerates ST-segment resolution in patients with

acute coronary syndrome. A prospective, randomized, controlled study. *Circulation* 2002; **105**: 2355–60.

21. Yip H-K, Chen M-C, Chang H-W, *et al.* Angiographic morphologic features of infarct-related arteries and timely reperfusion in acute myocardial infarction. *Chest* 2002; **122**: 1322–32.

22. Alp NJ, Gunn J, Channon KM. In-stent restenosis and atherosclerosis in a human saphenous vein graft. *Heart* 2003; **89**: 132.

23. Limbruno U, Micheli A, Petronio AS, *et al.* Adjunctive porous filter protection from distal embolization in primary percutaneous coronary intervention for acute myocardial infarction. ACC Scientific Sessions. Chicago, 31 March 2003 (Abstract).

24. Park CH, Salem M, Jauhar R, *et al.* Effect of distal protection or thrombectomy on corrected thrombolysis in myocardial infarction frame counts in stenting for acute myocardial infarction. ACC Scientific Sessions. Chicago, 31 March 2003 (Abstract).

25. Ito N, Nakamura M, Komatso H, *et al.* Thrombectomy with distal protection prior to stenting is a novel strategy to obtain optimal reperfusion in patients with acute myocardial infarction. ACC Scientific Sessions. Chicago, 31 March 2003 (Abstract).

12

Drug-eluting stents

Introduction

The introduction of drug-eluting stents may revolutionize percutaneous intervention. Restenosis following angioplasty has plagued interventional cardiology since its inception, but using drug-eluting stents we will be able to treat our existing patients more decisively and, perhaps more importantly, we will be able to broaden the range of patients treated by percutaneous intervention – in particular, diabetics and patients with multivessel disease.

It has been recognized for some years that the process of restenosis following balloon inflation is dominated by both initial recoil and late adverse remodelling of the vessel. In contrast, in-stent restenosis is caused exclusively by proliferation of vascular smooth muscle cells (SMCs) and matrix formation resulting in dense new neointimal formation |1|. Although some neointima formation following stent implantation is ubiquitous, diffuse, severe in-stent disease is particularly problematic as it is only treatable percutaneously using brachytherapy. Despite refinements to this technique, limitations of availability and long-term concerns about the safety of brachytherapy persist. Prevention of restenosis is clearly desirable but for many years and despite intensive research the solution evaded researchers worldwide. Using stents as a vehicle for local drug delivery to prevent restenosis has always been a potentially attractive solution but turning the idea into clinical reality has required a series of technology developments:

1. Identification of a drug. Despite encouraging results with *in vitro* small animal models successive antithrombotic and antiplatelet therapies have failed to influence the cascade of events that results in restenosis. In contrast, both rapamycin and paclitaxel have been shown to be potent inhibitors of vascular SMC proliferation in animal models and these encouraging results have now translated into benefits in man.

2. Development of a polymer. Moderating release of the drug over a pre-defined time course is an important component of drug-eluting stent technology. The biological cascade resulting in neointimal formation begins within seconds of vessel injury, but vascular SMC proliferation peaks within the first week and persists for up to 28 days. Maintaining drug concentrations throughout the 'healing phase' is essential. The polymer must also be resistant to cracking and damage during stent expansion and the process of applying the polymer/drug

combination must allow an even distribution of drug to prevent areas of either inadequate or excess drug delivery.

3. The stent. Many of the stents used in initial drug-eluting stent studies have been replaced by newer more advanced designs. Stent design which minimizes the neointimal reaction and provides maximal vessel support with optimal flexibility will always be an essential part of the ideal drug-eluting stent. |2–5|

The first study to be reported using drug-eluting stent technology was the 'randomized study with the sirolimus-eluting velocity balloon-expandable stent in the treatment of patients with *de novo* native coronary artery lesions' (RAVEL). When it was first presented at the European Cardiac Society meeting in Stockholm in 2001 the excitement was palpable. The reported 0% restenosis rate with the drug-eluting stent resulted in optimistic bravado suggesting that 'restenosis had been cured'. Inevitably, this is not the case. Drug-eluting stents have reduced, but not abolished, restenosis. Also their use will require changes in practice to obtain an optimal benefit. We concentrate principally on the published results in the literature, but some unpublished data will be discussed for completeness.

Initially, we consider the published data on sirolimus and then subsequently on paclitaxel and its derivatives (with and without polymer delivery).

Sirolimus

Sirolimus is a macrolide antibiotic with potent antifungal, immunosuppressive and antimycotic properties. It binds to specific cytosolic proteins and regulates FK506-binding protein 12. This binding protein complex binds to a specific cell-cycle regulatory protein, the mammalian Target Of Rapamycin (mTOR) and inhibits its activation. This inhibition of mTOR ultimately induces arrest of the cell cycle in the late G_1 phase and thus arrests SMC growth. Its effect on endothelial cells is similar to a control drug and thus it is not thought to impair endothelial recoverage following vascular injury |4|. The Cordis Cypher stent (Johnson and Johnson) is loaded with a fixed amount of sirolimus per unit of metal surface area (140 µg of sirolimus per cm^2). A layer of drug-free polymer is applied on top of the drug–polymer matrix as a diffusion barrier to prolong the release of the drug, and the stent is designed to release approximately 80% of the drug within 30 days after implantation.

A randomized comparison of a sirolimus-eluting stent with a standard stent for coronary revascularization: randomized study with the sirolimus-coated Bx Velocity balloon-expandable stent in the treatment of patients with *de novo* native coronary artery lesions (RAVEL study).

M C Morice, P W Serruys, J E Sousa, *et al. N Engl J Med* 2002; **346**(23): 1773–80.

BACKGROUND. RAVEL was a randomized, double-blind trial comparing bare metal stents with sirolimus drug-eluting stents for revascularization of short, single, *de novo* lesions in native coronary arteries. Two hundred and thirty-eight patients were enrolled at 19 centres. The primary end-point was in-stent late luminal loss. Secondary end-points included the percentage of in-stent stenosis of the luminal diameter and the restenosis rate. Standard clinical end-points of death, myocardial infarction (MI) and percutaneous or surgical revascularization at 1, 6 and 12 months were also assessed. There were no episodes of early stent thrombosis in either treatment group. At 6-month follow-up angiography, late luminal loss was significantly lower in the sirolimus stent than in the bare metal stent group (-0.01 ± 0.33 mm vs 0.80 ± 0.53 mm, $P <0.001$). Angiographic restenosis of >50% of the luminal diameter occurred in 0% of the patients in the sirolimus stent group, compared with 26.6 % of those in the bare metal stent group ($P <0.001$). During a follow-up period of up to 1 year, the overall rate of major cardiac events was 5.8% in the sirolimus stent group and 28.8% in the bare metal stent group ($P <0.001$). This difference was due entirely to a higher rate of revascularization of the target vessel in the bare metal stent group (caused by restenosis).

INTERPRETATION. The RAVEL study may be the single most important study in interventional cardiology to date. It demonstrates a clear difference in both angiographic and clinical outcomes between the sirolimus-coated and bare metal stents. The safety profile of both products was good although this was a low-risk population. It can be expected that benefits seen in this low-risk patient group are likely to be even greater in a higher risk population.

Comment

Principal criticism of the RAVEL study has been the higher than expected event rate in the bare metal stent group. A restenosis rate of over 25% in a study with relatively few diabetics, initially appeared surprising. Subsequent analysis of the expected angiographic restenosis rates suggests that it is not excessive, however. This is principally due to the relatively small vessel size.

The high event rate in the bare metal group cannot dilute the impact of almost complete inhibition of restenosis within the sirolimus stents. Indeed, the extent of the inhibition has caused concern. A mean late loss of 0 suggests that in some patients there must have been significant expansion of the vessel around the stent. The relevance of this at the time was uncertain but there were concerns as to whether it may

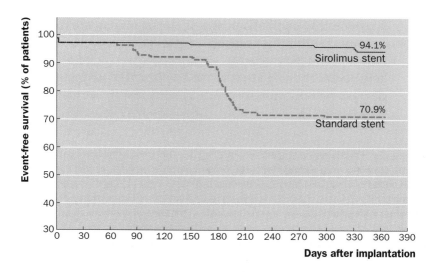

Fig. 12.1 Kaplan–Meier estimates of survival free of myocardial infarction and repeated revascularization among patients who received sirolimus-eluting stents and those who received standard stents. The rate of event-free survival was significantly higher in the sirolimus-stent group than in the standard-stent group ($P < 0.001$ by the Wilcoxon and log-rank tests). Source: Morice *et al.* (2002).

result in incomplete stent apposition to the vessel wall at follow-up and have clinical consequences.

Many of the safety concerns expressed about RAVEL are ameliorated by the relatively short duration of clopidogrel therapy. Clopidogrel was only used for two months following stent implantation and there was no evidence of stent thrombosis following drug withdrawal. This is very reassuring.

The final important point is the absence of any edge effect since the RAVEL study. There are positive effects on the edges of the treated segment adjacent to the stent with no evidence of excess neointima formation.

Intravascular ultrasound findings in the multicenter, randomized, double-blind RAVEL (randomized study with the sirolimus-eluting velocity balloon-expandable stent in the treatment of patients with *de novo* native coronary artery lesions) trial.

P W Serruys, M Degertekin, K Tanabe, *et al. Circulation* 2002; **106**(7): 798–803.

BACKGROUND. In a subset of 95 patients of the RAVEL trial (sirolimus-eluting stent = 48, uncoated stent = 47), motorized intravascular ultrasound pullback (0.5 mm/s) was performed at a 6-month follow-up. Stent volumes, total vessel volumes and plaque-behind-stent volumes were comparable. However, the difference in neointimal hyperplasia (2 ± 5 vs 37 ± 28 mm³) and percent of volume obstruction (1 ± 3% vs 29 ± 20%) at 6 months between the two groups was highly significant (P <0.001) demonstrating the almost complete abolition of neointimal proliferation by this drug-eluting stent. Analysis of proximal and distal edge volumes showed no significant difference between the two groups in external elastic membrane or lumen and plaque volume at the proximal and distal edges. There was also no evidence of intrastent thrombosis or persisting dissection at the stent edges. Although there was a higher incidence of incomplete stent apposition in the sirolimus group compared with the uncoated stent group (P <0.05), this was not associated with any adverse clinical events at 1-year follow-up.

INTERPRETATION. These data represent the intravascular ultrasound (IVUS) sub-study of the RAVEL trial. Although concerning a minority of the total patient population, the data conclusively demonstrate the effect of the drug-eluting stent. Neointimal hyperplasia is prevented without any evidence of adverse effects on the edges of the stent and no effect on the plaque burden behind the struts. The phenomenon of late-acquired stent malapposition (i.e. presence at IVUS follow-up of at least one stent strut separated from the vessel wall by blood speckles) is described, but in this small sub-study, no clinical sequelae arose from this finding.

Comment

Unfortunately, the investigators in the RAVEL study did not perform IVUS immediately following implantation of the stent. It, therefore, limits one's ability to interpret these findings. Differentiation between late-acquired malapposition and persistent malapposition without this data is impossible. This is clearly an important differentiation given the mode of action of sirolimus. Nevertheless, 21% late-acquired stent malapposition in the sirolimus-eluting stent group compared with only 4% in the bare stent-treated group caused some concern. Whether this possible inhibition of healing would progress leaving the stent floating in an enlarged arterial lumen was hypothesized. Similarly, the possibility of slow flow behind the stent inducing late-stent thrombosis was also suggested.

Table 12.1 IVUS measurements at 6-month follow-up in the RAVEL trial. A significant reduction of neointimal stent volume obstruction is clearly shown

Lesion parameters measured	Sirolimus-eluting stent (n = 48)			Uncoated stent (n = 47)		
	Proximal	Stent	Distal	Proximal	Stent	Distal
Total vessel volume	64 ± 27	280 ± 69	51 ± 24	59 ± 24*	280 ± 75*	49 ± 21*
Plaque and NIH	31 ± 15	152 ± 47	21 ± 12	30 ± 13*	183 ± 53†	24 ± 14*
Plaque behind stent	NA	150 ± 44	NA	NA	146 ± 43*	NA
Stent volume	NA	131 ± 35	NA	NA	132 ± 36*	NA
Neointimal volume	NA	2 ± 5	NA	NA	37 ± 28‡	NA
Lumen volume	33 ± 16	129 ± 34	30 ± 14	30 ± 15*	95 ± 41‡	25 ± 11*
% Stent volume obstruction	NA	1 ± 3	NA	NA	29 ± 20‡	NA

* Not significant; † $P < 0.05$; ‡ $P < 0.001$.
NA, not applicable.
Source: Serruys *et al.* (2002).

Subsequent analysis of this phenomenon, particularly in the TAXUS II study and in a large database |6|, has suggested that late-acquired stent malapposition occurs with both bare and drug-eluting stents. It is probably more common than previously recognized and at this stage it does not appear to be linked to clinical consequences.

Persistent inhibition of neointimal hyperplasia after sirolimus-eluting stent implantation: long-term (up to 2 years) clinical, angiographic, and intravascular ultrasound follow-up.

M Degertekin, P W Serruys, D P Foley, *et al. Circulation* 2002; **106**(13): 1610–13.

BACKGROUND. This study reported 2-year angiographic follow-up following implantation of sirolimus-eluting stents. Fifteen patients with *de novo* coronary artery disease were treated using 18-mm sirolimus-eluting Bx Velocity stents (Cordis) loaded with 140 μg sirolimus per cm^2 metal surface area. Quantitative coronary angiography (QCA) and IVUS were performed. During the in-hospital course, one patient died of cerebral haemorrhage after peri-procedural administration of abciximab, and one patient underwent repeat stenting after 2 h because of edge dissection that led to acute occlusion. Through 6 months and up to 2 years of follow-up, no additional events occurred. QCA analysis revealed no significant change in-stent minimal lumen diameter or percent diameter stenosis, and three-dimensional IVUS showed no significant

Table 12.2 Volumetric IVUS measurements

	Rotterdam (*n* = 10)		Sao Paulo (*n* = 14)*	
Follow-up period, mo	6	20	4	12
Stent volume	133 ± 31	132 ± 29	138 ± 21	127 ± 30
Lumen volume	132 ± 31	126 ± 28	137 ± 22	124 ± 30
NIH volume	1.4 ± 1.6	5.9 ± 5.3†	0.3 ± 0.9	2.5 ± 3.4
% Volume obstruction	1.1 ± 1.2	4.4 ± 3.1†	0.3 ± 0.8	2.2 ± 3.4

* Data from Sao Paulo (slow release formulation stent group).
† *P* <0.05, 6-month vs 20-month follow-up.
Source: Degertekin *et al.* (2002).

deterioration in lumen volume. In two patients, additional stenting was performed because of significant progression of disease remote from the area treated by the sirolimus-eluting stent.

INTERPRETATION. This data represents 2-year follow-up of the Dutch experience of the First-In-Man study using sirolimus-eluting stents. Reassuringly, new intimal hyperplasia remained inhibited at this late time point. This study employed the slow release formulation of the sirolimus. The safety profile continued to be excellent.

Comment

There has been extensive debate as to whether restenosis is truly prevented by drug-eluting stents. Sceptics have suggested that restenosis may be deferred and once the active agent has eluted from the stent it will then occur and 'catch up'. Initial long-term follow-up of the first patients to have sirolimus-eluting stents goes a long way to addressing this scepticism. Persistent inhibition of restenosis seen at 2 years is clearly highly reassuring, particularly when the time course of restenosis biologically is initiated in hours, cell division is essentially complete in a month and neointima volume is maximal by 6 months.

Two-year angiographic and intravascular ultrasound follow-up after implantation of sirolimus-eluting stents in human coronary arteries.

J E Sousa, M A Costa, A G Sousa, *et al. Circulation* 2003; **107**(3): 381–3.

BACKGROUND. This Brazilian study reported angiographic, IVUS and clinical outcomes of patients treated with sirolimus-eluting stents 2 years after implantation. It included 30 patients treated with sirolimus-eluting Bx Velocity stents (slow release [SR], *n* = 15, and fast release [FR], *n* = 15) in Sao Paulo, Brazil. Twenty-eight patients underwent 2-year angiographic and IVUS follow-up. No deaths occurred during the study period.

In-stent late loss was slightly greater in the FR group (0.28 ± 0.4 mm) than in the SR group (–0.09 ± 0.23 mm, *P* = 0.007). No patient had in-stent restenosis. At 2-year follow-up, only one patient (FR group) had a 52% diameter stenosis within the lesion segment, which required repeat revascularization. The target-vessel revascularization rate for the entire cohort was 10% (3/30) at 2 years. All other patients had ≤35% diameter stenosis. Angiographic lumen loss at the stent edges was also minimal (in-lesion late loss was 0.33 ± 0.42 mm [FR] and 0.13 ± 0.29 mm [SR]). In-stent neointimal hyperplasia volume, as detected by IVUS, remained minimal after 2 years (FR = 9.90 ± 9 mm³ and SR = 10.35 ± 9.3 mm³). This study demonstrates the safety and efficacy of sirolimus-eluting Bx Velocity stents 2 years after implantation in humans. In-stent lumen dimensions remained essentially unchanged at 2-year follow-up in both groups, although angiographic lumen loss was slightly higher in the FR group. There was no evidence of delayed restenosis and 'catch-up' at a later time point.

INTERPRETATION. This 2-year data on the Brazilian arm of First-In-Man study includes both angiographic and IVUS follow-up. Clinical end-points remain good with an excellent safety profile.

Comment

This study is particularly noteworthy because of the IVUS. Similar to the Dutch data there is persistent inhibition of neointima angiographically and this is confirmed by IVUS. Reassuringly, there are no major changes in vessel size at this late follow-up and no evidence of problems appearing either at the edges or behind the drug-eluting stents.

Sirolimus-eluting stent for the treatment of in-stent restenosis: a quantitative coronary angiography and three-dimensional intravascular ultrasound study.

J E Sousa, M A Costa, A Abizaid, *et al. Circulation* 2003; **107**(1): 24–7.

BACKGROUND. Twenty-five patients in São Paulo, Brazil, with in-stent restenosis were successfully treated with the implantation of one or two sirolimus-eluting Bx Velocity stents. Nine patients received two stents (1.4 stents per lesion). Angiographic and volumetric IVUS images were obtained after the procedure and at 4 and 12 months. All vessels were patent at the time of 12-month angiography. Angiographic late loss averaged 0.07 ± 0.2 mm in-stent and –0.05 ± 0.3 mm in-lesion at 4 months, and 0.36 ± 0.46 mm in-stent and 0.16 ± 0.42 mm in-lesion after 12 months. No patient had in-stent or stent margin restenosis at 4 months, and only one patient developed in-stent restenosis at 1-year follow-up. Intimal hyperplasia by three-dimensional IVUS was 0.92 ± 1.9 mm³ at 4 months and 2.55 ± 4.9 mm³ after 1 year. Percentage volume obstruction was 0.81 ± 1.7% and 1.76 ± 3.4% at the 4- and 12-month follow-up, respectively. The safety profile appeared to be excellent with no deaths, stent thrombosis or repeat revascularization, and no evidence of stent malapposition at follow-up IVUS imaging.

INTERPRETATION. This study looks at a well-defined, straightforward patient group with in-stent restenosis. Sirolimus-eluting stents were used to treat the restenotic lesions with good angiographic results initially and reassuring clinical, IVUS and angiographic results at 1 year. This study suggests that using drug-eluting stents as a treatment for in-stent restenosis is both rational and safe.

Comment

Clearly, it is desirable to find a simple solution for those patients with bare metal stents who present with symptomatic restenosis. These data in a straightforward patient group suggests that drug-eluting stents are likely to be beneficial. In this demanding patient group intimal hyperplasia was restricted with maintenance of good luminal areas for the majority of patients at follow-up. IVUS suggested no evidence of late stent malapposition.

Sirolimus-eluting stent for treatment of complex in-stent restenosis: the first clinical experience.

M Degertekin, E Regar, K Tanabe, *et al. J Am Coll Cardiol* 2003; **41**(2): 184–9.

BACKGROUND. Sixteen patients with severe, recurrent in-stent restenosis in native coronary arteries (average lesion length 18.4 mm) and objective evidence of ischaemia were included. They received one or more 18 mm *Cypher* stents (Cordis). Quantitative angiographic and three-dimensional IVUS follow-up was performed at 4 months, and clinical follow-up at 9 months. Four patients had recurrent restenosis despite brachytherapy, and three patients had totally occluded vessels prior to the procedure. At 4 months follow-up, one patient had died and three had angiographic evidence of restenosis (one in-stent and two in-lesion). In-stent late lumen loss averaged 0.21 mm and the volume obstruction of the stent by IVUS was 1.1%. At 9 months clinical follow-up, three patients had experienced four major adverse cardiac events (two deaths and one acute MI necessitating repeat target vessel angioplasty).

INTERPRETATION. These Dutch data look at a complex patient group with in-stent restenosis treated using sirolimus-eluting stents. Although for the majority of patients outcomes were good, there were clinical end-points within a short time following stent implantation. It appeared that these were not related to the use of the drug-eluting stents but more to the complex nature of the disease in these patients.

Comment

When first reported, these data caused some concern in the interventional community. Patient details were initially sparse and there was suggestion that perhaps drug-eluting stents (DES) were not as safe as initially considered. This paper presents the data clearly and it can be seen that this is an extremely complex patient group, particularly the presence of previous brachytherapy treatment. Although outcomes are not optimal, these results are balanced by more encouraging results from the Brazilian group who treated a more conventional patient subset.

Preliminary observations regarding angiographic pattern of restenosis after rapamycin-eluting stent implantation.

A Colombo, D Orlic, G Stankovic, *et al*. *Circulation* 2003; **107**: 2178–80.

B A C K G R O U N D . **This study evaluates the pattern of restenosis occurring after implantation of DES in unselected lesions. Between 15 April and 6 December 2002, they treated 368 patients with 735 lesions by using 841 rapamycin-eluting stents (Cypher, Cordis). Mean baseline lesion length was 17.48 ± 12.19 mm, and mean stent length was 27.59 ± 14.02 mm. Follow-up ischaemia-driven angiography was performed in 24 patients. Eleven patients had angiographic restenosis (≥50% diameter stenosis) in 14 stented segments (stent and 5 mm proximal and distal to the stent). The pattern of restenosis in all 14 in-stent segments was focal, and in 6 of them it was multifocal. Mean length of restenotic lesions was 5.62 ± 1.90 mm, with a range from 2.54 to**

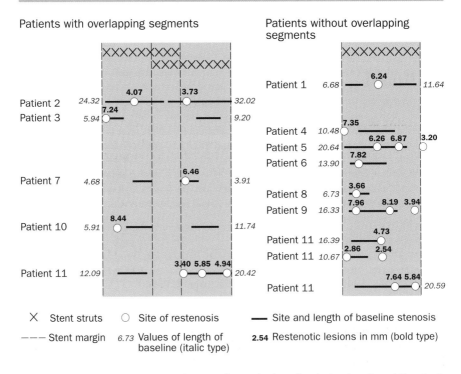

Fig. 12.2 Location of the restenosis according to the baseline lesion length and the stent length. Source: Colombo *et al.* (2003).

8.44 mm. One multifocal restenosis also involved the distal stent margin. IVUS evaluation at follow-up, performed in two patients, showed significant lumen obstruction attributable to in-stent hyperplasia in both cases.

INTERPRETATION. This study from a large group represents a single centre experience with DES in the real world. The data confirm that restenosis has not been cured completely but that DES have improved clinical outcome considerably. Importantly the pattern of restenosis in those few patients who did experience symptoms appears to be more treatable than the severe diffuse pattern of disease observed with bare metal stents.

Comment

These data are important as they confirm the benefits of DES in a large, almost unselected, patient group. The number of failures with DES overall is small. The pattern of in-stent restenosis also appears to have changed with no evidence of diffuse in-stent disease. Focal patterns of proliferation were noted although in some this was at a number of sites. This type of study will not document why these patients have 'broken through' the inhibition of restenosis. Further research into procedural details are required to assess implant details and patient characteristics need to be analysed. In the future, combinations of drug therapy mounted to the stent may be necessary particularly for treatment of diffuse in-stent disease

Paclitaxel

Paclitaxel (Taxol) is a hydrophobic, microtubule-stabilizing agent with potent anti-proliferative activity. The binding of paclitaxel to tubulin results in blockade of cell division in the G_0/G_1 and G_2/M phases of the cell cycle. When the compound is attached to tubulin it loses its flexibility and can no longer disassemble. This effect is obtained by altering the equilibrium between microtubules and α- and β-tubulin, favouring the formation of abnormally stable microtubules. Thus, unlike colchicine, paclitaxel shifts microtubule equilibrium towards assembly, leading to reduced proliferation, migration and signal transduction [4,5,7]. Paclitaxel has been shown to inhibit SMC proliferation and migration in a dose-dependent manner *in vitro* and to prevent neointima formation after balloon angioplasty and stenting in animal models. However, long-term studies in animals (rabbit iliac artery) have been inconsistent: in one study (rapid release with a biodegradable polymer loaded with 42.0 and 22.2 µg of drug) there was reduced neointima formation at 1 month with delayed healing, but the benefit was lost by 3 months [8]; in another using a non-biodegradable polymer loaded with 200 µg of drug (i.e. more than 4 µg/mm2 of stent), there was persistent neointimal inhibition for up to 6 months, but the neo-intimal tissue was incompletely healed [9]. A better result was obtained selecting a lower paclitaxel dosage (1 µg/mm2) [10].

To date, four different delivery platforms have been used in humans for the release of taxanes into vessel walls.

1. The QuaDDS system: a stainless-steel, 316 L slotted tube covered by multiple non-biodegradable polyacrilate sleeves that release the more hydrophobic derivative of paclitaxel, 7-hexanoyltaxol (QP2 or taxen). Approximately 800 μg of the drug are loaded per 2.4 sleeve length, with number of sleeves increasing according to the length of the stent (3 for 13-mm long stents and 4 for 17-mm long stents). The QuaDDS stent (Boston Scientific Corp.) was evaluated in the study to compare restenosis rate between QueST and QuaDS-QP2 (SCORE) trial.

2. The V-Flex Plus paclitaxel-eluting stent (no polymer, Cook Inc. license): evaluated in four different dosage regimens (from 0.2 to 2.7 μg/mm^2) versus control bare metal stent in the European ELUTES (EvaLUation of pacliTaxel Eluting Stent) trial in 190 patients. No polymer was employed in this study as the drug was bound directly to the stent. The ELUTES trial, presented at the America Heart Association congress in late 2001 but still unpublished, showed a significant decrease in percentage diameter stenosis and late loss between control and high dose arms and a trend towards a decrease in binary restenosis between control and high dose arms. Short-term safety at all doses was confirmed.

3. The Supra G™ paclitaxel-eluting stent (no polymer, Cook Inc. license), evaluated at two different dosages (1.3 and 3.1 μg/mm^2) in the ASian Paclitaxel-Eluting stent Clinical Trial (ASPECT trial). The same stent, called Achieve, (drug dosage 3 μg/mm^2) was evaluated in the Guidant DELIVER I study and DELIVER II registry (still unpublished). The DELIVER trial, which enrolled 1043 patients, was presented at the ACC 2003 Late Breakings trial but is still unpublished. The investigators failed to show any difference between the treatment groups regarding the main end-point of target vessel failure (a composite of death, infarction and target lesion revascularization) or binary restenosis.

4. The TAXUS programme: low dosages of paclitaxel (1–4 μg/mm^2), impregnated in a biocompatible polymer, were evaluated by Boston Scientific. The initial stent was the NIRx system for TAXUS I–III and the new Express stent for TAXUS IV–VI. Two different release kinetics have been evaluated: SR and moderate release (MR), which differ because of the presence of a 'burst' release of drug in the first two days with the MR system.

First clinical experience with a paclitaxel derivate-eluting polymer stent system implantation for in-stent restenosis: immediate and long-term clinical and angiographic outcome.

F Liistro, G Stankovic, C Di Mario, *et al. Circulation* 2002; **105**: 1883–6.

BACKGROUND. This is a single-centre registry reporting the first clinical experience of 7-hexanoyltaxol (QP2)-eluting polymer stent system (QuaDS) implantation for in-stent restenosis in 15 patients. Immediate results, along with 6- and 12-month follow-up are presented. Immediately, there was one post-procedural non-Q wave myocardial infarction (NQWMI). No other adverse events were observed during hospital stay. At 6 months follow-up, three patients had target lesion revascularization (20%). Two patients had restenosis (13.3%); one experienced restenosis in a gap between two DES, and the other had stent occlusion leading to NQWMI. However, minimal intimal hyperplasia was observed in all the segments covered by DES (late loss = 0.47 ± 1.01 mm with a loss index = 0.17 ± 0.39). At 12 months follow-up, one patient suffered from NQWMI, and eight of thirteen patients (61.5%) had angiographic restenosis (late loss = 1.36 ± 0.94 mm with a loss index = 0.62 ± 0.44). Thus, QuaDS–QP2 stent implantation for in-stent restenosis was associated with minimal intimal hyperplasia at the 6-month follow-up. However, the antiproliferative effect was not maintained at the 12-month follow-up, resulting in delayed occurrence of angiographic restenosis.

INTERPRETATION. This was the first reported experience of the use of paclitaxel-eluting stents for in-stent restenosis. Although the 6-month data looked encouraging, the 12-month data showed evidence of progressive renarrowing resulting in significant recurrent in-stent restenosis requiring therapy.

Comment

The data were clearly disappointing. The stent that was used (the Cook QuaDs stent) may have been the problem rather than the paclitaxel itself. Certainly the SCORE trial was stopped prematurely because of a high major adverse cardiac event (MACE) rate at 40 days using this stent. This stent employs drug-eluting polymer embedded on plastic sleeves mounted on the stent. It is possible that the high concentrations of the Taxus analogue were toxic to the vessel wall and that in retrospect this stent is a poor vehicle for drug delivery. Indeed, this stent design may produce a more proliferative response than conventional slotted tube stents. Its use has essentially now been abandoned.

Table 12.3 Cumulative in-hospital, 6-month and 12-month clinical outcome

	In-hospital (%)	6-month(%)	12-month(%)
Death	0	0	0
Q MI	0	0	0
Non-Q MI	1 (6.6)	2 (13.2)	3 (20)
CABG	0	1 (6.6)	1 (6.6)
Target lesion revascularization	0	3 (20)	9 (60)

CABG, coronary artery bypass graft.
Source: Liistro et al. (2002).

7-Hexanoyltaxol-eluting stent for prevention of neointimal growth: an intravascular ultrasound analysis from the study to compare restenosis rate between QueST and QuaDS-QP2 (SCORE).

T Kataoka, E Grube, Y Honda, *et al. Circulation* 2002; **106**(14): 1788–93.

BACKGROUND. The SCORE trial is a human, randomized, multicentre trial comparing 7-hexanoyltaxol (QP2)-eluting stents (qDES) with bare metal stents (BMS) in the treatment of *de novo* coronary lesions. The purpose of this sub-study was to evaluate the acute expansion property and long-term neointimal responses of qDES compared with BMS as assessed using IVUS. A total of 122 (qDES 66, BMS 56) patients were enrolled into the IVUS sub-study. At baseline, qDES achieved stent expansion similar to BMS. At 6-month follow-up, qDES showed reduced neointimal growth by 70% at the tightest cross-section and by 68% over the stented segment (*P* <0.0001 for both), resulting in a significantly larger lumen in qDES than in BMS. There was no evidence of negative edge effects, unhealed dissections or late stent-vessel wall malapposition over the stented and adjacent references segments in either group.

INTERPRETATION. These are the IVUS sub-study results at 6-month follow-up of the unpublished (and prematurely stopped) SCORE trial, evaluating the QuaDS stent in *de novo* coronary lesions. These favourable IVUS sub-study results with the QuaDS stent were not matched in the study as a whole as very high 6-month MACE rates were demonstrated.

Comment

The results of this study confirm that the high-dose paclitaxel can inhibit neointimal growth; however, the amount of reduction in neointimal tissue growth with the use of taxane-eluting stents is not so striking as in the RAVEL IVUS sub-study (approximately 70% reduction in neointimal volume in SCORE and ASPECT vs over 95% reduction in RAVEL). Reassuringly, in this study no significant stent malapposition, 'black holes' or edge effects were observed.

Paclitaxel coating reduces in-stent intimal hyperplasia in human coronary arteries: a serial volumetric intravascular ultrasound analysis from the ASian Paclitaxel-Eluting stent Clinical Trial (ASPECT).

M K Hong, G S Mintz, C W Lee, *et al. Circulation* 2003; **107**(4): 517–20.

BACKGROUND. The aim of this study was to use serial volumetric IVUS to evaluate the effect of a paclitaxel coating on in-stent intimal hyperplasia (IH). Patients were randomly allocated to receive placebo (bare metal stents) or one of two doses of paclitaxel (low dose: 1.28 μg/mm²; high dose: 3.10 μg/mm2). Complete post-stent implantation and follow-up IVUS were available in 81 patients, including 25 control patients and in 28 receiving a low dose and 28 receiving a high dose. Volumetric analysis of the stented segment and of both reference segments was performed. Baseline stent measurements and both reference measurements were similar among the groups. With increasing doses, there was a stepwise reduction in IH accumulation within the stented segment (31 ± 22 mm^3 in control, 18 ± 15 mm^3 in low dose and 13 ± 14 mm^3 in high dose, $P <0.001$). *Post hoc* analysis showed less IH accumulation when low- and high-dose patients were compared with control ($P = 0.009$ and $P <0.001$, respectively), but not when low-dose patients were compared with high-dose patients ($P = 0.2$). Focal late malapposition was seen in one high-dose patient. With increasing doses, there was no significant change in the reference segments.

INTERPRETATION. This is the IVUS sub-study of the ASPECT trial: this trial evaluated the Cook Supra G™ paclitaxel-eluting stent at two different dosages for the prevention of restenosis in *de novo* coronary lesion. In this stent, the drug is bound directly to the stent struts and there is no eluting polymer.

Comment

The IVUS results are comparable with the SCORE IVUS results, showing a consistent reduction in neointimal growth, but not abolition. Again, no adverse effects (stent malapposition, 'black holes' or edge effect) were seen during IVUS imaging.

A paclitaxel-eluting stent for the prevention of coronary restenosis. The ASian Paclitaxel-Eluting stent Clinical Trial (ASPECT).

S J Park, W H Shim, D S Ho, *et al*. *N Engl J Med* 2003; **348**(16): 1537–45.

BACKGROUND. This study is a multicentre, randomized, controlled, triple-blind study to evaluate the ability of a paclitaxel-eluting stent to inhibit restenosis. At three centres, 177 patients with discrete coronary lesions (<15 mm in length, 2.25–3.5 mm in diameter) underwent implantation of the Cook Supra G™ paclitaxel-eluting stent (low dose, 1.3 µg/mm^2, or high dose, 3.1 µg/mm^2) or control stents. In this stent, the drug is released directly by the stent struts, and there is no eluting polymer. Antiplatelet therapies included aspirin with ticlopidine (120 patients), clopidogrel (18 patients) or cilostazol (37 patients). At angiographic follow-up (4–6 months), the high-dose group, compared with the control group, had significantly better results for the degree of stenosis (mean $\pm$ SD, 14 ± 21 vs $39 \pm 27\%$; $P <0.001$), late loss of luminal diameter (0.29 ± 0.72 vs 1.04 ± 0.83 mm, $P <0.001$) and restenosis of >50% (4 vs 27%, $P <0.001$). IVUS analysis demonstrated a dose-dependent reduction in the volume of intimal hyperplasia (31, 18 and 13 mm^3, in the high-dose, low-dose and control groups, respectively). There was a higher rate of major cardiac events in patients receiving cilostazol than in those receiving ticlopidine or clopidogrel. Among patients receiving ticlopidine or clopidogrel, event-free survival was 98 and 100% in the high-dose and control groups, respectively, at 1 month, and 96% in both groups at 4–6 months.

Table 12.4 Angiographic measures, according to the dose of paclitaxel*

Variable	Dose of paclitaxel			P value (high dose vs control)
	3.1 µg/mm^2	1.3 µg/mm^2	0 µg/mm^2	
Lesion length (mm)	10.9 ± 3.6	11.2 ± 3.2	10.5 ± 3.1	0.52
Diameter of reference vessel (mm)	2.94 ± 0.39	2.93 ± 0.38	2.88 ± 0.36	0.69
Stenosis (% of luminal diameter)				
Before procedure	79.4 ± 9.0	80.1 ± 8.0	80.9 ± 9.9	0.14
After procedure	1.87 ± 5.38	3.27 ± 5.03	3.77 ± 8.42	0.67
At follow-up	14 ± 21	23 ± 25	39 ± 27	<0.001
Minimal luminal diameter (mm)				
Before procedure	0.64 ± 0.29	0.57 ± 0.25	0.54 ± 0.33	0.19
After procedure	2.85 ± 0.34	2.84 ± 0.39	2.82 ± 0.42	0.92
At follow-up	2.53 ± 0.72	2.28 ± 0.83	1.79 ± 0.86	<0.001
Late loss (mm)	0.29 ± 0.72	0.57 ± 0.71	1.04 ± 0.83	<0.001
Average loss or gain (mm)	0.13 ± 0.33	0.26 ± 0.34	0.46 ± 0.37	<0.001
Restenosis (% of patients)	4	12	27	<0.001

* The numbers of patients for whom there were measurements before and after the procedure were as follows: 58 in the high-dose group, 57 in the low-dose group, and 57 in the control group. For follow-up measurements, the numbers were 50 in the high-dose group, 50 in the low-dose group, and 55 in the control group. Plus/minus values are means ± SD.
Source: Park et al. (2003).

INTERPRETATION. The data initially appeared to support the use of paclitaxel-eluting stents in *de novo* short coronary lesions. This was important as the paclitaxel was not mounted on a polymer. Unfortunately, the actual numbers in each treatment arm were quite small.

Comment

This was essentially preliminary data using the Cook stent. Although the results are encouraging at first glance, it is apparent that the actual time prior to restudy is short in many patients and that drug treatment does vary considerably both in drug dosage on the stent and on the antiplatelet agent used following the procedure. These relatively small patient numbers may explain the divergent results seen with subsequent studies using this drug/stent combination – DELIVER I and DELIVER II.

TAXUS III trial: in-stent restenosis treated with stent-based delivery of paclitaxel incorporated in a slow-release polymer formulation.

K Tanabe, P W Serruys, E Grube, *et al. Circulation* 2003; **107**(4): 559–64.

BACKGROUND. The TAXUS III trial was a single-arm, two-centre study that enrolled 28 patients with in-stent restenosis meeting the criteria of lesion length ≤30 mm, 50–99% diameter stenosis, and vessel diameter 3.0–3.5 mm. They were treated with one or more TAXUS NIRx paclitaxel-eluting stents (actually, approximately half of the patients received two stents). Twenty-five patients completed the angiographic follow-up at 6 months, and 17 of these underwent IVUS examination. No subacute stent thrombosis occurred up to 12 months, but there was one late chronic total occlusion, and an additional three patients showed angiographic restenosis. The mean late loss was 0.54 mm, with neointimal hyperplasia volume of 20.3 mm³. The MACE rate was 29% (eight patients; one non-Q wave MI, one coronary artery bypass grafting and six target lesion revascularization [TLR]). Of the patients with TLR, one had restenosis in a bare stent implanted for edge dissection and two had restenosis in a gap between two paclitaxel-eluting stents. Two patients without angiographic restenosis underwent TLR as a result of the IVUS assessment at follow-up (one incomplete apposition and one insufficient expansion of the stent).

INTERPRETATION. TAXUS III is an observational study (registry) evaluating the performance of the paclitaxel-coated NIRx stent in only 28 patients with in-stent restenosis. The results show a near 30% MACE rate at 6 months, principally driven by TLR. However, there is a detailed discussion in the paper, elucidating that only one of these TLR was actually due to an intimal regrowth in a paclitaxel-covered segment. Moreover, this single restenosis occurred after placement of the study stent for treating restenosis within a PTFE-covered stent that was itself previously used for treating restenosis in a gold-covered stent! In the other paclitaxel-covered segments, minimal neointimal growth was seen.

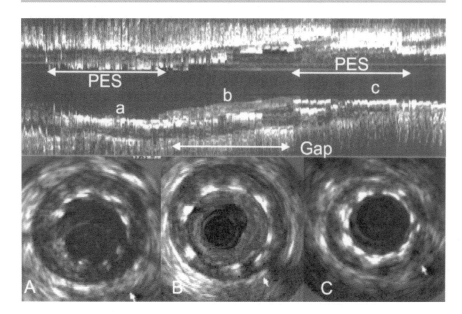

Fig. 12.3 Example of IVUS from the TAXUS III trial. The IVUS images at follow-up of a patient who showed restenosis in a gap between the 2 paclitaxel-eluting stents (PES). Minimal neointimal hyperplasia was observed within the PES (A and C), whereas neointimal hyperplasia was noted in a gap (B). The cross-sectional views (A, B and C) correspond to the a, b and c sections of the longitudinal views. Source: Tanabe *et al.* (2003).

Comment

The principal issues with this study were whether the occurrence of symptom-driven target lesion revascularization was due to failure of the drug/stent platform. Close analysis suggests that there were areas of geographical miss during stent placement and that these may explain the areas of breakthrough of new intimal growth. Importantly the safety profile is good.

TAXUS I: six- and twelve-month results from a randomized, double-blind trial on a slow-release paclitaxel-eluting stent for *de novo* coronary lesions.

E Grube, S Silber, K E Hauptmann, *et al. Circulation* 2003; **107**(1): 38–42.

BACKGROUND. The TAXUS I trial was a prospective, double-blind, three-centre study randomizing 61 patients with *de novo* or restenotic *de novo* lesions (≤12 mm) to receive

a TAXUS (n = 31) versus control (n = 30) stent (diameter 3.0 or 3.5 mm).
Demographics, lesion characteristics and clinical outcomes were comparable between
groups. The 30-day MACE rate was 0% in both groups (P = NS). No stent thromboses
were reported at 1, 6, 9 or 12 months. At 12 months, MACE rate was 3% (one event) in
the TAXUS group and 10% (four events in three patients) in the control group (P = NS).
Six-month angiographic restenosis rates were 0% for TAXUS versus 10% for control
(P = NS) patients. There were significant improvements in minimal lumen diameter
(2.60 ± 0.49 mm vs 2.19 ± 0.65 mm), diameter stenosis (13.56 ± 11.77 mm vs
27.23 ± 16.69 mm) and late lumen loss (0.36 ± 0.48 mm vs 0.71 ± 0.48 mm) in the
TAXUS group (all P <0.01). No evidence of edge restenosis was seen in either group.
IVUS analysis showed significant improvements in normalized neointimal hyperplasia in
the TAXUS (14.8 mm^3) group compared with the control group (21.6 mm^3) (P <0.05).

INTERPRETATION. The TAXUS I trial was the first in-human experience evaluating safety
and feasibility of the TAXUS NIRx stent system compared with bare NIR stents (control) for
treatment of coronary lesion. In this feasibility trial, the stent performed well, with a late
lumen loss of 0.36 mm.

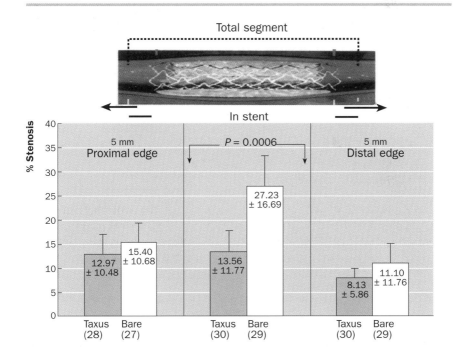

Fig. 12.4 Six-month percentage diameter stenosis comparing in-stent and edge results.
There is a significant improvement in the % DS within the stented area with no differences
at the proximal and distal edges (5 mm from the stent margins) between the TAXUS and
control groups. Source: Grube *et al.* (2003).

Comment

The data suggest that the Boston stent and its polymer paclitaxel can be used safely to prevent restenosis in *de novo* lesions. The amount of late loss is clearly greater than seen with sirolimus. Although this may be considered disadvantageous, it could also be argued that less potent inhibition of healing may be a safer long-term solution as long as there is no late 'catch up' subsequently.

The antiplatelet regime for this study was 6 months of clopidogrel. It is currently unclear whether this duration of therapy could be shortened.

Conclusion

Inevitably, in a review like this the published data are almost immediately outdated by new data presented at international meetings. We now have encouraging results from SIRIUS in the USA (Fig 12.5), C-SIRIUS in Canada (Fig 12.6), and E-SIRIUS (Fig 12.7) in Europe, with each trial showing a major reduction in 9-month MACEs. Ongoing work continues, particularly bifurcations and diabetics using the Cypher stent, and a further comparison with coronary surgery for patients with multivessel disease is underway (the ARTS-II study).

The TAXUS II study 12-month results have been formally reported (Fig 12.8). This study compares the Boston polymer; the NIR stent and paclitaxel with a bare metal NIR stent. The results show impressive differences in clinical end-points, principally

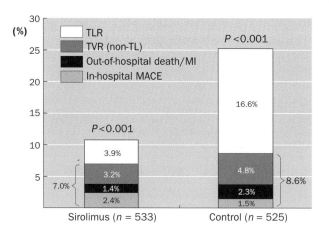

Fig. 12.5 Comparison of clinical events in the sirolimus and control arms of SIRIUS trial. A significant difference is observed, principally driven by a striking reduction in target lesion revascularization (TLR). TVR, target vessel revascularization. MACE, major adverse cardiac event. Source: J W Moses, presented at TCT 2002, accessed at www.TCTMD.com.

target lesion revascularization, which translates in better MACE-free survival. The safety profile is excellent, although the reduction of late loss and IVUS-measured volumetric obstruction is less striking than in the sirolimus trials. We expect more interesting data from the ongoing TAXUS II two-year angiographic follow-up and from the American TAXUS IV and European TAXUS VI trials, which have randomized very complex patients.

Both the Cypher stent and Taxus stent are now available commercially in Europe and the Cypher stent has now been made available in the USA. FDA approval for the Taxus stent is pending.

Clinical F/U: 100%	Control stent (n = 50)	Sirolimus-eluting stent (n = 50)	P
MACE* n (%)	9(18%) ● ●	2(4%) ○ ○	0.05
Death	0	0	1.00
Q MI	0	0	1.00
Non-Q MI (WHO)	2 ● ●	1 ○	ns
TLR-PCI	9(18%) ● ●	2(4%) ○ ○	0.05
TLR-CABG	0	1 ○	ns
TVF	9 ● ●	2 ○ ○	0.05
Subacute closure	0	1 ○	ns
Late-stent thrombosis	1 ●	0	ns

All events per patient ● ● ○ ○

*Death, MI, emergent CABG, clinically driven TLR

Fig. 12.6 The Canadian C-SIRIUS Study included patients (mean age 60.5 years) who had stable or unstable angina or documented silent ischaemia. Lesion lengths were ≥15 mm and ≤32 mm in vessels of ≥2.5 mm and ≤3.0 mm. Actual baseline angiographic lesion lengths were a mean of 14.5 mm for sirolimus-eluting stents (SES) and 12.6 mm for controls—therefore, longer lesion and smaller vessel than in the SIRIUS trial. Most patients received 1 (SES 54%, control 66%) or 2 stents (SES 34%, control 30%). Patients received clopidogrel for 2 months. At 8 months, angiographic follow-up was completed in 88% of patients (43/49 controls and 43/49 SES). The in-stent MLD for patients in the SES arm was 2.46 mm as compared with 1.50 mm for bare metal stent controls (a 64% increase). Late loss was 0.09 mm for SES and 1.01 for controls (a 91% increase for controls). Restenosis was 0% for the SES arm and 41.9% for controls. All differences were statistically significant ($P < 0.001$). These differences translate in the significant reduction in MACE events showed here, even if only 100 patients were randomized. Source: E Schampaert, presented at the ACC 2003 Congress, accessed at www.TCTMD.com.

Future studies, particularly using rapamycin analogues, are well advanced. Head to head comparisons between the DES platforms are also scheduled.

In our opinion it seems likely that using DES will actually change our interventional techniques. Stent lengths will inevitably increase, as there is a need to cover all the atheroma within the DES. This will result in increased use of glycoprotein IIb/IIIa inhibitors. Leaving mild to moderate disease at the stent edges is inadvisable and will lead to clinical consequences. Similarly making sure that stents overlap properly appears to be best practice. Optimization of stent expansion remains important and this may require increased usage of both IVUS and the pressure wire technology. Increasing numbers of bifurcations will be covered but we still await an optimal management plan for treating challenging bifurcational disease.

A consistent reduction in the coronary artery bypass grafting referrals (more than 20% in some analysis |11|) is also likely to affect the cardiac surgeons' practice.

DES will shift the time of intervention to an earlier point in the disease process. It will be more logical to treat intermediate stenosis with DES than with bare stents and angiography with revascularization will be mandatory for all patients with ischaemic heart disease, not just those with symptoms that persist despite medical therapy. New

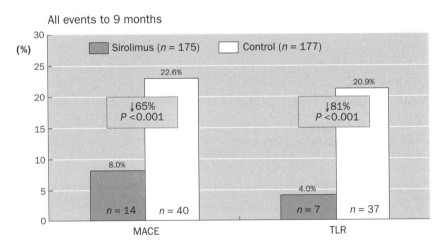

Fig. 12.7 The European E-SIRIUS enrolled a higher risk population (353 points) compared to SIRIUS: more previous MI, more smokers, longer lesion and smaller vessels (2.55 vs 2.8 mm, $P < 0.001$). Moreover, direct stenting was allowed at investigator's discretion. The primary end-point (maintenance of in-stent MLD) was achieved, with a mean late loss of 0.2 mm in the sirolimus arm vs 1.05 mm in the bare stent arm. Differently from SIRIUS, no proximal edge effect was observed. The clinical results were very similar to the main SIRIUS study, with a significant reduction in 9-month clinical events, mainly driven by TLR reduction. Source: J Schofer, presented at the CRF Drug-Eluting Stent Symposium of ACC 2003, accessed at www.TCTMD.com.

techniques allowing detection of the so-called 'vulnerable plaques' are under evaluation, and DES may play a role in the difficult decision of sealing a non-obstructive
but dangerous plaque, due to their intrinsic low-risk of restenosis.

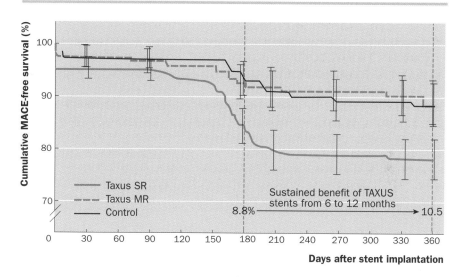

Days after stent implantation

Fig. 12.8 The TAXUS II was designed to assess the safety and efficacy of Boston
Scientific's paclitaxel-eluting coronary stent implanted for reducing restenosis in *de novo*
lesions up to 12 mm in length. The stent employed, a 15-mm polymer-coated NIRx™
Conformer Stent, delivers 1μg/mm^2 of paclitaxel in either a slow-release (SR) or
moderate-release (MR) formulation. Patients ($n = 536$) were randomized in 2 cohorts
(4 arms) to the SR group or bare metal stent controls or the MR group or controls. Controls
were combined in analyses. Antiplatelet therapy with clopidogrel was prescribed for 6
months. Lesions were relatively short, with means ranging between 10.2 and 10.6 mm for
the groups. Analysis of 6-month IVUS end-points had shown highly significant reductions in
the primary end-point of percent net volume obstruction at 7.85% for both SR and MR as
compared with 21.89% for controls. QCA showed binary restenosis of the stented
segment at 2.3% and 4.7% for the SR and MR groups versus 19.0% for controls
($P <0.0001$). Three clinical end-points significantly favoured the paclitaxel-eluting stent at
6 months: MACE, TLR and TVR. MACE was 8.5% for SR and 7.8% for MR as compared with
the combined controls—10.8%. Also, TLR was 4.6% for SR, 3.1% for MR, and 13.3% for
combined controls. TVR overall was 7.7% and 6.2% for SR and MR, respectively, and
16.0% for bare metal stent controls. The 12-month analysis, recently presented, has
shown significant benefits for the paclitaxel-eluting stent, with MACE at 10.9% and 9.9%
for SR and MR, and at 21.7% for controls. The other benefits, mostly significant, were in
TVR overall at 10.1% (NS) and 6.9% versus 17.5% for bare metal controls, and in TLR at
4.7% and 3.8% for SR and MR, as compared with 14.4% for controls. No deaths were
reported in patients receiving drug-eluting stents (2 in controls). Source: A Colombo,
presented at EURO-PCR 2003, accessed at www.TCTMD.com.

References

1. Bennett MR. In-stent restenosis: pathology and implications for the development of drug eluting stents. *Heart* 2003; **89**(2): 218–24.

2. Sousa JE, Serruys PW, Costa MA. New frontiers in cardiology: drug-eluting stents: Part I. *Circulation* 2003; **107**: 2274–9.

3. Sousa JE, Serruys PW, Costa MA. New frontiers in cardiology: drug-eluting stents: Part II. *Circulation* 2003; **107**: 2383–9.

4. Chieffo A, Colombo A. Drug-eluting stents. *Minerva Cardioangiol* 2002; **50**: 419–29.

5. Guagliumi G, Musumeci G, Vassileva A, Tespili M, Valsecchi O. Through the drug-eluting stent labyrinth. *Ital Heart J* 2003; **4**: 236–45.

6. Shah VM, Mintz G S, Apple S, Weissman NJ. Background incidence of late malapposition after bare-metal stent implantation. *Circulation* 2002; **106**: 1753–5.

7. Sonoda S, Honda Y, Kataoka T, *et al*. Taxol-based eluting stents from theory to human validation: clinical and intravascular ultrasound observations. *J Invasive Cardiol* 2003; **15**: 109–14.

8. Farb A, Heller PF, Shroff S, *et al*. Pathological analysis of local delivery of paclitaxel via a polymer-coated stent. *Circulation* 2001; **104**: 473–9.

9. Drachman DE, Edelman ER, Seifert P, *et al*. Neointimal thickening after stent delivery of paclitaxel: change in composition and arrest of growth over six months. *J Am Coll Cardiol* 2000; **36**: 2325–32.

10. Heldman AW, Cheng L, Jenkins GM, *et al*. Paclitaxel stent coating inhibits neointimal hyperplasia at four weeks in a porcine model of coronary restenosis. *Circulation* 2001; **103**: 2289–95.

11. Ferreira AC, Peter AA, Salerno TA, Bolooki H, de Marchena E. Clinical impact of drug-eluting stents in changing referral practices for coronary surgical revascularization in a tertiary care center. Ann Thorac Surg 2003; **75**: 485–9.

13

Intravenous ultrasound in percutaneous coronary intervention

Introduction

Intravascular ultrasound (IVUS) examination of human coronary arteries has significantly increased our knowledge in mechanisms of balloon angioplasty, stent implantation and (in-stent) restenosis. Serial IVUS studies in humans showed that stents exhibit almost no early or chronic recoil, that in-stent restenosis was almost entirely due to neointimal hyperplasia (NIH) and that neointimal thickness appeared to be independent of stent size |**1**|.

IVUS has shown that stent implantation is quite often associated with angiographically undetected underexpansion of the stent, which is thought to be a significant source of late in-stent restenosis |**2**|. Several studies have suggested that IVUS-guided stent implantation offered superior results compared to angiographic guidance |**3,4**|, although the Opticus Trial and Resist did not show any difference |**5,6**|.

Ongoing studies reported here provided further evidence of the clinical use of IVUS.

Is adjunctive balloon post-dilatation necessary after coronary stent deployment? Final results from the POSTIT trial.

B R Brodie, C Cooper, M Jones, P Fitzgerald, F Cummins. *Catheter Cardiovasc Interv* 2003; **59**: 184–92.

BACKGROUND. Early-generation balloon-expandable stents required post-dilatation with non-compliant balloons at high pressure to optimize stent deployment. The need for adjunctive balloon post-dilatation with modern stent delivery systems is unknown. Patients undergoing elective stenting were randomized to Boston Scientific NIR, Guidant Tri-Star/Tetra, and Medtronic AVE S670 stents. The primary end-point was optimum stent deployment defined as a minimal stent diameter (MSD) ≥90% of the average reference lumen diameter assessed by IVUS performed immediately following stent deployment. If, by operator assessment, the primary end-point was not achieved with the stent delivery system, adjunctive post-dilatation with non-compliant balloons was performed. Of 256 patients with IVUS studies adequate for core laboratory analysis, only 29% achieved optimum stent deployment with the stent delivery system. None of the baseline clinical or angiographic variables predicted optimum stent deployment. Of the procedural variables, the type of stent and nominal stent size were not predictors, but higher deployment pressures were associated with a higher frequency of optimum stent deployment (<12 atm 14% vs ≥12 atm 36%; $P = 0.007$). The inability to achieve optimum stent deployment was not due to undersizing the stent delivery balloon, but rather to an inability of the stent delivery balloon to expand fully the stent to nominal size. In patients who underwent post-dilatation, the frequency of achieving optimum stent deployment increased from 21 to 42%, minimal stent area increased from 6.6 ± 2.2 to 7.8 ± 2.3 mm^2, and MSD increased from 2.6 ± 0.5 to 2.8 ± 0.4 mm.

INTERPRETATION. These data stress the continued need for adjunctive balloon post-dilatation with modern stent delivery systems.

Comment

With newer generation stents, the practice of high-pressure balloon dilatation (which was mandatory with the optimal deployment of the Palmaz-Schatz stent) has diminished leading to the majority of stents being under-expanded. This has implications for the incidence of restenosis. This small randomized trial confirms the large incidence of under-expansion with routine stent deployment and demonstrates the value of post-stent dilatation with a non-compliant balloon.

Preliminary observations regarding angiographic pattern of restenosis after rapamycin-eluting stent implantation.

A Colombo, D Orlic, G Stankovic, *et al. Circulation* 2003; **107**: 2178–80.

BACKGROUND. Restenosis after implantation of drug-eluting stents is a rare phenomenon, occurring more frequently peri-stent. We evaluated the pattern of restenosis occurring after implantation of a drug-eluting stent in unselected lesions. Between 15 April and 6 December 2002, we treated 368 patients with 735 lesions by using 841 sirolimus-eluting stents (Cypher, Cordis). Mean baseline lesion length was 17.48 ± 12.19 mm, and mean stent length was 27.59 ± 14.02 mm. Follow-up ischaemia-driven angiography was performed in 24 patients. Eleven patients had angiographic restenosis (≥50% diameter stenosis) in 14 stented segments (stent and 5 mm proximal and distal to the stent). The pattern of restenosis in all 14 stented segments was focal, and in 6 of them it was multifocal, occurring inside the stents. Mean length of restenotic lesions was 5.62 ± 1.90 mm, with a range of 2.54–8.44 mm. One multifocal restenosis involved also the distal stent margin. Intravascular ultrasound evaluation at follow-up, performed in two patients, showed significant lumen obstruction attributable to in-stent hyperplasia in both cases.

INTERPRETATION. The pattern of restenotic lesions after sirolimus-eluting stent implantation was focal and mostly inside the stent.

Comment

A total of 841 sirolimus-eluting stents were deployed in unselected lesions (735) over 6 months with extensive lesion coverage of around 5 mm each side of the lesion. Mean reference diameter was 2.69 mm. Follow-up angiography was driven by either a recurrence of symptoms or a positive stress test in 21 patients with 11 patients having angiographic restenosis (>50% diameter stenosis) at 5 months. This equated to 14 focal in-stent restenosis lesions with a mean length of 5.6 mm. These lesions were in the body of the stent in contrast to the RAVEL or SIRIUS trials in which the majority were at the stent edges or at gaps. IVUS was not used routinely for deployment or in-stent restenosis assessment. The authors believe that this may be because of the extensive coverage of lesions from normal to normal vessel.

Sirolimus-eluting stent for treatment of complex in-stent restenosis: the first clinical experience.

M Degertekin, E Regar, K Tanabe, *et al. J Am Coll Cardiol* 2003; **41**: 184–9.

BACKGROUND. The treatment of in-stent restenosis remains a therapeutic challenge, since many pharmacological and mechanical approaches have shown disappointing results. Sirolimus-eluting stents have been reported to be effective in *de novo* coronary lesions. Sixteen patients with severe, recurrent in-stent restenosis in a native coronary artery (average lesion length 18.4 mm) and objective evidence of ischaemia were included. They received one or more 18 mm Bx VELOCITY sirolimus-eluting stents (Cordis Waterloo, Belgium). Quantitative angiographic and three-dimensional IVUS follow-up was performed at 4 months, and clinical follow-up at 9 months. The sirolimus-eluting stent implantation (*n* = 26) was successful in all 16 patients. Four patients had recurrent restenosis following brachytherapy, and three patients had totally occluded vessels pre-procedure. At 4 months follow-up, one patient had died and three patients had angiographic evidence of restenosis (one in-stent and two in-lesion). In-stent late lumen loss averaged 0.21 mm and the volume obstruction of the stent by IVUS was 1.1%. At 9 months clinical follow-up, three patients had experienced four major adverse cardiac events (MACE; two deaths and one acute myocardial infarction [MI] necessitating repeat target vessel angioplasty).

INTERPRETATION. The sirolimus-eluting stent implantation in patients with severe in-stent restenosis lesions effectively prevents neointima formation and recurrent restenosis at four months angiographic follow-up.

Comment

Sirolimus-eluting stents (*n* = 26) were used to treat recurrent in-stent restenosis in 16 patients with an average lesion length of 18 ± 13 mm. There was intravascular ultrasound follow-up at post-procedure and 4 months, and clinical follow-up at 9 months. The patient group was fairly heterogeneous with four having had previous brachytherapy, five unstable and one heart transplant recipient. Only three lesions were focal in-stent restenosis, and one patient had a difficult-to-expand lesion. Two additional patients had >50% restenosis, one with a gap between the drug-eluting stents, the other was a non-flow-limiting proximal edge restenosis. Volumetric IVUS confirmed a neointimal volume of 1.5 mm^3 at 4 months equivalent to a volume obstruction of 1%. Two of the patients had significant co-morbidity and died within the follow-up period. The outcomes in this group compare with an angiographic restenosis of 45% in a similar complex lesion group treated with bare-metal stents. It is felt that patients with failed brachytherapy in whom there is sustained endothelial dysfunction should receive prolonged clopidogrel treatment. The whole area of balloon injury should be covered with drug-eluting stents and overlapped carefully where appropriate.

Paclitaxel coating reduces in-stent intimal hyperplasia in human coronary arteries: a serial volumetric intravascular ultrasound analysis from the ASian Paclitaxel-Eluting stent Clinical Trial (ASPECT).

M K Hong, G S Mintz, C W Lee, *et al. Circulation* 2003; **107**: 517–20.

B A C K G R O U N D . The aim of this study was to use serial volumetric IVUS to evaluate the effect of a paclitaxel coating on in-stent intimal hyperplasia (IH). Patients were randomized to placebo (bare metal stents) or one of two doses of paclitaxel (low dose: 1.28 μg/mm^2; high dose: 3.10 μg/mm^2). Complete post-stent implantation and follow-up IVUS were available in 81 patients, including 25 control patients and in 28 receiving a low dose and 28 receiving a high dose. Volumetric analysis of the stented segment and of both reference segments was performed. Baseline stent measurements and both reference measurements were similar among the groups. With increasing doses, there was a step-wise reduction in IH accumulation within the stented segment (31 ± 22 mm^3 in control, 18 ± 15 mm^3 in low dose and 13 ± 14 mm^3 in high dose, *P* <0.001). *Post hoc* analysis showed less IH accumulation when low- and high-dose patients were compared with control (*P* = 0.009 and *P* <0.001, respectively), but not when low-dose patients were compared with high-dose patients (*P* = 0.2). Focal late malapposition was seen in one high-dose patient. With increasing doses, there was no significant change in the reference segments.

I N T E R P R E T A T I O N . Paclitaxel-coated stents are effective in reducing in-stent neointimal tissue proliferation in humans. They are not associated with edge restenosis or significant late malapposition.

Comment

Serial volumetric IVUS was performed in a subgroup of 81 patients from ASPECT which was the first randomized trial of paclitaxel-eluting stents (with low- and high-dose drug concentrations). Stent deployment was IVUS guided with adjunctive balloon post-dilatation required in a total of nine patients across the trial. There was a step-wise reduction in NIH with the increasing dose of paclitaxel. One patient in the high-dose group had late stent malapposition due to positive remodelling of the vessel. The angiographic restenosis rate was 27% in controls and 4% in the high-dose group. The issue of late-stent malapposition (i.e. not present by IVUS at the time of deployment) has been raised since the IVUS follow-up of RAVEL confirmed a rate of 21%. The IVUS in this sub-study suggests that it is not a major issue. Furthermore, the 'candy-wrapper' effect of increased neointimal at the stent edges seen with intra-coronary brachytherapy was not seen in this trial, suggesting a beneficial effect of paclitaxel on the adjacent reference segments.

Stenting of culprit lesions in unstable angina leads to a marked reduction in plaque burden: a major role of plaque embolization? A serial intravascular ultrasound study.

F Prati, T Pawlowski, R Gil, *et al. Circulation* 2003; **107**: 2320–5.

BACKGROUND. IVUS studies have shown that a mechanism of plaque compression/embolization contributes to the post-stenting increase in lumen area. The aim of this IVUS study was to compare the mechanisms of lumen enlargement after coronary stenting in 54 consecutive patients with unstable angina (group 1) and 56 with stable angina (group 2) to verify whether plaque embolization plays a major role in the former. Both groups underwent the IVUS assessment (speed, 0.5 mm/s) before the intervention and after stent implantation. The lumen area, the external elastic membrane area, and the plaque + media area (PA) were measured at 0.5-mm intervals. PA reduction in the lesion site was significantly greater in group 1 (−2.50 ± 1.97 vs −0.53 ± 1.43 mm^2, P <0.001). After stenting, 47% of the lumen area increase in group 1 was obtained by means of PA reduction, and 53% was attributable to external elastic membrane area increase; the corresponding figures in group 2 were 13 and 87% (P <0.05). Decrease in PA after stenting was the only significant predictor of the MB fraction of creatinine kinase (CK-MB) release in a multiple regression model (P = 0.047).

INTERPRETATION. Serial volumetric IVUS assessment revealed in unstable angina lesions a marked post-stenting reduction in plaque volume, which is significantly greater than in stable angina and is associated with post-procedural CK-MB release. The decrease in PA during the procedure predicts CK-MB release in a multiple regression model. These findings suggest that stent deployment is often associated with plaque embolization in patients with unstable angina.

Comment

Previous work has shown that stable and unstable coronary plaques have different degrees of remodelling associated with the vascular inflammatory process. Arterial compliance is also greater in unstable lesions. In this study, a comparison was made of the effect of intracoronary stenting on both types of lesion using IVUS to measure the morphometric changes involved with an assessment of plaque embolization and myocardial injury. A total of 110 patients were enrolled with pre-procedural clopidogrel load or glycoprotein IIb/IIIa receptor blockade. Stents were deployed after predilatation with IVUS before and after intervention. Volumetric analysis of thirty-two 13-mm length stents across both groups was carried out to enable a more accurate assessment of plaque dimensions at the stent site and the reference segments. A total of 63% of the unstable group has Braunwald class IIIB with a higher prevalence of lipid pools demonstrated in unstable lesions, 38 versus 25% ($P < 0.05$). As noted previously, positive remodelling was higher in the unstable group (70 vs 49%) with negative remodelling more prevalent in stable lesions (31 vs 14%). IVUS revealed that 47% of the post-stenting lumen enlargement in the unstable group was attributable to plaque reduction and 53% to vessel wall expansion compared with 13 and 87%, respectively in the stable group. The interpretation of the greater reduction in plaque volume in the unstable group (36 vs 11 mm^3) was interpreted as plaque embolization, with acknowledgment that a slight axial plaque shift was seen in the reference segments. The unstable group had a higher mean CK-MB level at 12 h post-procedure, 50 versus 24 IU/ml ($P < 0.01$), with 15% of the unstable patients having a CK-MB level >3 times upper limit of normal (none in the stable group). By multivariate analysis, this CK-MB release correlated with the decrease in plaque area (and plaque burden by univariate analysis). It was felt that that thrombus associated with ulcerated plaque favours distal embolization although it was conceded that plaque compression may be an alternative explanation. The significant correlation between the decrease in the plaque area and CK-MB release does suggest an embolic process. The need for an aggressive anti-thrombotic strategy and the use of distal protection devices is strongly suggested by this non-randomized observational study.

Intravascular ultrasound-guided balloon angioplasty compared with stent: immediate and 6-month results of the multicenter, randomized Balloon Equivalent to Stent Study (BEST).

F Schiele, N Meneveau, M Gilard, *et al. Circulation* 2003; **107**: 545–51.

B A C K G R O U N D. Balloon angioplasty guided by IVUS makes it possible to choose the balloon size according to the true vessel diameter and to detect suboptimal results requiring subsequent stent implantation. The Balloon Equivalent to Stent (BEST) study aimed to assess whether this strategy would give the same results as systematic stenting. A total of 132 of 254 patients were randomized to IVUS-guided percutaneous transluminal coronary angioplasty (aggressive PTCA), and 122 were randomized to stenting (stent group). We hypothesized that a difference of <8% in the 6-month angiographic restenosis rate (primary end-point) could be considered non-inferior. The aggressive PTCA procedure was longer and had a greater use of contrast medium than stenting. In the aggressive PTCA group, cross-over to stent was needed in 58 patients

(44%). At 6 months, 20 of 119 patients (16.8 ± 6.7%) in the aggressive PTCA group and 21 of 116 patients (18.1 ± 7.0%) in the stent group had restenosis. The difference was −1.3%, with an upper limit of 95% confidence interval of 7.1% (i.e. less than the non-inferiority boundary). The in-stent restenosis rate was higher in the stent group (15.5 vs 5%, P = 0.02). The differences in minimum lumen diameter (MLD), lumen cross-section area and 1-year event rate were not significant.

INTERPRETATION. A strategy of IVUS-guided angioplasty with provisional stenting is feasible and safe. At the cost of a more complex procedure, it reduces the stent rate by half, with similar 6-month angiographic IVUS and clinical outcome compared with stent implantation.

Comment

IVUS may be used to guide balloon angioplasty to get the best acute result and can also be used to guide a provisional stenting strategy. The BEST trial is a randomized, three-centre, non-inferiority trial of IVUS guided balloon angioplasty against stenting in 254 patients. The non-inferiority boundary was set at 8% with angiographic restenosis at 6 months the primary end-point. Recent acute coronary syndromes and lesions >20 mm in length were excluded. In the 'aggressive' balloon angioplasty group, the balloon size was selected closest to the vessel diameter at the lesion. Post-dilatation IVUS was used to assess the need for adjunctive balloon dilatation. The indications for cross-over to stenting (44% of cases) was flow-limiting dissection (18% of cases), >30% residual stenosis by angiography or a >30% IVUS area stenosis associated with a minimum lumen area <6 mm². Baseline demographics were not significantly different between the groups although the study population accounted for only 4.2% of all interventions taking place in the units at the time. The IVUS-guided PTCA group were associated with a longer procedure (51 vs 39 min), with longer screening times and more contrast use. Immediate procedural outcomes were no different. Larger balloon sizes (3.85 vs 3.75 mm) were used in the aggressive PTCA group, but with lower inflation pressures (13.3 vs 14.5 atm). The decision to cross-over to stenting was based on angiography in 29% and on IVUS in 16% of patients. A total of 93% had angiographic follow-up at 6 months which showed an angiographic restenosis of 16.8 and 18.1% in the PTCA and stent groups, respectively. This fell within the non-inferiority boundary. IVUS follow-up was carried out in 85%—the average minimum lumen area was 5.1 and 5.2 mm in both groups, respectively. Interestingly, there was a trend towards greater late loss in the stent group but there was a higher in-stent restenosis rate, 15.5 vs 5.0%, in the PTCA group. Clinical events at 12 months were similar at 16 and 20% in the PTCA and stent groups respectively. The study is interesting as it shows the feasibility of a provisional stenting strategy based on a more complex and longer procedure based on IVUS guidance. This results in a reduction in the stent rate by >50%. The study is limited to a wider application because there was not an angiography-guided provisional stenting group. Nonetheless, the value of IVUS in improving the quality of intervention is still clear if procedure time is not limited.

Two-year angiographic and intravascular ultrasound follow-up after implantation of sirolimus-eluting stents in human coronary arteries.

J E Sousa, M A Costa, A G Sousa, et al. *Circulation* 2003; **107**: 381–3.

BACKGROUND. The safety and efficacy of sirolimus-eluting stenting have been demonstrated, but the outcome of patients treated with this novel technology beyond the first year remains unknown. We sought to evaluate the angiographic, IVUS and clinical outcomes of patients treated with sirolimus-eluting stents 2 years after implantation. This study included 30 patients treated with sirolimus-eluting Bx VELOCITY stenting (slow release [SR], *n* = 15, and fast release [FR], *n* = 15) in Sao Paulo, Brazil. Twenty-eight patients underwent 2-year angiographic and IVUS follow-up. No deaths occurred during the study period. In-stent late loss was slightly greater in the FR group (0.28 ± 0.4 mm) than in the SR group (–0.09 ± 0.23 mm, *P* = 0.007). No patient had in-stent restenosis. At 2-year follow-up, only one patient (FR group) had a 52% diameter stenosis within the lesion segment, which required repeat revascularization. The target vessel revascularization rate for the entire cohort was 10% (3/30) at 2 years. All other patients had ≤35% diameter stenosis. Angiographic lumen loss at the stent edges was also minimal (in-lesion late loss was 0.33 ± 0.42 mm FR and 0.13 ± 0.29 mm SR). In-stent NIH volume, as detected by IVUS, remained minimal after 2 years (FR = 9.90 ± 9 mm^3 and SR = 10.35 ± 9.3 mm^3).

INTERPRETATION. This study demonstrates the safety and efficacy of sirolimus-eluting Bx Velocity stents 2 years after implantation in humans. In-stent lumen dimensions remained essentially unchanged at 2-year follow-up in the two groups, although angiographic lumen loss was slightly higher in the FR group. Restenosis 'catch-up' was not found in our patient population.

Comment

Angiographic and IVUS follow-up was performed in 28 of 30 patients receiving a sirolimus-eluting stent at 2-year follow-up. All patients received one 18 mm stent with half receiving fast-release (<15 days) and half receiving slow-release (≥28 days) formulations. The slow-release formulations had an extra layer of polymer and are similar to those used in RAVEL and SIRIUS. The in-segment (within 5 mm either side) and in-stent restenosis were calculated. One patient sustained a vessel occlusion at 14-month follow-up. Although both negligible, the late loss was least in the slow release group, with no patient in this group having >0.2 mm late loss. One patient did develop a 52% diameter stenosis lesion proximal to the stent. The IVUS examination confirmed a small amount of NIH with 9.9 and 10.4 mm^3 in the fast-release and slow-release groups respectively. Two-year lumen diameters were virtually unchanged from post-implantation diameters. There was even a slight increase in the MLD between 1 and 2 years in the slow-release group. Because of the potential for in-segment restenosis, it is important that the entire length ballooned is covered with a drug-eluting stent to avoid the development of lesions just outside the stent edges.

Relative contributions of intimal hyperplasia and vascular remodelling in early cardiac transplant-mediated coronary artery disease.

SK Mainigi, L R Goldberg, B M Sasseen, V Y See, R L Wilensky. *Am J Cardiol* 2003; **91**: 293–6.

B A C K G R O U N D . The relative contribution of IH and vascular remodelling in early transplant coronary artery disease (TxCAD) is unknown. This study was designed to determine the contributions of vascular remodelling and IH in the initial year after transplantation by IVUS. Twenty-five patients underwent baseline (<6 weeks after transplant) and 1-year angiography and IVUS to evaluate total vessel, luminal and intimal + medial areas in ≥3 segments of the coronary artery. Nine patients had donor atherosclerotic disease on baseline study (23% of segments), and at 1-year, 21 patients (84%) had IH (70% of segments). Fourteen patients had positive remodelling in all arterial segments, whereas the remaining 11 had positive and negative remodelling in the same vessel. Mean plaque area and total vessel area increased significantly (*P* = 0.0001) in proximal, mid and distal segments, whereas total vessel area was most pronounced in distal segments. Luminal area did not change over time. Of the 87 segments evaluated, 68 (78%) had an increase in total vessel area, 57 (66%) had intimal growth and 54 (62%) had an increase in luminal area.

I N T E R P R E T A T I O N . Although changes in total vessel and luminal area were closely correlated, a decrease in luminal area was associated with positive and negative remodelling. In conclusion, luminal area is generally maintained during the initial transplant year despite significant IH due to positive remodelling. Reduction in the luminal area results from either inadequate positive remodelling or negative remodelling without intimal growth and often occurs in the same artery.

Comment

IVUS demonstrates transplant coronary artery disease well before angiography is abnormal, with 90% of patients demonstrating disease within 5 years of transplantation. Transplant IVUS also allows observation of the atherosclerotic process at its earliest stage. The role of vascular remodelling (vessel expansion and constriction) was investigated in 25 transplant recipients at baseline and after 1 year. Proximal, mid and distal segments were studied in each artery along with segments demonstrating intimal plaque at initial IVUS (donor disease, seen in nine patients, was defined as plaque >500 μm). The remodelling index was calculated as the change in vessel area at the lesion site relative to the change in intimal area (>1 = positive remodelling, 0–1 = positive remodelling inadequate for intimal growth, and <0 = negative remodelling). Plaque and vessel area increased in all segments over the year and was most marked in the distal segments, with overall preservation of lumen area. Positive vascular remodelling with an associated increase in lumen area occurred both in the absence and presence of intimal growth, with a mean remodelling index of 1.9 ± 0.4 suggesting an over-compensation for intimal growth. Positive and negative remodelling was present within the same artery. Lumen area decreased when plaque area reached 40% of vessel area. The presence of baseline disease influenced remodelling and luminal area. Segments with baseline disease had less positive remodelling and demonstrated a decrease in luminal area rather than increase, suggesting that established donor disease may prevent necessary compensatory changes after transplantation. Thus, when coronary angiography shows decreased lumen dimensions, it can occur through excessive IH, inadequate positive remodelling in response to increased IH or negative remodelling.

Predictors and implications of residual plaque burden after coronary stenting: an intravascular ultrasound study.

F Alfonso, P Garcia, G Pimentel, *et al. Am Heart J* 2003; **145**: 254–61.

BACKGROUND. Residual plaque burden after coronary stenting may be visualized by use of IVUS. Determinants and implications of residual atherosclerotic plaque burden after coronary stenting are not well established. In particular, the implications of residual plaque burden, after adjusting for confounding factors, are still unknown. Sixty-two consecutive patients (age 56 ± 9 years) undergoing coronary stenting under IVUS imaging guidance were prospectively studied. In total 616 slices were analysed (every 2 mm of stent length) from motorized pull-back recordings. Residual plaque burden was calculated as residual plaque/vessel area × 100. In 565 slices (89%), both residual plaque area and stent area could be measured. Mean residual plaque burden was 46.5 ± 6%. By use of multiple regression analysis, lesion plaque area and reference segment plaque burden were identified as independent predictors of residual plaque burden after stenting. In addition, a significant correlation was found between residual plaque burden and most relevant angiographic parameters at follow-up (including MLD, per cent diameter stenosis and loss index), which persisted after adjustment. Furthermore, stents with a residual plaque burden ≥46% had a higher restenosis rate (relative risk [RR] 4.4, 95% confidence interval [CI] 1.09–18.2, $P = 0.03$). On logistic regression analysis, residual plaque burden (RR 4.8, 95% CI 4.1–5.6, $P = 0.01$) and diabetes (RR 4.3, 95% CI 3.6–5.1, $P = 0.03$) emerged as the only independent predictors of restenosis.

INTERPRETATION. The amount of residual plaque burden after coronary stenting plays an independent role on the late angiographic outcome of these patients.

Comment

IVUS can be used to quantify the plaque area outside the stent within the vessel wall after stent deployment. The 62 patients represent a cohort undergoing IVUS-guided stent deployment with late angiographic follow-up. Three stent types were used (NIR [$n = 29$], Multilink [$n = 12$] and the Wallstent [$n = 21$]). The gain settings of the IVUS catheter were adjusted to allow delineation of the external elastic lamina which is the outer limit of the vessel wall. The MUSIC criteria of optimal stent expansion were used to guide stent deployment (minimum stent area [MSA] >100% distal reference, MSA >90% proximal reference segment) but left to the operator's discretion. A total of 65% of the patients fulfilled the criteria as a result of this. The lesion site before intervention was selected as the image slice showing the smallest lumen area (or the greatest plaque area where the catheter obstructed the lumen). Lesion length was 14 ± 9 mm in reference vessels of 3.3 ± 0.7 mm. The mean stent length was 20 ± 7 mm and the mean maximum pressure was 15 ± 2 atm with a balloon:artery ratio of 1.1 ± 0.16. In total, 565 of 616 slices could be analysed. The mean residual plaque burden was $46 \pm 6\%$ with a MSA of 9.0 ± 3.0 mm^2. Both absolute plaque area at the lesion site and plaque burden at the reference segment were independent predictors of the residual plaque burden after stenting as one would have predicted, albeit with a low correlation coefficient. Interestingly, the residual plaque burden after stenting predicted MLD and loss index at follow-up. This and diabetes were the only independent predictors of angiographic restenosis. Intuitively based on this and pre-existing data, one might expect that a debulking strategy before stenting could lead to a lower restenosis rate although this has not been proven directly in a clinical trial. The data has to be interpreted carefully as both balloon-expandable and self-expanding stents were used and calcified lesions were excluded. Nonetheless, residual plaque burden after stenting appears to have a major and independent influence on the late angiographic outcome of these patients.

Conclusion

IVUS also remains useful to assess stent deployment with the currently available stent technology. Low-pressure balloon dilatation with current stent often leads to stent underexpansion, as was clearly shown by IVUS control. This should alert operators to use high-pressure dilatation more often.

IVUS has been shown to be an extremely reliable tool to assess the amount, severity and pattern of in-stent neo-intimal hyperplasia. The neo-intimal hyperplasia after rapamycin-eluting stent is limited and angiographic restenosis occurs in less than 5%. The in-stent restenosis pattern was focal and almost exclusively inside the stent.

Several other studies using IVUS to assess the neo-intimal response after drug-eluting stent with either Sirolimus or Paclitaxel demonstrated limited in-stent NIH, no edge restenosis, and no clinically significant late stent-malapposition at 6-month and 2-year follow-up.

IVUS has elucidated the mechanisms of lumen enlargement after balloon angioplasty and stent implantation. Of interest was the recent finding that distal plaque embolization after stent implantation of an unstable plaque played an undesired role in the lumen enlargement which was often associated with creatine kinase release.

IVUS guidance may play a beneficial role as guidance of an initial aggressive PTCA strategy with cross-over to stenting compared to systematic stenting. Using this approach the stenosis rate was almost similar in both strategies (17% versus 18%).

IVUS examination provided superior insights to coronary angiography when assessing the incidence and progression of transplant coronary artery disease. It demonstrated that the progression of intimal hyperplasia is often associated with preserved lumen due to expansive remodelling, whereas reduction of lumen is due to either progression of disease with inadequate remodelling or to constrictive remodelling only.

Several IVUS parameters including minimum in-stent cross-section and reference vessel cross-section have predictive value for late in-stent restenosis. In a recent study it appeared that residual plaque burden, in addition to stent area, confers independent predictive value for late in-stent restenosis.

In conclusion, IVUS examination is useful to elucidate pathophysiologic mechanisms, and is a predictor of late in-stent restenosis. Whether IVUS should be routinely used remains a matter of debate, but in case of doubt of optimal stent implantation, IVUS may play a significant and decisive role. The value of IVUS to quantify in-stent NIH is beyond any doubt and is the primary end-point of many restenosis studies.

References

1. Mehran R, Dangas G, Abizaid AS, *et al*. Angiographic patterns of in-stent restenosis: classification and implications for long-term outcome. *Circulation* 1999; **100**: 1872–8.

2. Mintz GS, Popma JJ, Pichard AD, *et al*. Intravascular ultrasound predictors of restenosis after percutaneous transcatheter coronary revascularization. *J Am Coll Cardiol* 1996; **27**: 1678–87.

3. Fitzgerald PJ, Oshima A, Hayase M, *et al*. Final results of the Can Routine Ultrasound Influence Stent Expansion (CRUISE) Study. *Circulation* 2000; **102**: 523–33.

4. Frey AW, Hodgson JM, Muller C, Bestehorn HP, Roskamm H. Ultrasound-guided strategy for provisional stenting with focal balloon combination catheter: results from the randomized Strategy for Intracoronary Ultrasound-Guided PTCA and Stenting (SIPS) Trial. *Circulation* 2000; **102**: 2497–502.

5. Schiele F, Meneveau N, Vuillemenok A, *et al*. Impact of intravascular ultrasound guidance in stent deployment on 6-month restenosis rate: a multicenter, randomized study comparing two strategies—with and without intravascular ultrasound guidance. *J Am Coll Cardiol* 1998; **32**: 320–8.

6. Mudra H, di Mario C, de Jaegere P, *et al*. Randomized comparison of coronary stent implantation under ulstrasound or angiographic guidance to reduce stent restenosis (OPTICUS Study). *Circulation* 2001; **104**: 1343–9.

14

Atherectomy

Introduction

Atherectomy, directional or rotational, has so far met only limited use in the practice of percutaneous interventional cardiology. The debulking effects of atherectomy were believed to improve initial results of balloon angioplasty, or stenting, while it appeared that stand-alone atherectomy might only be successful in a minority of procedures. The availability of coronary athero-sclerotic tissue retrieved from directional atherectomy for scientific purposes to gain further understanding of athero-sclerosis is still a significant reason for investigators to perform this procedure. Although many studies have been published, the precise role of atherectomy is still evolving. The value of atherectomy is discussed in the Conclusion.

Treatment of diffuse in-stent restenosis with rotational atherectomy followed by radiation therapy with a rhenium 188 mercaptoacetyltrigycine.
S W Park, M K Hong, D H Moon, *et al. J Am Coll Cardiol* 2001; **38**: 631–7.

BACKGROUND. This study indicates the feasibility and safety of intracoronary β-irradiation combined with rotational atherectomy for the treatment of diffuse in-stent restenosis (ISR) (length >10 mm) in native coronary arteries. Fifty consecutive patients were enrolled.

INTERPRETATION. No adverse event, including myocardial infarction (MI), death or stent thrombosis, occurred during the follow-up period (mean 10.3 ± 3.7 months). Binary angiographic restenosis was seen in five patients; thus the overall angiographic restenosis rate was 10.4%. The late loss was 0.17 ± 0.31. The pattern of restenosis included two focal ISR and three edge restenosis (one in the proximal and two in the distal edge). The results of this study suggest that β-radiation using rhenium 188 mercaptoacetyltrigycine (^{188}Re-MAG 3) combined with rotational atherectomy may be a synergic strategy for patients with diffuse ISR.

Comment

Rotational atherectomy is a technique with limited application for treatment of *de novo* lesions. The only large randomized multicentre trial of ISR (ARTIST) |**1**| is still struggling to pass the comments and criticisms of the reviewers but undoubtedly shows that new recurrences are extremely high and restenosis occurs in >50% of cases both after percutaneous transluminal coronary angioplasty (PTCA) and rotational atherectomy for the treatment of diffuse restenosis. The leading group of the Asian Medical Center combines rotational atherectomy with brachytherapy and obtains a 10.4% angiographic restenosis rate, unexpected for restenotic lesions longer than 20 mm, in 58% of cases and with an average reference diameter of 2.89 mm. A possible explanation may be the achievement of a large initial gain, due to the combined effect of debulking and intravascular ultrasound (IVUS)-guided balloon dilatation using oversized balloons (1.23 balloon-to-artery ratio) but the main reason is the minimal late loss (0.37 mm, with a loss index of 0.17). The radioactive balloons used, a regular balloon filled with radioactive rhenium, are unlikely to become a standard for brachytherapy; the risk of balloon rupture, and the uneven dose if air is mixed with the liquid radioactive source eliminates the advantages of placing the source in contact with the vessel wall. Unlike for *de novo* lesions, and possibly because longer balloons were used that fully covered the lesion in most cases, edge restenosis is more rare (3/50%). Excellent results have been reported for a balloon-like delivery system with a solid P34 source, the Radiance balloon, with a restenosis rate below 10% in the initial oral presentation.

Recurrent unstable angina after directional coronary atherectomy is related to the extent of initial coronary plaque inflammation.

M Meuwissen, J J Piek, A C van der Wal, *et al. J Am Coll Cardiol* 2001; **37**: 1271–6.

BACKGROUND. A positive correlation between coronary plaque inflammation and angiographic restenosis has been reported. A total of 110 patients underwent directional coronary atherectomy (DCA). One-year clinical follow-up was completed in all 110 patients. Recurrent angina occurred in 33 patients (30%), of these patients, 17 presented with stable angina at a mean interval of 5.7 ± 2.8 months (range 3–12 months) and 16 presented with unstable angina at a mean interval of 4.9 ± 3.7 months (range 2–11 months).

INTERPRETATION. This study showed that the immunopositive areas of macrophages and the number of T lymphocytes in the initial atherectomy specimens were significantly larger in patients who developed recurrent unstable angina than in those presenting with recurrent stable angina ($P = 0.02$ and $P = 0.0001$, respectively). Univariate analysis demonstrated a positive and significant correlation between the number of T lymphocytes/mm^2 atherectomy tissue ($P = 0.002$) and percent macrophage area ($P = 0.005$) in recurrent unstable angina. Multivariate logistic regression analysis identified percent macrophage area (odds ratio [OR] 1.04, 95% confidence interval [CI] 0.996–1.087, $P = 0.079$) and T lymphocytes/mm^2 (OR 1.055, 95% CI 1.008–1.103, $P = 0.020$) as independent predictors of recurrent unstable angina. The present findings strongly suggest that the chronic inflammatory process at the side of the culprit lesion is not eradicated by atherectomy, so that the smouldering effects of the inflammatory may again destabilize the repair tissue after coronary interventions.

Comment

This elegant study relies on the experience of one of the best cardiac pathologists, Anton Becker, to identify plaques with inflammatory changes: infiltration of macrophages and T lymphocytes have been reported to weaken the fibrous cap and facilitate intraluminal rupture of the necrotic core, inducing thrombus formation and distal embolism. A possible explanation for the efficacy of percutaneous coronary intervention (PCI) in unstable angina is the fibrotic response induced, so that balloon dilatation of haemodynamically non-significant plaques to induce plaque sealing has been proposed. According to this study, a favourable modification of the plaque substrate does not occur in some cases after DCA. Quantitative immunohistochemistry showed a higher presence of macrophages and T lymphocytes/mm^2 in patients with unstable presentation at follow-up and suggests that ongoing inflammation is responsible for those recurrences. The applicability of these findings to current practice is limited as most patients receive a stent after DCA and lipid-lowering agents are universally used, possibly affecting the inflammatory response of the unstable atherosclerotic plaque (myocardial ischaemia reduction with aggressive cholesterol lowering [MIRACL]) |2|.

Elective stenting of unprotected left main coronary artery stenosis: effect of debulking before stenting and intravascular ultrasound.
S J Park, M K Hong, C W Lee, et al. J Am Coll Cardiol 2001; **38**: 1054–60.

B a c k g r o u n d . **A total of 127 consecutive patients with unprotected left main coronary artery (LMCA) stenosis and normal left ventricular function were treated by elective stenting. The long-term outcomes were evaluated between two groups: debulking/stenting ($n = 40$) and stenting only ($n = 87$). Angiographic follow-up data were obtained for 100 of the 106 eligible patients (follow-up rate 94%). Angiographic restenosis was documented in 19 (19%) of these 100 patients. The angiographic restenosis rate was statistically different at the cut-off level of 3.6 mm for the reference artery size: 13% (9/68) for a reference artery size >3.6 mm compared with 31% (10/32) for a reference artery size <3.6 mm ($P = 0.032$). The angiographic restenosis rate was 13% (1/8) in the debulking/stenting group compared with 40% (8/20) in the stenting only group for a reference vessel size <3.5 mm ($P = 0.159$), and 7% (2/28) in the debulking/stenting group compared with 18% (8/44) in the stenting only group for a reference vessel size >3.5 mm ($P = 0.187$). Four patients died during the follow-up period (mean 12.0 ± 10.7 months). One died of an extensive MI after elective coronary artery bypass graft (CABG) for the treatment of restenosis (at 3.5 months); one died of**

sepsis (at 12.6 months); and the other two died of cancer (at 5 and 27 months). Debulking before stenting seems to be effective in reducing the restenosis rate.

INTERPRETATION. The major findings of this study are: (1) stenting of unprotected LMCA stenosis may be safe and have a high procedural success rate in selected patients with normal left ventricular function; (2) the overall long-term survival and major cardiac event-free survival rates are good; (3) IVUS guidance may help to achieve excellent initial outcomes; (4) debulking before stenting results in lower restenosis rates; and (5) the reference artery diameter is an independent predictor of angiographic restenosis.

Comment

Treatment of left main (LM) disease remains a questionable indication to PCI: the use of stents has reduced the risk of immediate complications but late restenosis can have ominous consequences such as sudden death. In no other location does optimization of immediate and long-term results have greater clinical relevance. Hong *et al.* |3| pioneered percutaneous treatment of LM disease and report their consecutive cumulative experience with 127 patients (100 with angiographic follow-up). Atherectomy was performed in 40/127 patients prior to stent implantation, mainly for treatment of distal bifurcational LM lesions. A dramatic difference in restenosis rate was observed (8.3% in the debulking + stent group vs 25 % in the group with stenting alone). This was not a randomized study, and the lesions had different location and characteristics. However, vessel size was similar in the two groups and the greater plaque burden observed with ultrasound confers a higher *a priori* risk for the group with debulking before stenting.

Relation between pre-intervention remodelling and late arterial responses to coronary angioplasty or atherectomy.

G S Mintz, T Kimura, M Nobuyoshi, G Dangas, M Leon. *Am J Cardiol* 2001; **87**: 392–6.

BACKGROUND. The purpose of the SURE (Serial Ultrasound REstenosis trial) study was to use serial IVUS before intervention, and immediately, and 1 and 6 months after PTCA ($n = 35$) or DCA ($n = 26$) to confirm the presence and define the time course of the changes in external elastic membrane and plaque + media areas. Stenoses were divided into three groups: positive remodelling, intermediate remodelling and negative remodelling. In the first month after intervention, there was an increase in plaque + media area that was accompanied by an equal or greater increase in external elastic membrane area in positive ($r = 0.78$, $P < 0.0001$), intermediate ($r = 0.69$, $P < 0.0001$) and negative ($r = 0.59$, $P = 0.0003$) remodelling lesions. During the subsequent 5 months (from the first to sixth month) pre-intervention positive and intermediate remodelling stenoses behaved differently from pre-intervention negative remodelling stenoses. At 6 months decrease in external elastic membrane area was inversely correlated with the early increase in plaque + media area in positive ($r = 0.77$,

$P = 0.0002$) and intermediate ($r = 0.45$, $P = 0.0003$), but not in negative ($r = 0.02$, $P = 0.9$) remodelling lesion.

INTERPRETATION. Positive remodelling lesions have an exaggerated early increase in external elastic membrane area, and especially an exaggerated late decrease in external elastic membrane area after PTCA and DCA.

Comment

Histopathological studies have indicated that during *de novo* stenosis formation, enlargement of the diseased arterial wall occurs to compensate for the accumulation of atherosclerotic plaque. These studies suggest that, on average, lumen compromise is delayed until the atherosclerotic lesion occupies more than 40–50% of the cross-sectional area within the internal elastic lamina. This compensatory mechanism has been termed positive remodelling. The clinical characteristics of patients have associations with plaque remodelling: smokers have negative/intermediate remodelling and patients with positive remodelling have hypercholesterolaemia and unstable angina. The observations in this study may help to explain why positively remodelled lesions have a higher rate of target lesion revascularization.

This study suggests that arterial responses to non-stent interventions are greater in positively remodelled lesions and explains the increased clinical restenosis when positively remodelled lesions are treated without stents.

Results of the study to determine rotablator and transluminal angioplasty strategy (STRATAS).

P L Whitlow, T A Bass, R M Kipperman, *et al.* for the STRATAS Investigators.
Am J Cardiol 2001; **87**: 699–705.

BACKGROUND. This study reports the outcome of 500 patients randomized to either an aggressive rotablation strategy (burr/artery ratio >0.70 followed by no angioplasty, or angioplasty <1 atm) versus routine rotablation (maximum burr/artery ratio <0.70, followed by routine balloon angioplasty ≥4 atm). Fifteen per cent routine and 16% aggressive strategy patients had a restenotic lesion treated. However, the present study confirms a dichotomous restenosis rate of >50%, even with a very aggressive rotational atherectomy strategy. Results suggest that the burr/artery ratio has little impact on the high restenosis rate seen after rotational atherectomy in complex lesions in vessels averaging 2.6 mm. Lesion length in the Study to Determine Rotablator System and Transluminal Angioplasty Strategy (STRATAS) was 13–14 mm. Creatinine kinase-myocardial band (CK-MB) was >5 times normal in 7% of the routine versus 11% of the aggressive group. At 6 months, 22% of the routine patients compared with 31% of the aggressive strategy patients had target lesion revascularization.

INTERPRETATION. Multivariable analysis indicated that left anterior descending and operator reported excessive speed decreases >5000 rpm (OR 1.74, $P = 0.01$) were significantly associated with restenosis. STRATAS establishes that today's rotational atherectomy technique may also be related to 6-month restenosis. Technique is theoretically controllable by the operator; thus, the more aggressive rotablator strategy, as used in this study, did not confer any benefit to the patient.

Comment

The design of this study (moderate vs aggressive rotational atherectomy) was conceived to determine whether less complete ablation followed by increased barotrauma with balloon stretching aggravates late loss and restenosis.

However, the only difference between the two groups was a higher incidence of slow flow in the aggressive strategy of group (15.7 vs 7.7%, $P = 0.008$), whereas no improvement was observed in long-term angiographic and clinical results. This trial is a survivor of the prehistory of interventional cardiology, belongs to the pre-stent era and its conclusions are not, therefore, applicable to current practice. The only interest of this trial is the final confirmation that strategies aimed at minimizing wall damage to parted restenosis are not effective. Previous reports have shown (Kobayashi, Colombo) |4| that aggressive rotablator followed by aggressive stenting can improve long-term outcome. In this study, however, following this principle, a very conservative dilatation at very low pressure was performed after atherectomy, with the net effect that the final minimum lumen diameter (MLD) was similar in the two groups.

Long-term outcome of patients with proximal left anterior descending coronary artery in-stent restenosis treated with rotational atherectomy.

R Moreno, E Garcia, J Soriano, J Acosta, M Abeytua. *Cathet Cardiovasc Intervent* 2001; **52**: 435–42.

B A C K G R O U N D . The study population comprised 42 patients with proximal left anterior descending ISR treated with rotational atherectomy (RA). Restenosis length was 16.5 ± 9.2 mm, and restenosis was diffuse (>10 mm in length) in 30 patients (71.4%). Eighteen patients (42%) underwent IVUS evaluation. An angiographic evaluation was performed at 6.5 ± 2.7 months in 32 patients (76.2%). Angiographic restenosis was documented in 17 (53%). Diffuse ISR was associated with a nearly twofold angiographic restenosis rate. Two patients with restenosis were initially referred for CABG, fourteen underwent new percutaneous re-intervention (three of whom were finally sent to CABG) and one patient was managed medically. The restenosis rate in patients with diffuse or non-diffuse ISR was 61.9 and 36.4%, respectively ($P = 0.16$). They found no death, Q wave infarction, or new target vessel revascularization during hospitalization, except for a non-Q wave peri-procedural infarction. The rate of surgical revascularization at 6 months, 1 year and 3 years was 4.8, 7.4 and 18% respectively.

I N T E R P R E T A T I O N . The use of RA is associated with a very good long-term outcome, with few patients undergoing surgical revascularization.

Comment

The approach to proximal left anterior descending (PLAD) ISR is usually CABG. Balloon angioplasty for ISR is associated with high restenosis rate of almost 40%, especially with diffuse ISR (length >10 mm). Some studies suggest that rotational atherectomy may be a better treatment for diffuse ISR than balloon PTCA. Dauerman *et al.* |5| showed that patients with IRS treated with debulking had lower restenosis and major adverse cardiac event (MACE) rates at 1 year than those treated with balloon angioplasty. Usually, RA achieved a higher acute lumen gain and lower clinical recurrence than balloon angioplasty. In the experimental study by McKenna *et al.* |6|, RA produced less intimal hyperplasia than balloon PTCA for ISR; this may partly explain the beneficial effect of RA for ISR.

This technique for the treatment of diffuse ISR may also be used in patients with left ventricular dysfunction and multivessel disease.

Clinical recurrence after RA has ranged from 28 to 50%, with an angiographic restenosis rate up to 45%. In one study, 28% of target lesion revascularization (TLR) occurred after RA with adjunctive PTCA compared with 46% with PTCA alone.

This study was performed in a small number of patients and has limited power to detect some clinical characteristics and procedural details able to predict the outcome. The main limitation of this report is the absence of a comparison group of patients with PLAD ISR managed with CABG.

Coronary angioplasty and rotablator atherectomy trial (CARAT): immediate and late results of a prospective multicenter randomized trial.

R D Safian, T Feldman, D W M Muller, *et al. Catheter Cardiovasc Intervent* 2001; **53**: 213–20.

BACKGROUND. This study aimed to compare immediate and late outcomes after rotablator using two treatment strategies: large burrs (burr/artery ratio >0.7) to achieve maximal debulking (lesion debulking strategy) or small burrs (burr/artery ratio <0.7) to modify lesion compliance (lesion modification strategy). A total of 222 patients at 6 centres were enrolled in this prospective multicentre trial. Quantitative angiographic results were similar for the two groups (debulking vs modification): final stenosis diameter 27 ± 17% and 23 ± 18%, respectively; rotational angiographic complications occurred in 31 lesions (12.1%) after rotablator (dissection, no-reflow and perforation), including 12.7% after a large burr and 5.1% after a small burr (*P* <0.05). In-hospital MACE occurred in 18 patients (8.1%), and included death, Q wave MI or emergency CABG in six patients (2.7%). Late MACE (death, MI and TLR) occurred in 73 patients (34.4%). Target vessel revascularization was required in 25% of patients.

INTERPRETATION. This study suggests that small burrs (burr/artery ratio <0.7) achieved similar immediate lumen enlargement and late target vessel revascularization as a more aggressive debulking strategy (burr/artery ratio >0.7) but with fewer angiographic complications.

Comment

Mechanical rotational atherectomy uses a high-speed rotablator burr to enlarge the lumen by plaque pulverization and embolization, rather than tissue removal. This study did not address the routine use of other adjunctive devices (directional atherectomy, stents) or pharmacological agents (glycoprotein IIb/IIIa inhibitors).

Data from randomized trials comparing PTCA with RA suggested that despite greater immediate lumen enlargement after RA, there is a paradoxical incidence of angiographic restenosis and target lesion revascularization. Retrospective analysis from a single-centre experience suggests that the greatest lumen enlargement and lowest target lesion revascularization rates were achieved when the burr/artery ratio was >0.6–0.8; burr/artery ratio <0.6 and 0.8 achieved inferior results. However, application of the maximal debulking strategy was limited by technical problems (failure to access target lesions because of severe tortuosity), angiographic complications (dissection) and severe arrhythmias (severe brachycardia), all of which precluded the use of larger burrs. These data coming from the STRATAS trial demonstrated no advantage for an aggressive rotablator strategy in *de novo* lesions.

Three-year follow-up after rotational atherectomy for the treatment of diffuse in-stent restenosis: predictors of major adverse cardiac events.

R W Radke, J vom Dahl, R Hoffman, *et al. Cathet Cardiovasc Intervent* 2001; **53**: 334–40.

BACKGROUND. In this study, RA with adjunct angioplasty for ISR was performed in 84 patients. Angiographic follow-up at 6 months was performed in 90% of patients. Restenosis was observed in 34/76 lesions (45%) with the need for target vessel revascularization in 27/84 (32%) patients. Overall, MACE rate at 6 months was 35% (29/84). Predictor of MACE by univariate analysis at 3-year follow-up was small vessel size. The only independent predictor of MACE within 3 years, as assessed by multivariate logistic regression analysis, however, was in-stent lesion length. Clinical follow-up over a period of 3 years documented a significant decline in the MACE rate after the first 6 months post intervention. Angiographic restenosis rate was 45% in patients with diffuse lesions characterized by rotational atherectomy of ISR. In-stent lesion length was the only independent predictor of adverse events.

Comment

Patients treated in this study had a mean small vessel diameter <2.5 mm. As vessel size was a predictor of MACE by univariate analysis, restenosis rate may potentially be lower than 45% when treating vessels of diameter >3.5 mm. This study reflects a single-centre experience in a consecutive series of patients and there was no control group. Limited experience with excimer laser angioplasty (ELA) and rotational atherectomy have shown that, although these strategies are safe and effective in discrete lesions, they have had high rates of recurrence when applied to diffuse lesions. It is of interest that use of mechanical treatment modalities seems to result in a high and rather unsatisfying clinical restenosis rate of 30% or more. In the conclusion to the largest, non-randomized comparative study (PTCA, ELA, rotablation and stent) by Mehran *et al.* |7|, the term great equalizer has been created to characterize the uniformly unsatisfactory clinical outcome following treatment for diffuse ISR.

Impact of pre-stent plaque debulking for chronic coronary total occlusion on restenosis reduction.

E Tsuchikane, S Otsuji, N Awata, *et al.* *J Invasive Cardiol* 2001; **13**(8): 584–9.

B A C K G R O U N D . **This study examined the pre-stent plaque debulking strategy with high-speed RA for 50 patients with chronic total occlusion (thrombolysis in myocardial infarction [TIMI] flow grade 0; estimated occlusive duration, >3 months). The angiographic follow-up results were compared with those for 120 consecutive patients with chronic total occlusion recanalized using primary stenting in which RA could be indicated retrospectively. RA could be performed safely in all lesions without any major complication. Quantitative coronary angiography revealed that diameter stenosis was smaller at follow-up (36.2 ± 20.0 vs 52.2 ± 26.7%, *P* = 0.0003) as well as post procedure (7.8 ± 11.5 vs 17.8 ± 13.6%, *P* < 0.0001) compared with the control group. Angiographic restenosis was also significantly reduced (29.2 vs 52.5%, *P* = 0.0061).**

I N T E R P R E T A T I O N . Plaque debulking of chronic total occlusion facilitates subsequent stent expansion and may reduce the restenosis rate.

Comment

Despite recanalization of chronic coronary total occlusion, restenosis remained high at >50%, RA may be a safe procedure in selected cases.

Directional atherectomy prior to stenting in bifurcation lesions: a matched comparison study with stenting alone.

E Karvouni, C Di Mario, T Nishida, *et al. Catheter Cardiovascular Interv* 2001; **53**(1): 12–20.

B A C K G R O U N D . **This study aimed to assess the acute and long-term outcome after the treatment of bifurcation lesions using DCA plus stenting in comparison with stenting alone. Thirty-one consecutive patients treated for bifurcation coronary lesions (62 lesions) were evaluated between two groups: debulking/stenting versus stenting alone. In-hospital MACE occurred only in the DCA group (13 vs 0%, *P* = 0.03) and was mainly non-Q wave MI. After the procedure, MLD and acute gain were significantly greater (*P* = 0.004 and 0.05, respectively) and percent diameter stenosis was significantly lower (*P* = 0.05) in the main branch in the DCA group. At follow-up angiogram, MLD in**

the main branch was still significantly greater in the DCA group than the non-DCA group. Restenosis rate was 28.8% in the DCA group compared with 43.5% in the non-DCA cohort ($P = 0.13$), and the incidence of follow-up MACE was 29% in the DCA group compared with 48.4% in the non-DCA group.

INTERPRETATION. Restenosis rate and follow-up MACE were lower following DCA and stenting, without reaching any statistical significance.

Conclusion

Debulking with atherectomy may play a role in various clinical settings to reduce the restenosis rate. It may be effective in the treatment of (a) diffuse ISR followed by radiation therapy, (b) stenting of left main, (c) ISR, (d) chronic total occlusion, or (e) bifurcation lesions by reducing late restenosis.

However, a large randomized trial demonstrated no benefit to reduce restenosis compared to coronary angioplasty and there appeared to be no difference in the restenosis rate using an aggressive versus a moderate rotablation strategy, whereas the technique was less effective in long in-stent lesions. Recurrent unstable angina occurs more often in plaques with extensive inflammation, as was shown in the retrieved atherectomy specimens, and the clinical restenosis was increased after atherectomy of lesions with expansive remodelling.

In conclusion: atherectomy may have some additional value as a debulking procedure. The impact is rather small and many investigators will not be inclined to use the technique except in severe calcified lesions, ostial lesions or need of tissue specimens for scientific purposes.

References

1. Gruberg L, Grenadier E, Miller H, Peled B, Rougin A, Markiewicz W, Beyar R. First clinical experience with the pre-mounted balloon-expandable serpentine stent: acute angiographic and intermediate-term clinical results. *Catheter Cardiovasc Intervent* 1999; **46**(2): 249–53.

2. Ahsan CH, Shah A, Ezekowitz M. Acute statin treatment in reducing risk after acute coronary syndrome: the MIRACL (Myocardial Ischaemia Reduction with Aggressive Cholesterol Lowering) Trial. *Curr Opin Cardiol* 2001; **16**(6): 390–3.

3. Hong MK, Park SW, Lee CW, *et al.* Intravascular ultrasound findings in stenting of unprotected left main coronary artery stenosis. *Am J Cardiol* 1998; **82**: 670–3.

4. Kobayashi Y, De Gregorio J, Kobayashi N, Akiyama T, Reimers B, Moussa I, Di Mario C, Finci L, Colombo A. Lower restenosis rate with stenting following aggressive versus less aggressive rotational atherectomy. *Catheter Cardiovasc Interv* 1999; **46**:(4) 406–14.

5. Dauerman HL, Baim DS, Cutlip DE, Sparano AM, Gibson CM, Kuntz RE, Carrozza JP, Garber GR, Cohen DJ. Mechanical debulking versus balloon angioplasty for the treatment of diffuse in-stent restenosis. *Am J Cardiol* 1998; **82**: 277–84.

6. McKenna CJ, Wilson SH, Camrud AR, Berger PB, Holmes DR, Schwartz RS. Neointimal response following rotational atherectomy compared to balloon angioplasty in a porcine model of coronary in-stent restenosis. *Cathet Cardiovasc Diagn* 1998; **45**: 332–6.

7. Mehran R, Dangas G, Mintz GS, Waksman R, Hong MK, Abizaid A, Abizaid AS, Kornowski R, Lansky AJ, Laird IR Jr, Kent KM, Pichard AD, Satler LF, Stone GW, Leon MB. In-stent restenosis: 'the great equalizer' – disappointing clinical outcomes with all interventional strategies. *J Am Coll Cardiol* 1999; **33**: 1129–91.

15

Contrast agent optimization

Introduction

Optimization of contrast media is a very intense field of current imaging research. Although contrast agents are also utilized for X-ray angiography, ultrasound and computed tomography, this review concentrates on contrast media for magnetic resonance imaging (MRI) because of the rapid advances and developments in this area of cardiovascular imaging.

Why do we need improved contrast agents for interventional cardiology? The MR contrast agents, which are clinically used and currently available worldwide, offer sufficient satisfactory properties to achieve quality images with MR angiography in most parts of the body. These extracellular compounds, however, are limited for imaging a rapidly moving organ with small vessels due to their fast wash-out effect and their relatively low relaxivity. Optimal contrast depends also on the imaging technology (hard- and software, power injector, etc.), which improves continuously and alters the requirements for new vascular contrast agents. To enable MR interventions in cardiology both aspects, equipment and contrast agents, need to evolve.

Several encouraging reports appeared in 2001 with emphasis on the two major imaging areas in cardiology: vessels and myocardium. Two papers concentrate on contrast media application and optimization of image acquisition. The other reports look at different extracellular and intravascular contrast agents either for coronary MR angiography (CMRA) or perfusion imaging of the myocardium. Most of the studies with intravascular contrasts agent were performed in animals indicating that there is still a lack of intravascular compounds on the market for cardiovascular imaging.

Two different ultra-small particles of iron oxides (USPIO) are presented as intravascular (blood pool) compounds showing their unique capabilities for comprehensive cardiovascular analysis. MRI of early atherosclerotic changes in the aorta has been described as a functional imaging approach by monitoring the macrophagosytation of iron particles.

Gadolinium (Gd)-based macromolecules are a different subgroup of blood pool contrast agents and are capable of improving steady-state CMRA. Two important studies have looked at two different kinds of macromolecules, each of them compared with an extracellular contrast agent.

There is still no definite agreement on which kind of contrast agent we should use to improve detection of microvascular damage of the myocardium. Considering changes in the vessel wall, there is a theoretical suggestion that macromolecular contrast agents could improve specificity. One study evaluated whether MRI using a small molecular contrast agent is able to detect early reduction of perfusion in still viable myocardium. This would be an indirect parameter of vascular stenosis and may be a valuable adjunct tool to assess vascular changes.

Contrast agents with a strong protein-binding effect reveal a higher relaxivity and are also able to remain within the vascular space for longer. It has been shown in previous studies that these compounds offer improved vascular characteristics in many applications.

Breath-hold 3D MR coronary angiography with a new intravascular contrast agent (feruglose)—first clinical experiences.

J J Sandstede, T Pabst, C Wacker, *et al. Magn Reson Imaging* 2001; **19**: 201–5.

BACKGROUND. This study reports the initial results of breath-hold 3D coronary MR angiography with patients using a superparamagnetic intravascular contrast agent. Feruglose (NC100150) belongs to the class of USPIOs. Contrast-enhanced 3D MR coronary angiography was performed in five patients with coronary artery disease after administration of NC100150 feruglose in three different doses (0.5 [n = 3], 2 and 5 mg/kg). MR coronary angiography was performed with an electrocardiogram (ECG)-triggered 3D-FLASH-sequence during breath-hold at 1.5 T (TR 6.8 ms, TE 2.5 ms, flip-angle 30°). To reduce data acquisition time, only the two anterior elements of the phased-array body coil were activated. The data acquisition window within the cardiac cycle ranged between 217 and 326 ms, depending on the matrix. Signal-to-noise (SNR) and contrast-to-noise (CNR) ratios of the coronary arteries were analysed, and the results for the detection of coronary artery stenoses were compared with those obtained using conventional coronary angiography.

INTERPRETATION. SNR and CNR revealed an improved image quality at a dose of 2 mg/kg compared with the lower dose, but no further improvement was obtained by increasing the dose to 5 mg/kg. Except for the left circumflex artery of one patient, the proximal parts of all four main coronary arteries at the very least could be imaged for all patients. Within the visible parts of the coronary arteries, six of eight significant coronary stenoses were identified correctly. Imaging of the proximal parts of the coronary arteries, including detection of stenoses, is possible during breath-hold using a USPIO.

Comment

This is a useful study in a small population (*n* = 5) that evaluates important aspects of vascular imaging with an USPIO. NC100150 has already been used successfully in the abdominal and pelvic region |**1**|. Delineation of the distal part of coronary arteries remains difficult. These superparamagnetic compounds are challenging for the

Table 15.1 Signal-to-noise ratio and contrast-to-noise ratio of the coronary arteries at three different doses

Dose	SNR	CNR (myocardium)	CNR (fat)
Unenhanced	8.6 ± 3.8	1.4 ± 5.4	–2.3 ± 6.5
0.5 mg Fe/kg BW*	15.9 ± 9.0	6.1 ± 1.8	5.3 ± 13.1
2 mg Fe/kg BW	24.1 ± 9.1	12.5 ± 5.8	14.8 ± 8.3
5 mg Fe/kg BW	26.5 ± 9.0	12.9 ± 8.2	14.8 ± 7.1

All data are presented as mean ± SD. *n = 3; SNR, signal-to-noise ratio; CNR, contrast-to-noise ratio of coronary artery/myocardium or of coronary artery/fat; BW, body weight.
Source: Sandstede *et al.* (2001).

research community because of the need to optimize sequence parameters (TE, TR, flip angle), and appropriate dosing to further improve SNR and CNR values [2]. The dose bandwidth for USPIOs is fairly small (Table 15.1) compared with extracellular, paramagnetic Gd-based contrast agents. Currently, image post processing for evaluation of the degree of vascular stenoses is carried out using maximum intensity projection (MIP) and multiplanar reconstruction (MPR) techniques. Advanced post-processing methods are needed to improve delineation of vascular stenoses and to reduce secondarily caused artefacts. Intravascular contrast agents are useful to enable comprehensive imaging of the heart, including functional analysis such as myocardial perfusion, as well as interventional procedures.

Gadolinium-enhanced, vessel-tracking, two-dimensional coronary MR angiography: single-dose arterial-phase vs delayed-phase imaging.

V B Ho, T K Foo, A E Arai, S D Wolff. *J Magn Reson Imaging* 2001; **13**: 682–9.

BACKGROUND. The authors investigated the benefits of using a single dose of an extracellular contrast agent for CMRA and determined the relative benefits of first-pass versus delayed-phase image acquisition. Only the right coronary artery was imaged in 10 healthy adults using a breath-hold, two-dimensional, fast-gradient echo pulse sequence designed for vessel tracking (multiphase, multislice image acquisition). Pre- and post-contrast CMRA was performed. Post-contrast imaging consisted of first-pass and delayed-phase CMRA following a 15 ml bolus (single dose) of contrast media and of a further delayed-phase imaging following a cumulative contrast dose of 45 ml (triple dose). Contrast-enhanced CMRA provided a significantly higher (P <0.001) SNR and CNR than non-contrast CMRA (Table 15.2). CNR was highest for single-dose, first-pass CMRA (13.1 ± 4.5) and triple-dose, delayed-phase CMRA (13.0 ± 4.8), followed by single-dose, delayed-phase CMRA (8.4 ± 3.5) and non-contrast CMRA (4.2 ± 1.8). Single-dose, first-pass CMRA provided the best visualization of the distal right coronary artery and was preferred for blinded physician assessments.

Table 15.2 Quantitative measurements of signal-to-noise and contrast-to-noise rations in the right coronary artery (RCA)

	Non-contrast	Single-dose arterial phase	Single-dose delayed phase	Triple-dose delayed phase
SNR	13.9 ± 4.6	23.1 ± 4.8	20.2 ± 4.5	26.5 ± 5.0
CNR	4.3 ± 1.5	13.5 ± 4.6	8.4 ± 3.7	13.0 ± 4.8
RCA length	6.4 ± 4.0	10.0 ± 4.2	8.2 ± 3.9	7.5 ± 3.6
	(6.9 ± 4.8*)	(11.9 ± 3.6*)	(9.4 ± 4.0*)	(8.5 ± 4.0*)

*Measurements excluding the three subjects in whom only the proximal RCA (initial 5–6 cm) was included within the 2D imaging line.
Source: Ho *et al.* (2001).

INTERPRETATION. Utilization of a single dose of an extracellular Gd-chelate improves CMRA, especially if timed for first-pass imaging.

Comment

This is an elaborate study that considers several different imaging aspects of contrast-enhanced CMRA. Other groups also analysed first-pass CMRA using an extracellular contrast agent but with segmented echo-planar imaging (SEPI) |**3**|. In this area of research, several imaging protocols have been described for different kinds of sequence design, dosing, injection rate, contrast media type, etc. |**4**|. In this study with healthy volunteers ($n = 10$) an ECG-gated vessel tracking pulse sequence was added to further improve image quality. Standard extracellular Gd-chelates (e.g. Gd-DTPA) improve first-pass imaging but are less useful for the steady-state phase which requires high dosing. Steady-state CMRA with advanced contrast agents like USPIO or strong protein-binding Gd-based chelates has been performed by other groups |**5,6**|. Additional studies may be warranted to investigate if first-pass CMRA could benefit from contrast agents with a higher T_1-relaxivity. The authors leave unanswered the question of how this encouraging technique can be applied if more than one vascular territory has to be imaged.

Slow clearance gadolinium-based extracellular and intravascular contrast media for three-dimensional MR angiography.
J Bremerich, J M Colet, G B Giovenzana, *et al. J Magn Reson Imaging* 2001; **13**: 588–93.

BACKGROUND. Two new, slow-clearance, contrast media with extracellular and intravascular distribution for magnetic resonance angiography (MRA) were assessed in animals. Extracellular Gd-DTPA-BC(2)glucA and intravascular Gd(DO3A)(3)-lys(16) were developed within the European Biomed2 MACE Program and compared with two reference compounds, intravascular CMD-A2-Gd-DOTA and extracellular Gd-DOTA, in 12 rats. Pre- and post-contrast three-dimensional MR (TR/TE = 5 ms/2.2 ms; isotropic voxel size 0.86 mm^3) was acquired for 2 h. Signal-to-noise enhancement (ΔSNR) was calculated. Two minutes after injection, all contrast media provided strong vascular signal enhancement. The ΔSNR for Gd-DTPA-BC(2)glucA, Gd(DO3A)(3)-lys(16), CMD-A2-Gd-DOTA and GdDOTA were 13.0 ± 1.8, 25.0 ± 3.2, 25.0 ± 4.0, and 18.0 ± 3.4, respectively. Gd-DTPA-BC(2)glucA, Gd(DO3A)(3)-lys(16), and CMD-A2-Gd-DOTA cleared slowly from the circulation, whereas GdDOTA cleared rapidly. Vascular ΔSNR at 2 hours were 2.9 ± 0.6, 25.0 ± 3.2, 25.0 ± 4.0, and 0.4 ± 1.0.

INTERPRETATION. Gd(DO3A)(3)-lys(16) provided strong vascular and minor background enhancement, and thus may be useful for MRA or perfusion imaging. Gd-DTPA-BC(2)glucA produces persistent enhancement of extracellular water, and thus may allow quantification of extracellular distribution volume and assessment of myocardial viability.

Comment

Currently, several groups are investigating different types of contrast agents for MRA of the coronary arteries, especially with blood pool contrast agents [7,8]. Although

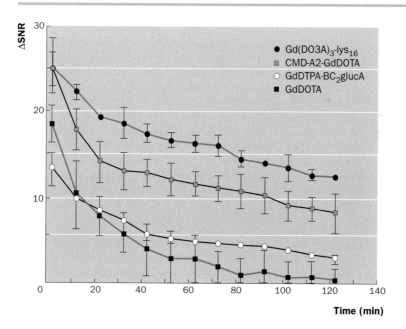

Fig. 15. 1 Change in signal-to-noise ratio (ΔSNR) of blood plotted over time after injection of Gd(DO3A)3-lys16, CMD-A2-Gd-DOTA, GdDTPA-BC2glucA or Gd-DOTA in a tail vein ($n = 3$ for each compound). Source Bremerich et al. (2001).

extracellular contrast agents like Gd-DTPA and its derivates are utilized with excellent safety records and established quality in clinical routine imaging, to date, no intravascular agent has been on the market. This interindividual animal study ($n = 12$) investigated a dextran, polylysine and glucose-coupled macromolecule. Dextran compounds have a favourable biocompatibility, solubility, versatility of chemical activation and are available at different molecular masses, but have the disadvantage of polydispersity. Highest SNR values were found for the polylysine complex (Fig. 15.1). The authors provide information on the blood half-life of the glucose-based compound (289 min) and the dextran (carboxymethyl-dextran polymer) complex (>182 min), but not on the polylysine compound which could be a major drawback for safety issues in humans, as already reported in the literature. Image acquisition time was 2 h which seems rather long for a practical application. An intra-individual study design, also for animal studies, may help to further optimize a standardized comparison.

Arterial first-pass gadolinium-CM dynamics as a function of several intravenous saline flush and Gd volumes.

M Boos, K Scheffler, R Haselhorst, *et al. J Magn Reson Imaging* 2001; **13**: 568–76.

BACKGROUND. This study was performed to evaluate the contrast enhancement dynamics of an arterial first-pass Gd contrast agent bolus at the descending aorta (DAo), depending on various saline flush and Gd volumes. Several saline flush volumes (15, 30 and 60 ml) were applied following the administration of 10 ml Gd (single dose) to a group of four normal volunteers using a mechanical MR injector (injection rate = 3.0 ml/s). Also, when performing a second test series, the saline volume remained constant, while the Gd volumes were varied from half doses to triple doses (5, 10, 20 and 30 ml Gd were given to every volunteer of the group). The signal intensity versus time (SI/T) curve at a measured region of interest (ROI) within the DAo was calculated. The bolus arrival time, the maximal SNR ratio (SNR_{max}), the bolus time length (BTL; 75 and 80% maximum intensity duration), the slope of the SI/T curve, and the areas below the SI/T curve for both the 80 and 75% maximum intensity duration level ($INT_{80\%}$ and $INT_{75\%}$) were calculated.

INTERPRETATION. The arterial bolus length benefits from increasing Gd and saline flush volumes due to increased venous bolus length and wash-out effects of Gd within the injection site of the vein. Doses larger than a single dose are not needed to increase the SNR in contrast-enhanced magnetic resonance angiography images of the thoracic aorta.

Comment

This study provides a very detailed analysis in healthy volunteers ($n = 8$) of the characteristics of signal intensity patterns in the DAo after changing the application protocol for an intravenous injection of MR contrast media (Fig. 15.2). Previous studies looked at different injection rates and Gd doses, but not at higher saline volumes |9|. A post-contrast media volume of 15–20 ml of saline has been used almost like a paradigm. The increase in saline flush volume from 30 to 60 ml caused significant bolus lengthening of approximately 50% (mean BTL = 9.5, 10.3 and 15.4 s for 15, 30 and 60 ml saline flush volumes, respectively, measured as SI/T duration at the 75% SNR_{max} level). Using saline flush volumes $\geq$30 ml increased the slope of the SI/T curve. A continuous increase of $INT_{75\%/80\%}$ using higher saline flush volumes was found. Different saline and Gd volumes did not affect the SNR_{max} and the bolus arrival time. Only the low dose (0.05 mmol/kg Gd) showed a 17–21.6% significantly lower SNR_{max}. The BTL and INT increased mainly by increasing applied Gd volume from single to double dose ($BTL_{75\%}$ and $INT_{75\%}$ were 9.6 s and 1305, 12.3 s and 2121, 38.5 s and 6181 and 37.8 s and 6613 for 5, 10, 20 and 30 ml applied Gd volume, respectively). This study shows that image quality is improved to a certain extend (up to 0.2 mmol/kg BW) by increasing the maximum signal intensity and the bolus length. Optimizing the duration of the bolus length can also be improved by higher saline volumes reducing dose and therefore costs.

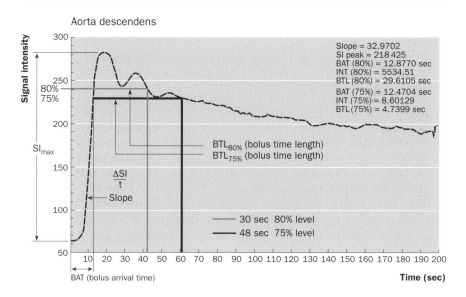

Fig. 15.2 Evaluation of the signal intensity (SI)/time (T) curve in the aorta descendens. Detailed analysis of the bolus arrival time (BAT), SI_{max} and the bolus time length (BTL) at the 80 and 75% maximum level. The repeated increase of SI is due to the second passage of the contrast medium through the aorta after passage through the lung and kidneys. Source: Boos *et al.* (2001).

Magnetic resonance imaging of atherosclerotic plaque with ultrasmall superparamagnetic particles of iron oxide in hyperlipidemic rabbits.

S G Ruehm, C Corot, P Vogt, S Kolb, J F Debatin. *Circulation* 2001; **103**: 415–22.

B A C K G R O U N D . USPIOs are phagocytosed not only by cells of the reticuloendothelial system (RES), but also by the mononuclear phagocytic system (MPS). AMI-27 (Combidex) was administered to evaluate its use as a marker of atherosclerosis-associated inflammatory changes in the vessel wall before luminal narrowing is present. Experiments were conducted on six heritable hyperlipidaemic and three New Zealand White rabbits. Three-dimensional MRA of the thoracic aorta was performed on all rabbits using a conventional paramagnetic contrast agent that failed to reveal any abnormalities. One week later, all rabbits except one of the hyperlipidaemic animals were injected with ferumoxtran at a dose of 1 mmol Fe/kg.

I N T E R P R E T A T I O N . USPIOs are phagocytosed by macrophages in atherosclerotic plaques of the aortic wall of hyperlipidaemic rabbits in a quantity sufficient to cause darkening (susceptibility) effects detectable by MRI.

Comment

Why do we need new contrast agents to detect atherosclerotic changes? Plaque imaging in clinical patients is currently a domain for computed tomography and to some extend for ultrasound, but overall it is still quite underdeveloped. MRI also shows promising results for high spatial resolution imaging of plaques |**10**|. This is a fascinating paper showing early-stage atherosclerotic changes in the aortic wall based on functional MRI using a recently introduced USPIO. The daily follow-up of the SNR values (Fig. 15.3) demonstrated how contrast enhancement characteristics can change over time after a single intravenous injection if the contrast agent does not only follow the usual excretion pathways.

Three-dimensional MRA images were acquired subsequently over 5 days and showed that the SI in the aortic lumen increased, whereas in the aortic wall a decrease in atherosclerosis-associated inflammatory changed vessels was noted. Whereas the aortic wall in the control rabbits remained smooth and bright, marked susceptibility (darkening) effects became evident in the aortic walls of hyperlipidaemic rabbits. Histology and electron microscopy confirmed marked uptake of iron in macrophages embedded in atherosclerotic plaque of the hyperlipidaemic rabbits. Morphological and functional MR open new strategies, ranging from the screening of high-risk patients for early detection and treatment to the monitoring of target areas for pharmacological intervention. This useful study would benefit from a larger number of animals and suggests that human applications are conceivable with a modified imaging technique.

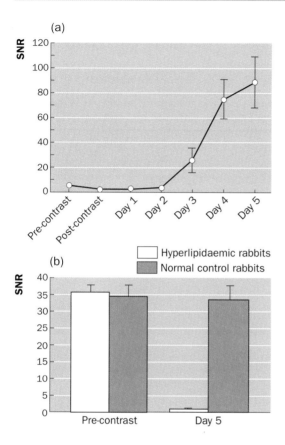

Fig. 15.3 Measurements of signal-to-noise ratio (SNR) of the aortic lumen and wall in hyperlipidaemic and healthy rabbits after intravenous administration of the USPIO AMI-227 (Sinerem) at a dose of 1 mmol Fe/kg. (a) Intraluminal signal intensity (SI) revealed an increase in SNR over time, with a maximum reached at day 5. The increase in SI is due to decreasing $T2^*$-effects. (b) SNR values based on three measurements of three regions of interest in the aortic wall. In normal rabbits, there is no difference between pre-contrast and 5-day post-contrast images. In hyperlipidaemic animals, a significant decrease in SNR corresponding to select USPIO uptake in plaque formations containing cells of the macrophagic system was noticed. Source: Ruehm *et al.* (2001).

Contrast-enhanced MR imaging of coronary arteries: comparison of intra- and extravascular contrast agents in swine.

D Li, J Zheng, H J Weinmann. *Radiology* 2001; **218**: 670–8.

BACKGROUND. The aim of this animal study was to compare the efficacy of the intravascular contrast agent Gadomer-17 and the extravascular agent gadopentetate dimeglumine (Gd-DTPA) for improved MRI of coronary arteries. The pigs (*n* = 8) underwent imaging after three injections: 0.2 mmol of Gd-DTPA/kg BW, 0.05 and 0.1 mmol of Gadomer-17/kg. Coronary images were acquired repeatedly after each injection using an inversion-recovery-prepared segmented three-dimensional sequence with either breath holding (*n* = 4) or respiratory gating (*n* = 4). Coronary artery-to-myocardium CNRs were compared between injections.

INTERPRETATION. Gadomer-17 provided greater and more persistent CNR improvements than did Gd-DTPA. SNR improvements even of larger volumes are possible with respiratory gating technique.

Comment

This animal study addresses an area of major interest in MRI of the coronary arteries by comparing a standard extracellular contrast agent (Gd-DTPA <1000 Da) with a

Table 15.3 Coronary artery signal-to-noise (SNR) and coronary artery–myocardium contrast-to-noise (CNR) at 3D breath-hold imaging in four pigs

Delay after contrast agent injection (min)	0.20 mmol/kg Gadopenetate dimeglumine	0.05 mmol/kg Gadomer-17	0.10 mm/kg Gadomer-17
Coronary artery SNR*			
0–10	7.4 ± 0.8	9.5 ± 0.8†	14.8 ± 1.3†
10–20	NA	7.5 ± 0.8	11.6 ± 0.8†
20–30	NA	6.0 ± 1.1	9.9 ± 0.9†
30–40	NA	NA	8.7 ± 1.2
40–50	NA	NA	5.3 ± 0.9
Coronary artery–myocardium CNR‡			
0–10	4.4 ± 0.6†	6.7 ± 0.9†	11.8 ± 1.0†
10–20	NA	5.1 ± 0.6†	8.7 ± 0.3†
20–30	NA	3.6 ± 0.6†	7.0 ± 0.9†
30–40	NA	NA	5.3 ± 0.8†
40–50	NA	NA	2.7 ± 0.6†

*The pre-contrast coronary artery SNR was 7.0 ± 0.8.
†Significantly higher than at pre-contrast imaging (*P* <0.05).
‡The pre-contrast coronary artery–myocardium CNR was 1.4 ± 0.9.
Source: Li *et al.* (2001).

macromolecular agent (Gadomer-17 = 35 kDa). Intravascular contrast agents enable a higher number of ECG-triggered acquisitions combined with respiratory gating and therefore, improve spatial resolution. At respiratory-gated imaging, a significant CNR improvement (P <0.05) over pre-contrast images was observed in images acquired up to 10, 30 and 50 min after gadopentetate dimeglumine and both Gadomer-17 injections, respectively. The CNR on the first images obtained after 0.1 mmol/kg Gadomer-17 injection was 168% (P <0.05) higher than that on the images obtained after gadopentetate dimeglumine injection (Table 15.3).

SNR computer simulations were performed to optimize parameters for the inversion recovery time. Further studies would probably benefit from a bigger delay between the application of different contrast agents. Results with this Gd-based macromolecule are encouraging to evaluate its utility for coronary imaging in humans.

Coronary magnetic resonance angiography: experimental evaluation of the new rapid clearance blood pool contrast medium P792.

M Taupitz, J Schnorr, S Wagner, *et al. Magn Reson Med* 2001; **46**: 932–8.

BACKGROUND. The signal-enhancing characteristics of a new monodisperse, monogadolinated, macromolecular MR contrast medium (P792) were evaluated for MRA of the coronary arteries. This contrast agent belongs to the group of rapid-clearance blood pool agents (RCBPAs) with a higher T1-relaxivity (R1) of approximately 39/s/M compared with Gd-DTPA (approximately 3.8/s/M) measured at 20 MHz in water. For comparison a weak protein binding Gd-chelate (gadobenate dimeglumine, Gd-BOPTA) was used. Gd-BOPTA has a T1-relaxivity in plasma almost twice as high as the R1 of standard Gd-chelates. In total, 15 cardiac examinations were performed in pigs ($n = 5$) at 1.5 T using a 3D gradient-echo sequence. Images were acquired during breath-hold before and up to 35 min after intravenous injection of Gd-DTPA (0.3 mmol Gd/kg), Gd-BOPTA (0.2 mmol Gd/kg) and P792 (13 μmol Gd/kg). An increase in the SNR of 97 ± 17, 108 ± 37 and 109 ± 31% in coronary arteries and of 82 ± 19, 82 ± 24 and 28 ± 18% in myocardium, respectively, was measured during the first post-contrast acquisition. The blood-to-myocardium signal-difference-to-noise ratio (SDNR) was significantly higher for P792 than for the other Gd compounds (P <0.05) for up to 15 min after injection. Qualitative assessment showed that visualization of the coronary arteries and their branches was significantly better for P792 than for the low molecular mass Gd compounds (P <0.05).

INTERPRETATION. The blood pool contrast medium P792 shows improved enhancement characteristics for blood pool MRA of the coronary arteries.

Comment

This relevant study compared three different contrast agents A, a gadolinium-based macromolecule (P792) B, a weak protein interacting Gd-chelate (Gd-BOPTA) and C, a low non-specific standard Gd-compound (Gd-DTPA), the latter are both extracellular contrast agents. Owing to the higher R1 values of P792, we would expect much higher SI values in the coronary arteries compared with the other two compounds. The similar results for the maximal increase in SNR of the left coronary artery may be due to the fact that Gd-DTPA was administered at a dose of 0.3 mmol/kg, whereas the applied dose for P792 (13 μmol Gd/kg) corresponds to a dose of only 0.1 mmol/kg Gd-DTPA in terms of R1. Gd-BOPTA shows highest SI values in the myocardium after 5 min owing to its properties. On delayed images, it was better suited to evaluated changes in the myocardium. The enhancement characteristics described for P792 in animals make it a potentially interesting compound for clinical trials. Although the increase in signal enhancement of this compound is not limited by T2*-effects that occur with USPIO higher dosing could be difficult as the higher viscosity requires a bigger volume ('double dose' = 60 ml/75 kg BW). Similar values for viscosity at 37°C are known for Gadomer-17 that is also a macromolecule presented in the previous paper by Li *et al.*

Contrast-enhanced coronary MR angiography: relationship between coronary artery delineation and blood T1.

J Zheng, D Li, F M Cavagna, *et al. J Magn Reson Imaging* 2001; **14**: 348–54.

BACKGROUND. Contrast-enhanced MR coronary angiography has become an important research technique for non-invasive cardiac imaging. However, the relationship between the quality of the coronary artery images and blood T1 has not yet been fully explored. In this study, the authors assessed this relationship in an animal model using a prototypical blood pool agent (mixed micelles) that has a R1 relaxivity of 23.1/mM/s. With accumulated injections of this agent, the blood T_1 would be analysed at different levels. The measured blood T1 values *in vivo* were 147 ± 3, 82 ± 6, 48 ± 4, 40 ± 3 and 30 ± 8 ms (*n* = 7). Fixed and variable flip-angle schemes were used in coronary artery imaging. The SNRs of coronary arteries were measured and the image quality was assessed.

INTERPRETATION. It was found that blood T1 <80 ms might be desired. No statistically significant difference was observed between two flip-angle schemes. There was better vessel definition using variable flip angle at blood T1 <50 ms. Understanding this relationship may be beneficial to optimizing image protocol and/or design of blood pool contrast agents for contrast-enhanced coronary angiography.

Comment

CMRA needs still to be optimized to gain clinical acceptance. There are many different intravascular contrast agents under investigation such as macromolecules (Gadomer-17, P792), particles (USPIO), strong protein binding Gd-chelates (MS-325, B-22956/1) and mixed micelles addressing only the main agent groups |**7,8**|. In this study, a potentially toxic contrast agent was used that stayed without any wash-out in the blood pool. These findings need to be revaluated for other types of contrast agents in humans to further improve clinical acceptance of CMRA.

Contrast agent distribution in microvascular damage of infarcted pig myocardium.

J Mark, G Dai, B Xiang, *et al. Acta Radiol* 2001; **42**: 515–20.

Background. The authors investigated whether reperfusion damage was sufficient to allow extravasation of a large molecular mass contrast agent into infarcted pig myocardium. Five pig hearts were subjected to *in situ* occlusion of the left anterior descending coronary artery (2 h) followed by reperfusion (1 h). The hearts were excised and perfused in the Langendorff mode for *ex vivo* MRI. Polylysine-Gd-DTPA (50 000 Da) and Gd-DTPA (500–700 Da) were injected into the aorta (alternately) and followed by measurements of T1 relaxation and mean transit time (MTT).

Interpretation. The results indicate that the permeability of capillaries to polylysine-Gd-DTPA was not significantly higher in infarcted regions of the myocardium than in normal tissue. However, infarcted myocardium displayed an increased permeability to the low molecular mass Gd-DTPA. It can be concluded that microvascular damage may not be sufficient to allow the extravasation of polylysine-Gd-DTPA in infarcted myocardium.

Comment

Do we need specific (targeted) contrast agents to answer the question of myocardial viability? This animal study ($n = 5$) follows this question comparing a 100 times bigger contrast molecule with the standard compound Gd-DTPA. In the normal myocardium, MTT of Gd-DTPA (56.8 ± 23.2 s) was significantly ($P = 0.02$) longer than that of polylysine-Gd-DTPA (29.0 ± 7 s) indicating 'trapping' of the small molecular contrast agent into the interstitial compartment. ΔT1 after administration of Gd-DTPA between normal and infarcted myocardium showed significant contrast enhancement in the damaged region. However, both normal and infarcted myocardium showed similar MTT (29.0 ± 7.0 vs 28.0 ± 5.0 s, $P > 0.05$) when using polylysine-Gd-DTPA (Table 15.4).

Table 15.4 T1 relaxation times of non-enhanced and Gd-DTPA or polylysine-Gd-DTPA enhanced myocardium

	T1 relaxation time (ms)		ΔT1 relaxation (ms)	
	Normal	**Infarct**	**Normal**	**Infarct**
No contrast agent	1824 ± 74	2050 ± 142*		
Polylysine-Gd-DTPA	1186 ± 89	1143 ± 152	637 ± 94	907 ± 231
Gd-DTPA	605 ± 169	476 ± 151*	1218 ± 200	1574 ± 197*

*Significantly different from normal myocardium, $P < 0.05$.
Source: Mark *et al.* (2000).

Studies looking at permeability changes in tumour vasculature are also evaluating small molecular (extracellular) contrast agents and macromolecules as well as strong protein binding compounds |11,12|. It is still not clear if the endothelial changes of the altered vasculature can be answered more specifically using larger molecules. Further studies could investigate whether prolonged imaging of severely damaged myocardium could show slow leakage of macromolecules from the intravascular in the extracellular space.

Limits of detection of regional differences in vasodilated flow in viable myocardium by first-pass magnetic resonance perfusion imaging.

F J Klocke, O P Simonetti, R M Judd, *et al. Circulation* 2001; **104**: 2412–16.

BACKGROUND. Perfusion imaging techniques intended to identify regional limitations in coronary flow reserve in viable myocardium need to consistently identify twofold differences in regional flow during coronary vasodilation. This study evaluated the suitability of current first-pass magnetic resonance approaches for evaluating such differences, which are one to two orders of magnitude less than in MI. Graded regional differences in vasodilated flow were produced in chronically instrumented dogs with either left circumflex (LCx) infusion of adenosine or partial LCx occlusion during global coronary vasodilation. First-pass myocardial signal intensity–time curves were obtained after right atrial injection of gadoteridol (0.025 mmol/kg) with an MRI inversion recovery true-FISP sequence. The area under the initial portion of the LCx curve was compared with that of a curve from a remote area of the ventricle. Relative LCx and remote flows were assessed simultaneously using microspheres. In this experimental model the ratio of LCx and remote MRI curve areas and the ratio of LCx and remote microsphere concentrations were identified which correlated highly and linearly related over a fivefold range of flow differences ($y = 0.96\ x \pm 0.07$, $P <0.0001$, $r^2 = 0.87$). The 95% confidence limits for individual MRI measurements were ± 35%. Regional differences of greater than or equal to twofold were consistently apparent in unprocessed MR images.

INTERPRETATION. Clinically relevant regional reductions in vasodilated flow in viable myocardium can be detected with 95% confidence over the range of 1–5 times resting flow. This suggests that MRI can identify and quantify limitations in perfusion reserve that are expected to be produced by stenoses of ≥70%.

Comment

Non-invasive assessment of a relative perfusion deficit in patients with known or suspected coronary artery disease, i.e. in viable myocardium is a major challenge. Recent studies indicate that contrast-enhanced MRI can identify viable areas in myocardium |13,14|. Although in this study the imaging protocol is optimized for contrast-enhanced detection of perfusion changes clinical relevance is still limited by a one slice acquisition. Evaluation of the potential usefulness of different kinds of blood pool contrast agents warrant further studies.

Conclusion

What can we expect from current developments in the field for MR contrast agents? Interventional cardiologists and radiologists still need to be patient until intravascular contrast agents are available for clinical procedures. Promising results have been reported for contrast-enhanced CMRA using USPIOs or macromolecules, but clinical availability of these agents will still take some time and there will be regulatory hurdles. Dosing still needs to be optimized in order to minimize T2*-effects and safety issues. Knowledge of the biodistribution after application of a contrast medium is also a key component of comprehensive MRI.

First-pass imaging is challenged by a very small time window and also requires further improvements in hard- and software design. The developments in cardiovascular contrast agents are very promising, but we are seeing only gradual advances. The most important development is that we will have a variety of different vascular agents available which possess uniquely different properties. Our challenge will be to use these agents in new ways and optimize image acquisition in order to leverage those moderate advances.

References

1. Weishaupt D, Ruhm SG, Binkert CA, Schmidt M, Patak MA, Steybe F, McGill S, Debatin JF. Equilibrium-phase MR angiography of the aortoiliac and renal arteries using a blood pool contrast agent. *Am J Roentgenol* 2000; **175**: 189–95.

2. Li D, Deshpande V. Magnetic resonance imaging of coronary arteries. *Top Magn Reson Imaging* 2001; **12**: 337–47.

3. Deshpande VS, Wielopolski PA, Shea SM, Carr J, Zheng J, Li D. Coronary artery imaging using contrast-enhanced 3D segmented EPI. *J Magn Reson Imaging* 2001; **13**: 676–81.

4. Bunce NH, Lorenz CH, Pennell DJ. MR coronary angiography: 2001 update. *Rays* 2001; **26**: 61–9.

5. Klein C, Nagel E, Schnackenburg B, Bornstedt A, Schalla S, Hoffmann V, Lehning A, Fleck E. The intravascular contrast agent Clariscan (NC100150 injection) for 3D MR coronary angiography in patients with coronary artery disease. *MAGMA* 2000; **11**: 65–7.

6. Stuber M, Botnar RM, Danias PG, McConnell MV, Kissinger KV, Yucel EK, Manning WJ. Contrast agent-enhanced, free-breathing, three-dimensional coronary magnetic resonance angiography. *J Magn Reson Imaging* 1999; **10**: 790–9.

7. Knopp MV, von Tengg-Kobligk H, Floemer F, Schoenberg SO. Contrast agents for MRA: future directions. *J Magn Reson Imaging* 1999; **10**: 314–16.

8. Saeed M, Wendland MF, Higgins CB. Blood pool MR contrast agents for cardiovascular imaging. *J Magn Reson Imaging* 2000; **12**: 890–8.

9. Frayne R, Grist TM, Swan JS, Peters DC, Korosec FR, Mistretta CA. 3D MR DSA: effects of injection protocol and image masking. *J Magn Reson Imaging* 2000; **12**: 476–87.

10. Corti R, Fuster V, Badimon JJ, Hutter R, Fayad ZA. New understanding of atherosclerosis (clinically and experimentally) with evolving MRI technology *in vivo*. *Ann NY Acad Sci* 2001; **947**: 181–95.

11. Turetschek K, Floyd E, Helbich T, Roberts TP, Shames DM, Wendland MF, Carter WO, Brasch RC. MRI assessment of microvascular characteristics in experimental breast tumors using a new blood pool contrast agent (MS-325) with correlations to histopathology. *J Magn Reson Imaging* 2001; **14**: 237–42.

12. Knopp MV, Giesel FL, Marcos H, von Tengg-Kobligk H, Choyke P. Dynamic contrast-enhanced magnetic resonance imaging in oncology. *Top Magn Reson Imaging* 2001; **12**: 301–8.

13. Stillman AE, Wilke N, Jerosch-Herold M. Myocardial viability. *Radiol Clin North Am* 1999; **37**: 361–78.

14. Al-Saadi N, Nagel E, Gross M, Schnackenburg B, Paetsch I, Klein C, Fleck E. Improvement of myocardial perfusion reserve early after coronary intervention: assessment with cardiac magnetic resonance imaging. *J Am Coll Cardiol* 2000; **36**: 1557–64.

List of Abbreviations

ACE	angiotensin converting enzyme
ACS	acute coronary syndromes
ADVANCE	additional value of the NIR stent for the treatment of long coronary lesions
AMI	acute myocardial infarction
ARTS	Arterial Revascularization Therapy Study
ASPECT	Asian Paclitaxel-Eluting stent Clinical Trial
ATP	adenosine 5′-triphosphate
AUC	area under the curve
AWESOME	Angina With Extremely Serious Operative Mortality Evaluation
BARI	Bypass Angioplasty Revascularization Investigation
BAT	bolus arrival time
BE-SMART	be-stent in small arteries
BEST	Balloon Equivalent to Stent Study
BIT	balloon inflation time
BMS	bare metal stents
BNP	brain natriuretic peptide
BRIE	Beta Radiation In Europe
BTL	bolus time length
BW	body weight
CABG	coronary artery bypass grafting
CABRI	Coronary Angioplasty versus Bypass Revascularization Investigation
CAD	coronary artery disease
CADILLAC	Controlled Abciximab and Device Investigation to Lower Late Angioplasty Complications
CAPTIM	Comparison of Angioplasty and Prehospital Thrombolysis In acute Myocardial infarction
CARAT	Coronary Angioplasty and Rotablator Atherectomy Trial
CFR	coronary flow reserve
CFVR	coronary flow velocity reserve
CHECKMATE	CHest pain Evaluation by Creatinine Kinase-MB, Myoglobin, And Troponin I
CI	confidence interval
CK-MB	creatinine kinase-MB
CMRA	coronary magnetic resonance angiography
CNR	contrast-to-noise
COAST	heparin-coated stent
CPB	cardiopulmonary bypass
C-PORT	Cardiovascular Patient Outcomes Research Team
CPTC	pulse transmission coefficient
CRP	C-reactive protein
CS	conventional stenting
CSA	cross-sectional area
cTnI	cardiac troponin I
cTnT	cardiac troponin T
DAo	descending aorta
DCA	directional coronary atherectomy
DEBATE	Doppler End-points Balloon Angioplasty Trial in Europe
DES	drug-eluting stents
DISCO	DIrect Stenting of COronary arteries
DPD	distal protection device
DS	direct stenting
EAST	Emory Angioplasty versus Surgery Trial

ECG	electrocardiogram	LIPS	Lescol Intervention Prevention Study
EEM	enlarged elastic membrane		
ELA	excimer laser angioplasty	LM	left main
EPISTENT	Evaluation of Platelet IIb/IIIa Inhibitor for Stenting Trial	LMCA	left main coronary artery
		LV	left ventricular
		LVEF	left ventricular ejection fraction
ESRD	end-stage renal disease		
FIRE	FIlterWiRE during transluminal intervention of saphenous vein grafts	MACCE	major adverse cardiac and cerebrovascular event
		MACE	major adverse cardiac event
FFR	fractional flow reserve	MCE	major clinical event
FR	fast release	MI	myocardial infarction
FRISC	Fast Revascularization during InStability in Coronary artery disease	MIP	maximum intensity projection
		MIRACL	myocardial ischaemia reduction with aggressive cholesterol lowering
Gd	Gadolinium		
Gp	glycoprotein		
GUSTO-IV	Global Use of STrategies to open Occluded coronary arteries IV	MLD	minimum lumen diameter
		MMI	minor myocardial injury
		MPR	multiplanar reconstruction
h-SRv	hyperaemic stenosis resistance indexes	MPS	mononuclear phagocytic system
HyR	hybrid revascularization	MR	moderate release
HPS	Heart Protection Study	MRA	magnetic resonance angiography
IA	intimal area		
ICUS	intracoronary ultrasound	MRI	magnetic resonance imaging
IH	intimal hyperplasia	MSA	minimum stent area
IMR	index of microcirculatory resistance	MSD	minimal stent diameter
		mTOR	mammalian Target Of Rapomycin
IRA	infarct-related arteries		
IRT	intracoronary radiation therapy	MTT	mean transit time
		MUSIC	MUlti-Spectral Infrared Camera
ISAR-SMART	Intracoronary Stenting or Angioplasty for Restenosis reduction in SMall ARTeries		
		NHLBI	National Heart, Lung, and Blood Institute
ISAR-STEREO-2	Intracoronary Stenting and Angiographic Results: Strut Thickness Effect on REstenosis Outcome trial	NIH	neointimal hyperplasia
		NQWMI	non-Q wave myocardial infarction
		NS	not significant
ISR	in-stent restenosis	NSTEACS	non-ST elevation acute coronary syndrome
ITT	intention-to-treat		
IVUS	intravascular ultrasound	NT-proBNP	N-terminal proBNP
LAD	left anterior descending coronary artery	OPTICUS	OPTimization with ICUS to reduce stent restenosis
LCx	left circumflex	OPUS-1	optimum percutaneous transluminal coronary angioplasty versus routine stent strategy trial
LDL	low density lipoprotein		
LIMA	left internal mammary artery		

OR	odds ratio	RLD	reference lumen diameter
PAMI	Primary Angioplasty in Myocardial Infarction	ROI	region of interest
		RR	relative risk
PARAGON	Platelet IIb/IIIa Antagonism for the Reduction of Acute Coronary Syndrome Events in a Global Organization Network	RT	received treatment
		SAFER	Saphenous vein graft Angioplasty Free of Emboli Randomized
		SBO	side branches occlusion
PAST	Platelet Activation in STenting study	SCORE	study to compare restenosis rate between QueST and QuaDS-QP2
PCI	percutaneous coronary intervention	SDNR	signal-difference-to-noise
PD	pre-dilatation	SEPI	segmented echo-planar imaging
PLAD	proximal left anterior descending coronary artery	SES	sirolemus-eluting stent
PLLA	poly-L-lactic acid	SIRIUS	A multicenter randomized double-blind study of the sirolimus-coated Bx Velocity™ stent in the treatment of patients with de novo coronary artery lesions
POBA	plain old balloon angioplasty		
PREDICT	PREdicting risk of Death In Cardiac disease Tool		
PS	pre-dilatation stenting		
PS	provisional stenting		
PTC	pulse transmission coefficient	SISA	stenting in small arteries
PTCA	percutaneous transluminal coronary angioplasty	SISCA	stenting in small coronary arteries
PURSUIT	Platelet glycoprotein IIb/IIIa in Unstable angina: Receptor Suppression Using Integrilin Therapy	SI/T	signal intensity/time
		SMC	smooth muscle cell
		SNR	signal-to-noise ratio
		SoS	Stent or Surgery trial
QCA	quantitative coronary angiography	SPECT	single photon emission scintigraphy
RAP	restenosis in arterias perquenas	SPS	stress perfusion scintigraphy
		SR	slow release
RAVEL	RAndomized study with the sirolimus-eluting VELocity balloon-expandable stent in the treatment of patients with de novo native coronary artery lesions	STEMI	ST-elevation myocardial infarction
		STRATAS	Study to determine Rotablator System And Transluminal Angioplasty Strategy
RCA	right coronary artery	SURE	Serial Ultrasound REstenosis
RCBPA	rapid-clearance blood pool agents	SVG	saphenous vein graft
		SWIBAP	Stent WIthout BAlloon Pre-dilatation
RD	reference diameter		
RES	reticuloendothelial system	SWP	stenting with pre-dilatation
RESIST	REStenosis after Ivus guided STenting	TACTICS	Treat angina with Aggrastat and determine Cost of Therapy with an Invasive or Conservative Strategy
RITA	Randomized Intervention Trial of unstable Angina		

TACTICS–TIMI	Treat angina with Aggrastat and determine Cost of Therapy with an Invasive or Conservative Strategy–Thrombolysis in Myocardial Infarction	UA/NSTEMI	unstable angina/non-ST-segment elevation myocardial infarction
TARGET	do Tirofiban And ReoPro Give similar Efficacy outcomes Trial	USPIO	ultra-small particles of iron oxides
		VAPOR	VAsodilator Prevention On no-Reflow
TIMI	Thrombolysis in Myocardial Infarction	VBT	vascular brachytherapy
		VINO	Value of first day angiography/angioplasty in evolving non-ST segment elevation myocardial infarction
TLR	target lesion revascularization		
TMR	true microcirculatory resistance	WRIST	Washington Radiation for In-Stent restenosis Trial
TVR	target vessel revascularization	X-TRACT	X-sizer for TReatment of thrombus and Atherosclerosis in Coronary interventions Trial
TxCAD	transplant coronary artery disease		

Index of Papers Reviewed

F Airoldi, C Di Mario, G Gimelli, AL Bartorelli, F Bedogni, C Briguori, A Frasheri, L Inglese, N Rubino, A Ferrari, B Reimers, A Colombo. A randomized comparison of direct stenting versus stenting with pre-dilatation in native coronary artery disease: results from the multicentric Crosscut study. *J Inv Cardiol* 2003; 15(1): 1–5. **77**

T Akasaka, A Yamamuro, N Kamiyama, Y Koyama, M Akiyama, N Watanabe, Y Neishi, T Takagi, E Shalman, C Barak, K Yoshida. Assessment of coronary flow reserve by coronary pressure measurement: comparison with flow- or velocity-derived coronary flow reserve. *J Am Coll Cardiol* 2003; 41: 1554–60. **114**

J Al Suwaidi, DN Reddan, K Williams, KS Pieper, RA Harrington, RM Califf, CB Granger, EM Ohman, DR Holmes Jr; GUSTO-IIb, GUSTO-III, PURSUIT. Global Use of Strategies to Open Occluded Coronary Arteries. Platelet Glycoprotein IIb/IIIa in Unstable Angina: Receptor Suppression Using Integrilin Therapy; PARAGON-A Investigators. Platelet IIb/IIIa Antagonism for the Reduction of Acute coronary syndrome events in a Global Organization Network. Prognostic implications of abnormalities in renal function in patients with acute coronary syndromes. *Circulation* 2002; 106: 974–80. **12**

F Alfonso, P Garcia, G Pimentel, R Hernandez, M Sabate, J Escaned, C Banuelos, C Fernandez, C Macaya. Predictors and implications of residual plaque burden after coronary stenting: an intravascular ultrasound study. *Am Heart J* 2003; 145: 254–61. **236**

D Antoniucci, R Valenti, A Migliorini, G Moschi, M Trapani, P Buonamici, G Cerisano, L Bolognese, GM Santoro. Relation of time to treatment and mortality in patients with acute myocardial infarction undergoing primary coronary angioplasty. *Am J Cardiol* 2002; 89: 1248–52. **28**

DT Ashby, G Dangas, EA Aymong, I Iakovou, F Kuepper, R Mehran, GW Stone, MB Leon, JW Moses. Effect of percutaneous coronary intervention for in-stent restenosis in degenerated saphenous vein grafts without distal embolic protection. *J Am Coll Cardiol* 2003; 41: 749–52. **197**

Y Atmaca, F Ertas, S Gulec, I Dincer, D Oral. Effect of direct stent implantation on minor myocardial injury. *J Invas Cardiol* 2002; 14(8): 443–6. **88**

T Aversano, LT Aversano, E Passamani, GL Knatterud, ML Terrin, DO Williams, SA Forman; Atlantic Cardiovascular Patient Outcomes Research Team (C-PORT). Thrombolytic therapy vs primary percutaneous coronary intervention for myocardial infarction in patients presenting to hospitals without on-site cardiac surgery. A randomized controlled trial. *JAMA* 2002; 287: 1943–51. **27**

RJ Aviles, AT Askari, B Lindahl, L Wallentin, G Jia, EM Ohman, KW Mahaffey, LK Newby, RM Califf, ML Simoons, EJ Topol, P Berger, MS Lauer. Troponin T levels in patients with acute coronary syndromes, with or without renal dysfunction. *N Engl J Med* 2002; 346: 2047–52. **8**

DS Baim, D Wahr, B George, MB Leon, J Greenberg, DE Cutlip, U Kaya, JJ Popma, KK, RE Kuntz; Saphenous vein graft Angioplasty Free of Emboli Randomized (SAFER) Trial Investigators. Randomized trial of a distal embolic protection device during percutaneous intervention of saphenous vein aorto-coronary bypass grafts. *Circulation* 2002; 105: 1285–90. **43, 193**

GJ Bech, B De Bruyne, NH Pijls, ED de Muinck, JC Hoorntje, J Escaned, PR Stella, E Boersma, J Bartunek, JJ Koolen, W Wijns. Fractional flow reserve to determine the appropriateness of angioplasty in moderate coronary stenosis. A randomized trial. *Circulation* 2001; 103: 2928–34. **95**

E Bonnefoy, F Lapostolle, A Leizorovicz, G Steg, EP McFadden, PY Dubien, S Cattan, E Boullenger, J Machecourt, JM Lacroute, J Cassagnes, F Dissait, P Touboul; Comparison of Angioplasty and Prehospital Thromboysis in Acute Myocardial Infarction Study Group. Primary angioplasty versus pre-hospital fibrinolysis in acute myocardial infarction: a randomized study. *Lancet* 2002; 360: 825–9. **29**

M Boos, K Scheffler, R Haselhorst, E Reese, J Frohlich, GM Bongartz. Arterial first-pass gadolinium-CM dynamics as a function of several intravenous saline flush and Gd volumes. *J Magn Reson Imaging* 2001; 13: 568–76. **256**

J Boschat, H Le Breton, P Commeau, B Huret, M Bedossa, M Gilard; Stent WIthout BAlloon Predilatation (SWIBAP) study group. Is coronary stent deployment and remodeling affected by pre-dilatation? An intravascular ultrasound randomized study stenting with or without pre-dilatation: an IVUS study. *Int J Cardiovasc Imaging* 2002; 18(6): 399–404. **85**

D Boulmier, M Bedossa, P Commeau, B Huret, M Gilard, J Boschat, P Brunel,

B Leurent, H Le Breton. Direct coronary stenting without balloon pre-dilation of lesions requiring long stents: immediate and 6-month results of a multicenter prospective registry. *Cath Cardiovasc Interv* 2003; 58(1): 51–8. **77**

J Bremerich, JM Colet, GB Giovenzana, S Aime, K Scheffler, S Laurent, G Bongartz, RN Muller. Slow clearance gadolinium-based extracellular and intravascular contrast media for three-dimensional MR angiography. *J Magn Reson Imaging* 2001; 13: 588–93. **254**

C Briguori, C Sarais, P Pagnotta, F Liistro, M Montorfano, A Chieffo, F Sgura, N Corvaja, R Albiero, G Stankovic, C Toutoutzas, E Bonizzoni, C Di Mario, A Colombo. In-stent restenosis in small coronary arteries: impact of strut thickness. *J Am Coll Cardiol* 2002; 40: 403–9. **131**

BR Brodie, C Cooper, M Jones, P Fitzgerald, F Cummins. Is adjunctive balloon post-dilatation necessary after coronary stent deployment? Final results from the POSTIT trial. *Cath Cardiovasc Interv* 2003; 59: 184–92. **227**

JM Brophy, P Belisle, L Joseph. Evidence for use of coronary stents. A hierarchical Bayesian meta-analysis. *Ann Intern Med* 2003; 138: 777–86. **40**

D Brosh, ST Higano, MJ Slepian, HI Miller, MJ Kern, RJ Lennon, DR Holmes, A Lerman. Pulse transmission coefficient: a novel non-hyperemic parameter for assessing the physiological significance of coronary artery stenoses. *J Am Coll Cardiol* 2002; 39: 1012–19. **115**

M Brueck, D Scheinert, A Wortmann, J Bremer, H von Korn, L Klinghammer, W Kramer, FA Flachskampf, WG Daniel, J Ludwig. Direct coronary stenting versus pre-dilatation followed by stent placement. *Am J Cardiol* 2002; 90(11): 1187–92. **78**

SA Chamuleau, RA Tio, CC de Cock, ED de Muinck, NH Pijls, BL van Eck-Smit,

M Degertekin, PW Serruys, DP Foley, K Tanabe, E Regar, J Vos, PC Smits, WJ van der Giessen, M van den Brand, P de Feyter, JJ Popma. Persistent inhibition of neointimal hyperplasia after sirolimus-eluting stent implantation: long-term (up to 2 years) clinical, angiographic, and intravascular ultrasound follow-up. *Circulation* 2002; **106**(13): 1610–13.   **208**

E Diderholm, B Andren, G Frostfeldt, M Genberg, T Jernberg, B Lagerqvist, B Lindahl, P Venge, L Wallentin; Fast Revascularization during Instability in coronary artery disease (FRISC II) Investigators. The prognostic and therapeutic implications of increased troponin T levels and ST depression in unstable coronary artery disease: the FRISC II invasive troponin T electrocardiogram substudy. *Am Heart J* 2002; **143**: 760–7.   **4**

A Diegeler, H Thiele, V Falk, R Hambrecht, N Spyrantis, P Sick, KW Diederich, FW Mohr, G Schuler. Comparison of stenting with minimally invasive bypass surgery for stenosis of the left anterior descending coronary artery. *N Engl J Med* 2002; **347**: 561–6.   **67**

DJ Drenth, NJ Veeger, JB Winter, JG Grandjean, MA Mariani, AJ van Boven, PW Boonstra. A prospective randomized trial comparing stenting with off-pump coronary surgery for high-grade stenosis in the proximal left anterior descending coronary artery: three-year follow-up. *J Am Coll Cardiol* 2002; **40**: 1955–60.   **64**

M Elbaz, E El Mokhtar, K Khalife, B Citron, K Izaaz, M Hamon, JM Juliard, F Leclercq, J Fourcade, J Lipiecki, R Sabatier, V Boulet, JP Rinaldi, S Mourali, M Fatouch, A Asmar, PG Steg, J Puel, D Carrie. Is direct coronary stenting the best strategy for long-term outcome? Results of the multicentric randomized benefit evaluation of direct coronary stenting (BET) study. *Am Heart J*; **144**(4): E7.   **80**

WF Fearon, LB Balsam, O Farouque, RC Robbins, PJ Fitzgerald, PG Yock, AC Yeung. Novel index for invasively assessing the coronary microcirculation. *Circulation* 2003; **107**: 3129–32.   **111**

WF Fearon, J Luna, H Samady, ER Powers, T Feldman, N Dib, EM Tuzcu, MW Cleman, TM Chou, DJ Cohen, M Ragosta, A Takagi, A Jeremias, PJ Fitzgerald, AC Yeung, MJ Kern, PG Yock. Fractional flow reserve compared with intravascular ultrasound guidance for optimizing stent deployment. *Circulation* 2001; **104**: 1917–22.   **103**

G Finet, NJ Weissman, GS Mintz, LF Satler, KM Kent, JR Laird, GA Adelmann, AE Ajani, MT Castagna, G Rioufol, AD Pichard. Mechanism of lumen enlargement with direct stenting versus pre-dilatation stenting: influence of remodelling and plaque characteristics assessed by volumetric intracoronary ultrasound. *Heart* 2003; **89**(1): 84–90.   **85**

KA Fox, PA Poole-Wilson, RA Henderson, TC Clayton, DA Chamberlain, TR Shaw, DJ Wheatley, SA Pocock; Randomized Intervention Trial of unstable Angina Investigators. Interventional versus conservative treatment for patients with unstable angina or non-ST elevation myocardial infarction: the British Heart Foundation RITA 3 randomized trial. Randomized Intervention Trial of unstable Angina. *Lancet* 2002; **360**: 743–51.   **45**

JM Garasic, ER Edelman, JC Squire, P Seifert, MS Williams, C Rogers. Stent and artery geometry determine intimal thickening independent of arterial injury. *Circulation* 2000; **101**: 812–18.   **126**

M Gasior, M Gierlotka, A Lekston, K Wilszek, E Zebik, J Szkodzinski, R Wojnar, L Polonski. Randomized comparison of direct stenting and stenting after pre-dilatation in acute myocardial infarction. In-hospital results of DIRAMI trial. *Eur Heart J* 2002; **390**: 2060.   **87**

R Gil, T Pawlowski, K Zmudka, *et al.* Reduction of restenosis rate for direct stenting with intracoronary ultrasound guidance. Results from the prospective, randomized trial. *Eur Heart J* 2002; **310**: 1661. **83**

R Glaser, HC Herrmann, SA Murphy, LA Demopoulos, PM DiBattiste, CP Cannon, E Braunwald. Benefit of an early invasive management strategy in women with acute coronary syndromes. *JAMA* 2002; **288**: 3124–9. **17**

MA Grise, V Massullo, S Jani, JJ Popma, RJ Russo, RA Schatz, EM Guarneri, S Steuterman, DA Cloutier, MB Leon, P Tripuraneni, PS Teirstein. Five-year clinical follow-up after intracoronary radiation: results of a randomized clinical trial. *Circulation* 2002; **105**(23): 2737–40. **177**

E Grube, S Silber, KE Hauptmann, R Mueller, L Buellesfeld, U Gerckens, ME Russell ME. TAXUS I: six- and twelve-month results from a randomized, double-blind trial on a slow-release paclitaxel-eluting stent for *de novo* coronary lesions. *Circulation* 2003; **107**(1): 38–42. **220**

L Gruberg, R Waksman, AE Ajani, HS Kim, RL White, EE Pinnow, LF Satler, AD Pichard, KM Kent, J Lindsay Jr. The effect of intracoronary radiation for the treatment of recurrent in-stent restenosis in patients with diabetes mellitus. *J Am Coll Cardiol* 2002; **39**(12): 1930–6. **166**

PA Gurbel, KP Callahan, AI Malinin, VL Serebruany, J Gillis. Could stent design affect platelet activation? Results of the Platelet Activation in Stenting (PAST) Study. *J Invas Cardiol* 2002; **14**: 584–9. **128**

KJ Harjai, GW Stone, J Boura, L Grines, E Garcia, B Brodie, D Cox, WW O'Neill, C Grines. Effects of prior beta-blocker therapy on clinical outcomes after primary coronary angioplasty for acute myocardial infarction. *Am J Cardiol* 2003; **91**: 655–60. **24**

JK Harjai, GW Stone, J Boura, L Mattos, H Chandra, D Cox, L Grines, O'Neill, C Grines; Primary Angioplasty in Myocardial Infarction Investigators. Comparison of outcomes of diabetic and non-diabetic patients undergoing primary angioplasty for acute myocardial infarction. *Am J Cardiol* 2003; **91**: 1041–5. **156**

M Haude, TF Konorza, U Kalnins, A Erglis, K Saunamaki, HD Glogar, E Grube, R Gil, A Serra, HG Richardt, P Sick, R Erbel; Heparin-COAted STents in Small Coronary Arteries Trial Investigators. Heparin-coated stent placement for the treatment of stenoses in small coronary arteries of symptomatic patients. *Circulation* 2003; **107**: 1265–70. **36**

Heart Protection Study Collaborative Group. MRC/BHF Heart Protection Study of cholesterol lowering with simvastatin in 20 536 high-risk individuals: a randomized placebo-controlled trial. *Lancet* 2002; **360**: 7–22. **141**

C Heeschen, CW Hamm, U Laufs, S Snapinn, M Bohm, HD White; Platelet Receptor Inhibition in Ischemic Syndrome Management (PRISM) Investigators. Withdrawal of statins increases event rates in patients with acute coronary syndromes. *Circulation* 2002; **105**: 1446–52. **146**

CA Herzog, JZ Ma, AJ Collins. Comparative survival of dialysis patients in the United States after coronary angioplasty, coronary artery stenting, and coronary artery bypass surgery and impact of diabetes. *Circulation* 2002; **106**: 2207–11. **158**

VB Ho, TK Foo, AE Arai, SD Wolff. Gadolinium-enhanced, vessel-tracking, two-dimensional coronary MR angiography: single-dose arterial-phase vs delayed-phase imaging. *J Magn Reson Imaging* 2001; **13**: 682–9. **253**

R Hoffmann, GS Mintz, PK Haager, T Bozoglu, E Grube, M Gross, C Beythien, H Mudra, J vom Dahl, P Hanrath. Relation of stent design and stent surface material to subsequent in-stent intimal hyperplasia in coronary arteries determined by intravascular ultrasound. *Am J Cardiol* 2002; 89: 1360–4. **120**

MK Hong, GS Mintz, CW Lee, JM Song, KH Han, DH Kang, JK Song, JJ Kim, NJ Weissman, NE Fearnot, SW Park, SJ Park; ASian Paclitaxel-Eluting stent Clinical Trial. Paclitaxel coating reduces in-stent intimal hyperplasia in human coronary arteries: a serial volumetric intravascular ultrasound analysis from the ASian Paclitaxel-Eluting stent Clinical Trial (ASPECT). *Circulation* 2003; 107(4): 517–20. **216, 230**

LF Hsu, KH Mak, KW Lau, LL Sim, C Chan, TH Koh, SC Chuah, R Kam, ZP Ding, WS Teo, YL Lim. Clinical outcome of patients with diabetes mellitus and acute myocardial infarction treated with primary angioplasty or fibrinolysis. *Heart* 2002; 88: 260–5. **156**

AJ IJsselmuiden, PW Serruys, A Scholte, F Kiemeneij, T Slagboom, LR van der Wieken, GJ Tangelder, GJ Laarman GJ. Direct coronary stent implantation does not reduce the incidence of in-stent restenosis or major adverse cardiac events. Six month results of a randomized trial. *Eur Heart J* 2003; 24(5): 421–9. **84**

T Jernberg, M Stridsberg, P Venge, B Lindahl. N-Terminal pro-brain natriuretic peptide on admission for early risk stratification of patients with chest pain and no ST-segment elevation. *J Am Coll Cardiol* 2002; 40: 437–45. **10**

E Karvouni, C Di Mario, T Nishida, V Tzifos, B Reimers, R Albiero, N Corvaja, A Colombo. Directional atherectomy prior to stenting in bifurcation lesions: a matched comparison study with stenting alone. *Catheter Cardiovascular Interven* 2001; 53(1): 12–20. **247**

T Kataoka, E Grube, Y Honda, Y Morino, SH Hur, HN Bonneau, A Colombo, C Di Mario, G Guagliumi, KE Hauptmann, MR Pitney, AJ Lansky, SH Stertzer, PG Yock, PF Fitzgerald. 7-Hexanoyltaxol-eluting stent for prevention of neointimal growth: an intravascular ultrasound analysis from the study to compare restenosis rate between QueST and QuaDS-QP2 (SCORE). *Circulation* 2002; 106(14): 1788–93. **216**

P Kaul, LK Newby, Y Fu, V Hasselblad, KW Mahaffey, RH Christenson, RA Harrington, EM Ohman, EJ Topol, RM Califf, F Van de Werf, PW Armstrong; PARAGON-B Investigators. Troponin T and quantitative ST-segment depression offer complementary prognostic information in the risk stratification of acute coronary syndrome patients. *J Am Coll Cardiol* 2003; 41: 371–80. **6**

EC Keeley, JA Boura, CL Grines. Primary angioplasty versus intravenous thrombolytic therapy for acute myocardial infarction: a quantitative review of 23 randomized trials. *Lancet* 2003; 361: 13–20. **30**

KE Kip, EL Alderman, MG Bourassa, MM Brooks, L Schwartz, DR Holmes, RM Califf, PL Whitlow, BR Chaitman, KM Detre. Differential influence of diabetes mellitus on increased jeopardized myocardium after initial angioplasty or bypass surgery. *Circulation* 2002; 105: 1914–20. **152**

FJ Klocke, OP Simonetti, RM Judd, RJ Kim, KR Harris, S Hedjbeli, DS Fieno, S Miller, V Chen, MA Parker. Limits of detection of regional differences in vasodilated flow in viable myocardium by first-pass magnetic resonance perfusion imaging. *Circulation* 2001; 104: 2412–16. **264**

A Konig, TM Schiele, J Rieber, K Theisen, H Mudra, V Klauss. Stent design-related coronary artery remodelling and patterns of neointima formation following

NH Pijls, B De Bruyne, L Smith, W Aarnoudse, E Barbato, J Bartunek, GJ Bech, F Van De Vosse. Coronary thermodilution to assess flow reserve: validation in humans. *Circulation* 2002; 105: 2482–6. **110**

NH Pijls, V Klauss, U Siebert, E Powers, K Takazawa, WF Fearon, J Escaned, Y Tsurumi, T Akasaka, H Samady, B De Bruyne; Fractional Flow Reserve (FFR) Post-Stent Registry Investigators. Coronary pressure measurement after stenting predicts adverse events at follow-up: a multicenter registry. *Circulation* 2002; 105: 2950–4. **102**

F Prati, T Pawlowski, R Gil, A Labellarte, A Gziut, E Caradonna, A Manzoli, A Pappalardo, F Burzotta, A Boccanelli. Stenting of culprit lesions in unstable angina leads to a marked reduction in plaque burden: a major role of plaque embolization? A serial intravascular ultrasound study. *Circulation* 2003; 107: 2320–5. **231**

R Prpic, PS Teirstein, JP Reilly, JW Moses, P Tripuraneni, AJ Lansky, JA Giorgianni, S Jani, SC Wong, RD Fish, S Ellis, DR Holmes, D Kereiakas, RE Kuntz, MA Leon. Long-term outcome of patients treated with repeat percutaneous coronary intervention after failure of gamma-brachytherapy for the treatment of in-stent restenosis. *Circulation* 2002; 106(18): 2340–5. **181**

PW Radke, J vom Dahl, R Hoffmann, HG Klues, M Hosseini, U Janssens, P Hanrath. Three-year follow-up after rotational atherectomy for the treatment of diffuse in-stent restenosis: predictors of major adverse cardiac events. *Cath Cardiovasc Intervent* 2001; 53: 334–40. **246**

SV Rao, EM Ohman, CB Granger, PW Armstrong, WB Gibler, RH Christenson, V Hasselblad, A Stebbins, S McNulty, LK Newby. Prognostic value of isolated troponin elevation across the spectrum of chest pain syndromes. *Am J Cardiol* 2003; 91: 936–40. **19**

E Regar, K Kozuma, G Sianos, VL Coen, WJ van der Giessen, D Foley, P de Feyter, B Rensing, P Smits, J Vos, AH Knook, AJ Wardeh, PC Levendag, PW Serruys. Routine intracoronary beta-irradiation. Acute and one year outcome in patients at high risk for recurrence of stenosis. *Eur Heart J* 2002; 23(13): 1038–44. **165**

FS Resnic, M Wainstein, MK Lee, D Behrendt, RV Wainstein, L Ohno-Machado, JM Kirshenbaum, CD Rogers, JJ Popma, R Piana. No-reflow is an independent predictor of death and myocardial infarction after percutaneous coronary intervention. *Am Heart J* 2003; 145: 42–6. **189**

FC Riess, R Bader, P Kremer, C Kuhn, J Kormann, D Mathey, S Moshar, T Tuebler, N Bleese, J Schofer. Coronary hybrid revascularization from January 1997 to January 2001: a clinical follow-up. *Ann Thorac Surg* 2002; 73: 1849–55. **70**

M Roffi, DJ Moliterno, B Meier, ER Powers, CL Grines, PM DiBattiste, HC Herrmann, M Bertrand, KE Harris, LA Demopoulos, EJ Topol; TARGET Investigators. Impact of different platelet glycoprotein IIb/IIIa receptor inhibitors among diabetic patients undergoing percutaneous coronary intervention. Do tirofiban and reopro give similar efficacy outcomes trial (TARGET) 1-year follow-up. *Circulation* 2002; 105: 2730–6. **155**

E Ronner, E Boersma, KM Akkerhuis, RA Harrington, AM Lincoff, JW Deckers, K Karsch, NS Kleiman, A Vahanian, EJ Topol, RM Califf, ML Simoons. Patients with acute coronary syndromes without persistent ST elevation undergoing percutaneous coronary intervention benefit most from early intervention with protection by a glycoprotein IIb/IIIa receptor blocker. *Eur Heart J* 2002; 23: 239–46 **47**

SG Ruehm, C Corot, P Vogt, S Kolb, JF Debatin. Magnetic resonance imaging of atherosclerotic plaque with ultrasmall superparamagnetic particles of iron oxide in hyperlipidemic rabbits. *Circulation* 2001; 103: 415–22. **258**

R Sabatier, M Hamon, QM Zhao, F Burzotta, E Lecluse, B Valette, G Grollier. Could direct stenting reduce no-reflow in acute coronary syndromes? A randomized pilot study. *Am Heart J* 2002; 143(6): 1027–32. **90**

RD Safian, T Feldman, DW Muller, D Mason, T Schreiber, B Haik, M Mooney, WW O'Neill. Coronary angioplasty and rotablator atherectomy trial (CARAT): immediate and late results of a prospective multicenter randomized trial. *Cath Cardiovasc Intervent* 2001; 53: 213–20. **245**

JJ Sandstede, T Pabst, C Wacker, F Wiesmann, V Hoffmann, M Beer, W Kenn, W Bauer, D Hahn. Breath-hold 3D MR coronary angiography with a new intravascular contrast agent (feruglose) – first clinical experiences. *Magn Reson Imaging* 2001; 19: 201–5. **252**

F Schiele, N Meneveau, M Gilard, J Boschat, P Commeau, LP Ming, P Sewoke, MF Seronde, M Mercier, S Gupta, JP Bassand JP. Intravascular ultrasound-guided balloon angioplasty compared with stent: immediate and 6-month results of the multicenter, randomized Balloon Equivalent to Stent Study (BEST). *Circulation* 2003; 107: 545–51. **232**

A Schomig, J Mehilli, H Holle, K Hosl, D Kastrati, J Pache, M Seyfarth, FJ Neumann, J Dirschinger, A Kastrati. Statin treatment following coronary artery stenting and one-year survival. *J Am Coll Cardiol* 2002; 40: 854–61. **144**

L Schwartz, KE Kip, RL Frye, EL Alderman, HV Schaff, KM Detre; Bypass Angioplasty Revascularization Investigation. Coronary bypass graft patency in patients with diabetes in the Bypass Angioplasty Revascularization Investigation (BARI). *Circulation* 2002; 106: 2652–8. **152**

SP Sedlis, DA Morrison, JD Lorin, R Esposito, G Sethi, J Sacks, W Henderson, F Grover, KB Ramanathan, D Weiman, J Saucedo, T Antakli, V Paramesh, S Pett, S Vernon, V Birjiniuk, F Welt, M Krucoff, W Wolfe, JC Lucke, S Mediratta, D Booth, E Murphy, H Ward, L Miller, S Kiesz, C Barbiere, D Lewis; Investigators of the Dept. of Veterans Affairs Cooperative Study #385, the Angina With Extremely Serious Operative Mortality Evaluation (AWESOME). Percutaneous coronary intervention versus coronary bypass graft surgery for diabetic patients with unstable angina and risk factors for adverse outcomes with bypass: outcome of diabetic patients in the AWESOME randomized trial and registry. *J Am Coll Cardiol* 2002; 40: 1555–66. **63, 160**

PW Serruys, P de Feyter, C Macaya, N Kokott, J Puel, M Vrolix, A Branzi, MC Bertolami, G Jackson, B Strauss, B Meier; Lescol Intervention Prevention Study (LIPS) Investigators. Fluvastatin for prevention of cardiac events following successful first percutaneous coronary intervention. *JAMA* 2002; 287: 3215–22. **144**

PW Serruys, M Degertekin, K Tanabe, A Abizaid, JE Sousa, A Colombo, G Guagliumi, W Wijns, WK Lindeboom, J Ligthart, PJ de Feyter, MC Morice; RAVEL Study Group. Intravascular ultrasound findings in the multicenter, randomized, double-blind RAVEL (randomized study with the sirolimus-eluting velocity balloon-expandable stent in the treatment of patients with *de novo* native coronary artery lesions) trial. *Circulation* 2002; 106(7): 798–803. **207**

GW Stone, C Rogers, S Ramee, C White, RE Kuntz, JJ Popma, J George, S Almany, S Bailey. Distal filter protection during saphenous vein graft stenting: technical and clinical correlates of efficacy. *J Am Coll Cardiol* 2002; **40**: 1882–8. **194**

LA Szczech, PJ Best, E Crowley, MM Brooks, PB Berger, V Bittner, BJ Gersh, R Jones, RM Califf, HH Ting, PJ Whitlow, KM Detre, D Holmes. Outcome of patients with chronic renal insufficiency in the bypass angioplasty revascularization investigation. *Circulation* 2002; **105**: 2253–8. **157**

H Tamai, K Igaki, E Kyo, K Kosuga, A Kawashima, S Matsui, H Komori, T Tsuji, S Motohara, H Uehata. Initial and 6-month results of biodegradable poly-L-lactic acid coronary stents in humans. *Circulation* 2000; **102**: 399–404. **133**

K Tanabe, PW Serruys, E Grube, PC Smits, G Selbach, WJ van der Giessen, M Staberock, P de Feyter, R Muller, E Regar, M Degertekin, JM Ligthart, C Disco, B Backx, ME Russell. TAXUS III trial: in-stent restenosis treated with stent-based delivery of paclitaxel incorporated in a slow-release polymer formulation. *Circulation* 2003; **107**(4): 559–64. **219**

M Taupitz, J Schnorr, S Wagner, D Kivelitz, P Rogalla, G Claassen, M Dewey, P Robert, C Corot, B Hamm. Coronary magnetic resonance angiography: experimental evaluation of the new rapid clearance blood pool contrast medium P792. *Magn Reson Med* 2001; **46**: 932–8. **261**

The SOS Investigators. Coronary artery bypass surgery versus percutaneous coronary intervention with stent implantation in patients with multivessel coronary artery disease (the Stent or Surgery trial): a randomized controlled trial. *Lancet* 2002; **360**: 965–70. **56**

T Timurkaynak, H Ciftci, M Ozdemir, A Cengel, Y Tavil, M Kaya, G Erdem, M Cemri, O Dortlemez, H Dortlemez. Sidebranch occlusion after coronary stenting with or without balloon pre-dilation: direct versus conventional stenting. *J Invas Cardiol* 2002; **14**(9): 497–501. **86**

T Timurkaynak, M Ozdemir, A Cengel, M Cemri, H Ciftci, R Yalcin, B Boyaci, O Dortlemez, H Dortlemez. Conventional versus direct stenting in AMI: effect on immediate coronary blood flow. *J Invas Cardiol* 2002; **14**(7): 372–7. **89**

E Tsuchikane, S Otsuji, N Awata, J Azuma, Y Nakaoka, H Uesugi, T Kobayashi, M Sakurai, T Kobayashi. Impact of pre-stent plaque debulking for chronic coronary total occlusion on restenosis reduction. *J Invas Cardiol* 2001; **13**(8): 584–9. **247**

F Unger, PW Serruys, MH Yacoub, C Ilsley, PK Paulsen, TT Nielsen, L Eysmann, F Kiemeneij. Revascularization in multivessel disease: comparison between two-year outcomes of coronary bypass surgery and stenting. *J Thorac Cardiovasc Surg* 2003; **125**: 809–20. **58**

E Van Belle, M Perie, D Braune, A Chmait, T Meurice, K Abolmaali, EP McFadden, C Bauters, JA Lablanche, ME Bertrand. Effects of coronary stenting on vessel patency and long-term clinical outcome after percutaneous coronary revascularization in diabetic patients. *J Am Coll Cardiol* 2002; **40**: 410–17. **154**

J vom Dahl, PK Haager, E Grube, M Gross, C Beythien, EP Kromer, N Cattelaens, CW Hamm, R Hoffmann, T Reineke, HG Klues. Effects of gold coating of coronary stents on neointimal proliferation following stent implantation. *Am J Cardiol* 2002; **89**: 801–5. **39, 122**

NN Wahab, EA Cowden, NJ Pearce, MJ Gardner, H Merry, JL Cox; ICONS Investigators. Is blood glucose an independent predictor of mortality in acute myocardial infarction in the thrombolytic era? *J Am Coll Cardiol* 2002; **40**: 1748–54. **15**

R Waksman, AE Ajani, E Pinnow, E Cheneau, L Leborgne, R Dieble, AB Bui, LF Satler, AD Pichard, KK Kent, J Lindsay. Twelve versus six months of clopidogrel to reduce major cardiac events in patients undergoing gamma-radiation therapy for in-stent restenosis: Washington Radiation for In-Stent Restenosis Trial (WRIST) 12 versus WRIST PLUS. *Circulation* 2002; **106**(7): 776–8. **169**

R Waksman, AE Ajani, RL White, RC Chan, LF Satler, KM Kent, AD Pichard, EE Pinnow, AB Bui, S Ramee, P Teirstein, J Lindsay. Intravascular gamma radiation for in-stent restenosis in saphenous-vein bypass grafts. *N Engl J Med* 2002; **346**(16): 1194–9. **179**

GS Werner, K Lang, H Kuehnert, HR Figulla. Intracoronary verapamil for reversal of no-reflow during coronary angioplasty for acute myocardial infarction. *Cath Cardiovasc Interv* 2002; **57**: 444–51. **191**

PL Whitlow, TA Bass, RM Kipperman, BL Sharaf, KK Ho, DE Cutlip, Y Zhang, RE Kuntz, DO Williams, DM Lasorda, JW Moses, MJ Cowley, DS Eccleston, MC Horrigan, RM Bersin, SR Ramee, T Feldman. Results of the study to determine rotablator and transluminal angioplasty strategy (STRATAS). *Am J Cardiol* 2001; **87**: 699–705. **243**

HK Yip, MC Chen, HW Chang, CL Hang, YK Hsieh, CY Fang, CJ Wu. Angiographic morphologic features of infarct-related arteries and timely reperfusion in acute myocardial infarction. *Chest* 2002; **122**: 1322–32. **190**

J Zheng, D Li, FM Cavagna, K Harris, FJ Klocke, F Maggioni, J Carr, O Simonetti, G Laub, JP Finn. Contrast-enhanced coronary MR angiography: relationship between coronary artery delineation and blood T1. *J Magn Reson Imaging* 2001; **14**: 348–54. **262**

General Index

4S trial 141

A

abciximab
  TARGET 155
  use in diabetic patients 154–5
  use in primary coronary angioplasty 25–6, 31
  see also antiplatelet therapy
ACE inhibitors, use in patients with acute
    coronary syndromes 148–9
Achieve paclitaxel-eluting stent 214
ACS RX Multilink stent, associated neointimal
    hyperplasia 130–1
acute coronary syndromes (ACS) 3
  early invasive strategy in women 17–19
  effect of statin discontinuation 146–7
  no-reflow 187
  use of secondary preventive drugs 148–9
  see also myocardial infarction; non-ST
      elevation acute coronary syndromes
      (NSTEACS); risk stratification in acute
      coronary syndromes; unstable angina
acute myocardial infarction *see* myocardial
    infarction
adenosine
  use in fractional flow reserve assessment 106–7
  use in no-reflow 188, 192, 199
  use during stent deployment 103–4
adenosine 5′-triphosphate (ATP), use in
    fractional flow reserve assessment 106–7
ADVANCE trial 41
allergy, association with in-stent restenosis
    125–6, 135
AMI-27 (Combidex), use in magnetic resonance
    imaging of atherosclerotic plaques 258–9
angina
  AWESOME (Angina With Extremely Serious
    Operative Mortality Evaluation) trial
    61–4
  comparison of coronary artery bypass grafting
    with stenting 60–1
  effect of epicardial stenosis on blood flow 93
  value of fractional flow reserve measurement
    95
  see also unstable angina

angiography
  predictive features for no-reflow in acute
    myocardial infarction 190–1
  timing in non-ST elevation acute coronary
    syndrome 36, 45–52
  use of glycoprotein IIb/IIIa antagonists in
    NSTEACS 47–9
  see also magnetic resonance imaging:
    angiography
angioplasty
  comparison with stenting in small coronary
    arteries 36–8
  outcome in diabetic patients 151–4, 161
  outcome in renal insufficiency 157–8
  primary *see* primary angioplasty
  see also balloon angioplasty; percutaneous
    coronary intervention (PCI)
antioxidant vitamins 142
antiplatelet therapy
  in ASPECT 217
  following brachytherapy 169–71
  see also abciximab; aspirin; clopidogrel;
    eptifibatide; glycoprotein (Gp)
    IIb/IIIa inhibitors; lamifiban;
    tirofiban
aortic stenosis, effect on dicrotic notch 116
arterial remodelling 242–3
  effect on mechanisms of stenting 85–6
ARTIST study of in-stent restenosis 239–40
ARTS (Arterial Revascularization Therapy Study)
    57, 58
ASPECT (ASian Paclitaxel-Eluting stent Clinical
    Trial) 214, 216–19
  intravascular ultrasound analysis 230–1
aspirin
  use in ASPECT 217
  use in patients with acute coronary syndromes
    148–9
  use with clopidogrel following brachytherapy
    169–71
  use with primary coronary angioplasty 23
atherectomy xii, 239, 248
  comparison of treatment strategies (CARAT)
    245–6
  directional 240–1

KEEPING UP TO DATE IN ONE VOLUME

The Year in Interventional Cardiology

———— ▬ ————

The Year in Interventional Cardiology
appears on a regular basis

———— ▬ ————

To receive more information about the next issue,
or to reserve a copy on publication,
please contact us at the address below:

Clinical Publishing
Oxford Centre for Innovation
Mill Street
Oxford OX2 0JX, UK

T: +44 1865 811116
F: +44 1865 251550
E: info@clinicalpublishing.co.uk
W: www.clinicalpublishing.co.uk

———— ▬ ————

KEEPING UP TO DATE IN ONE SERIES

"The Year in ..."

EXISTING AND FUTURE VOLUMES

The Year in Neurology 2001	ISBN 0 9537339 5 5
The Year in Rheumatic Disorders 2001	ISBN 0 9537339 1 2
The Year in Gynaecology 2001	ISBN 0 9537339 2 0
The Year in Hypertension 2001	ISBN 0 9537339 4 7
The Year in Diabetes 2001	ISBN 0 9527339 6 3
The Year in Dyslipidaemia 2002	ISBN 0 9537339 3 9
The Year in Interventional Cardiology 2002	ISBN 0 9537339 7 1
The Year in Rheumatic Disorders 2002	ISBN 0 9537339 9 8
The Year in Hypertension 2002	ISBN 1 904392 00 8
The Year in Gynaecology 2002	ISBN 1 904392 01 6
The Year in Neurology 2003	ISBN 1 904392 03 2
The Year in Diabetes 2003	ISBN 1 904392 02 4
The Year in Dyslipidaemia 2003	ISBN 1 904392 07 5
The Year in Allergy 2003	ISBN 1 904392 05 9
The Year in Rheumatic Disorders 2003	ISBN 1 904392 09 1
The Year in Respiratory Medicine 2003	ISBN 0 9537339 8 X
The Year in Hypertension 2003	ISBN 1 904392 13 X
The Year in Urology 2003	ISBN 1 904392 06 7
The Year in Infection 2003	ISBN 1 904392 12 1

To receive more information about these books and future volumes,
or to order copies, please contact the address below:

Clinical Publishing
Oxford Centre for Innovation
Mill Street
Oxford OX2 OJX, UK

T: +44 1865 811116
F: +44 1865 251550
E: info@clinicalpublishing.co.uk
W: www.clinicalpublishing.co.uk